Novel Medical and General Hebrew Terminology from the Middle Ages

Novel Medical and General Hebrew Terminology from the Middle Ages

VOLUME 7

By

Gerrit Bos

BRILL

LEIDEN | BOSTON

Cover illustration: Nathan ha-Me'ati's Hebrew translation of Avicenna's *Canon of Medicine*, Biblioteca Universitaria di Bologna, Ms 2197, fol. 402r: 'An Italian doctor visiting a patient'

The Library of Congress Cataloging-in-Publication Data is available online at https://catalog.loc.gov

Typeface for the Latin, Greek, and Cyrillic scripts: "Brill". See and download: brill.com/brill-typeface.

ISBN 978-90-04-69771-3 (hardback)
ISBN 978-90-04-69772-0 (e-book)
DOI 10.1163/9789004697720

This book is printed on acid-free paper and produced in a sustainable manner.

Contents

Sigla, Sources, and Abbreviations VII

Introduction 1

List of Terms 7

Bibliography 237
Corrections to BCD and NM 6 240
Index of Greek Terms 241
Index of Arabic/Persian Terms 243
Index of Latin/Romance Terms 254

Sigla, Sources, and Abbreviations

Sigla

a — Arabic text

ALC — Avicenna, *Liber Canonis*, ed. Venice 1507 (Repr., Hildesheim 2009).

BCD — G. Bos, *A Concise Dictionary of Novel Medical and General Hebrew Terminology of the Middle Ages* (Leiden 2019).

BM — E. Ben Yehuda, *Millon ha-Lashon ha-Ivrit: Thesaurus Totius Hebraitatis et Veteris et Recentioris*, 17 vols. (Repr., Tel Aviv 1948–1959).

BMA 2 — Maimonides, *On Asthma*, vol. 2: *Critical Editions of Medieval Hebrew* (ed. by G. Bos) *and Latin Translations* (ed. by M.R. McVaugh) (Provo, UT 2008).

BMCH 1 — Maimonides, *Commentary on Hippocrates'* Aphorisms: *A New Parallel Arabic-English Edition and Translation, with Critical Editions of the Medieval Hebrew Translations*, ed. and trans. by G. Bos, vol. 1 (Leiden 2020).

BMH — Maimonides, *On Hemorrhoids*: *A New Parallel Arabic-English Edition and Translation* (by G. Bos), *with Critical Editions of the Medieval Hebrew Translations* (by G. Bos) and *Medieval Latin Translations* (by M.R. McVaugh) (Provo, UT 2012).

BMMA — Maimonides, *Medical Aphorisms*: *A Parallel Arabic-English Edition*, 5 vols., ed. and trans. by G. Bos (Provo, UT 2004–2017).

BMMG — Maimonides, *Medical Aphorisms*: *Glossary & Indexes*, ed. by G. Bos (Leiden 2021).

BMMN — Maimonides, *Medical Aphorisms: Hebrew Translation by Nathan ha-Me'ati*, ed. by G. Bos (Leiden 2020).

BMMZ — Maimonides, *Medical Aphorisms: Hebrew Translation by Zeraḥyah ben Isaac ben She'altiel Ḥen*, ed. by G. Bos (Leiden 2020).

BMZ — G. Bos, G. Mensching, and J. Zwink, *Medical Glossaries in the Hebrew Tradition: Shem Tov ben Isaac*, Sefer Almansur, *with a Supplement on the Romance and Latin Terminology* (Leiden 2017).

BnF — Bibliothèque nationale de France (Paris).

CMM — Guigonis de Caulhiaco (Guy de Chauliac), *Inventarium sive Chirurgia Magna*, 2 vols. (vol. 1: *Text*; vol. 2: *Commentary*), ed. by M.R. McVaugh (Leiden 1997).

D — R. Dozy, *Supplément aux dictionnaires Arabes*, 2 vls. (Paris 1927).

DAN — G.H. Dalman, *Aramäisch-Neuhebräisches Handwörterbuch zu Targum, Talmud und Midrasch*, 2nd ed. (Frankfurt am Main 1922).

DBK — A. de Biberstein Kazimirski, *Dictionnaire Arabe-Français contenant toutes les racines de la langue Arabe*, 2 vols. (Paris 1960).

DDM	R.J. Durling, *A Dictionary of Medical Terms in Galen* (Leiden 1993).
DKT	P. de Koning, *Trois traités d'anatomie arabes*, ed. by F. Sezgin (Repr., Frankfurt am Main 1986).
DMLBS	R.E. Latham, D.R. Howlett, and R.K. Ashdowne (eds.), *Dictionary of Medieval Latin from British Sources*, 3 vols. (London 1975–2013).
DT	*Dioscurides Triumphans. Ein anonymer arabischer Kommentar (Ende 12. Jahr. n. Chr.) zur Materia medica*, vol. 2, ed. and trans. by A. Dietrich (Göttingen 1988).
DW	*Pedanii Dioscuridis Anazarbei De Materia Medica Libri Quinque*, ed. by M. Wellmann (Repr., 5 pts. in 1 vol., Berlin 1958).
DWB	*Pedanius Dioscorides of Anazarbus: De materia medica*, trans. by L.Y. Beck, 2nd rev. and enl. ed. (Hildesheim 2011).
EI^2	*The Encyclopaedia of Islam: New Edition*, ed. by H.A.R. Gibb, J.H. Kramers, et al., 11 vols., 1 suppl. (Leiden 1954–2002).
EM	Abraham Even-Shoshan, *Ha-Millon he-Ḥadash* (Repr., 7 vols., Jerusalem 1983).
FA	A. Fonahn, *Arabic and Latin Anatomical Terminology Chiefly from the Middle Ages* (Kristiana 1922).
FAB	J. Feliks, *The Animal World of the Bible* (Tel Aviv 1962).
FAQ	I. Fellmann, *Das Aqrābādīn al-Qalānisī: Quellenkritische und begriffsanalytische Untersuchung zur arabisch-pharmazeutischen Literatur* (Beirut 1986).
FEW	W. von Wartburg, *Französisches Etymologisches Wörterbuch* (Bonn 1922–).
FL	G.W. Freytag, *Lexicon Arabico-Latinum*, vols. 1–4 (Halis Saxonum 1830–1837).
HCD	A. Heschel, *A Concise Dictionary of Hebrew Philosophical Terms* (Cincinnati 1941).
HIM	W. Hinz, *Islamische Maße und Gewichte umgerechnet ins metrische System* (Repr., Leiden 1970).
HLA	J. Hirschberg and J. Lippert (trans.), *Die Augenheilkunde des Ibn Sina aus dem Arabischen übersetzt und erläutert.* (Repr. in: F. Sezgin (ed.), *Augenheilkunde im Islam*, vol. 1, Frankfurt am Main 1986, 9–194).
IBF	Ibn al-Bayṭār, *Traité des simples*, trans. by L. Leclerc, 3 vols. (Paris 1877–1883).
IJZ 1–2	Ibn al-Jazzār, *Zād al-musāfir wa-qūt al-ḥāḍir (Provisions for the Traveller and Nourishment for the Sedentary): Books I and II—Diseases of the Head and the Face: A Parallel Arabic-English Edition and Translation* (by G. Bos and F. Käs) *with Critical Editions of the Medieval Hebrew Translations* (by G. Bos) *and the Medieval Latin Translation* (by M.R. McVaugh) (Leiden 2022).

IJZ 7	Ibn al-Jazzār, *Zād al-musāfir wa-qūt al-ḥāḍir* (*Provisions for the Traveller and Nourishment for the Sedentary*): *Book 7* (*7–30*): *Critical Edition of the Arabic Text with English Translation and Critical Edition of Moses ibn Tibbon's Hebrew Translation* (Ṣedat ha-Derakhim), ed. and trans. by G. Bos (Leiden 2015).
JAD	A.S.G. Jayakar (trans.), *Ad-Damīrī's Ḥayāt al-Ḥayawān* (*A Zoological Lexicon*), 2 vols. (London 1906–1908).
JD	M. Jastrow, *A Dictionary of the Targumim, the Talmud Bavli and Yerushalmi, and the Midrashic Literature* (Repr., 2 vols., New York 1950).
KB	L. Koehler and W. Baumgartner, *The Hebrew and Aramaic Lexicon of the Old Testament*, rev. by W. Baumgartner and J.J. Stamm, with assistance from B. Hartmann, Z. Ben-Hayyim, E.Y. Kutscher, and Ph. Reymond, ed. and trans. under the supervision of M.E.J. Richardson, 5 vols. (Leiden 1994–2000).
KM	F. Käs, *Die Mineralien in der arabischen Pharmakognosie: Eine Konkordanz zur mineralischen Materia medica der klassischen arabischen Heilmittelkunde nebst überlieferungsgeschichtlichen Studien*, 2 vols. (Wiesbaden 2010).
KTA	S. Krauss, *Talmudische Archäologie*, 3 vols. (Leipzig 1910–1912).
L	Latin text
Lane	E.W. Lane, *Arabic-English Lexicon*, 8 vols. (London 1863–1879).
LF	I. Löw, *Die Flora der Juden*, 4 vols. (Repr., Hildesheim 1967).
LFF	P.B. Lewicka, *Food and Foodways of Medieval Cairenes: Aspects of Life in an Islamic Metropolis of the Eastern Mediterranean* (Leiden 2011).
Low	A. Lowinger, A., 'Register of Hebrew and Aramaic Terms,' ed. and trans. by S. Paley, in: J. Preuss, *Biblisch-talmudische Medizin: Beiträge zur Geschichte der Heilkunde und der Kultur überhaupt* (Repr., New York 1971).
LSG	H.G. Liddell and R. Scott, *A Greek-English Lexicon*, rev. and augm. by H.S. Jones, a.o., with a supplement (Repr., Oxford 1989).
LZ	L. Lewysohn, *Zoologie des Talmuds* (Frankfurt am Main 1858).
MD	A.M. Masie, *Dictionary of Medicine and Allied Sciences: Latin-English-Hebrew*, ed. by S. Tchernichowsky (Jerusalem 1934).
MIG	Marwān ibn Janāḥ, *On the Nomenclature of Medicinal Drugs* (*Kitāb al-Talkhīṣ*): *Edition, Translation, and Commentary with Special Reference to the Ibero-Romance Terminology*, by G. Bos, F. Käs, M. Lübke, and G. Mensching, 2 vols. (Leiden 2020).
MM	A.F. Maʿluf, *Muʿjam al-Ḥayawān* (Cairo 1932).
MMT	M. Meyerhof (ed.), *The Book of the Ten Treatises on the Eye Ascribed to Ḥunain ibn Isḥāq* (*809.877* A.D.) (Cairo 1928), and *Al-morchid fi'l kohhl ou le guide d'oculiste: Ouvrage inédit de l'oculiste arabe-espagnol Mohammad*

ibn Qassoûm ibn Aslam al-Ghâfiqî (Barcelona 1933) (Repr. in: F. Sezgin (ed.), *Augenheilkunde im Islam*, vol. 2, Frankfurt am Main 1986).

MSh — Maimonides, *Sharḥ asmāʾ al-ʿuqqār: Un glossaire de matière médicale composé par Maïmonide*, ed. by M. Meyerhof (Repr. in: F. Sezgin (ed.), *Islamic Medicine*, vol. 63, Frankfurt am Main 1996); English trans.: *Moses Maimonides' Glossary of Drug Names: Translated and Annotated from Max Meyerhof's French Edition*, by F. Rosner (Haifa 1995).

NA — N. Nasrallah (trans.), *Annals of the Caliphs' Kitchens: Ibn Sayyār al-Warrāq's Tenth-Century Baghdadi Cookbook*, with introduction and glossary (Leiden 2007).

ND — J. Norri, *Dictionary of Medical Vocabulary in English, 1375–1550: Body Parts, Sicknesses, Instruments, and Medicinal Preparations*, 2 vols. (Abingdon 2016).

NM 1 — G. Bos, *Novel Medical and General Hebrew Terminology from the 13th Century: Translations by Hillel ben Samuel of Verona, Moses ben Samuel ibn Tibbon, Shem Tov ben Isaac of Tortosa, and Zeraḥyah ben Isaac ben She'altiel Ḥen*, = *Journal of Semitic Studies*, suppl. 27 (Oxford 2011).

NM 2 — G. Bos, *Novel Medical and General Hebr. Terminology from the 13th Century*, vol. 2, = *Journal of Semitic Studies*, suppl. 30 (Oxford 2013).

NM 3 — G. Bos, *Novel Medical and General Hebrew Terminology: Hippocrates'* Aphorisms *in the Hebrew Tradition*, = *Journal of Semitic Studies*, suppl. 37 (Oxford 2016).

NM 4 — G. Bos, *Novel Medical and General Hebrew Terminology from the 13th Century*, vol. 4 (Leiden 2019).

NM 5 — G. Bos, *Novel Medical and General Hebrew Terminology from the Middle Ages*, vol. 5 (Leiden 2022).

NM 6 — G. Bos, *Novel Medical and General Hebrew Terminology from the Middle Ages*, vol. 6 (Leiden 2023).

NT — N. Nasrallah (trans.), *Treasure Trove of Benefits and Variety at the Table: A Fourteeenth-Century Egyptian Cookbook*, with introduction and glossary (Leiden 2018).

PESHAT — *Premodern Philosophic and Scientific Hebrew Terminology in Context: An Online Thesaurus*, ed. by R. Leicht and G. Veltri (Database: https://peshat.org).

SCP — F.A. Steingass, *A Comprehensive Persian-English Dictionary: Including the Arabic Words and Phrases to be Met with in Persian Literature* (Repr., London 1984).

SDA — M. Sokoloff, *A Dictionary of Jewish Babylonian Aramaic of the Talmudic and Geonic Period*, 2nd ed. (Ramat Gan 2020).

SHS 1 — G. Bos, M. Hussein, G. Mensching, and F. Savelsberg (eds.), *Medical Synonym Lists from Medieval Provence: Shem Tov ben Isaac of Tortosa*, Sefer

	ha-Shimmush, Book 29—*Part 1: Edition and Commentary of List 1* (*Hebrew-Arabic-Romance/Latin*) (Leiden 2011).
SUD	J. Schönfeld (ed. and trans.), *Über die Steine: Das 14. Kapitel aus dem* Kitāb al-Muršid *des Muḥammad ibn Aḥmad at-Tamīmī, nach dem Pariser Manuskript herausgegeben, übersetzt und kommentiert* (Freiburg im Breisgau 1976).
UW	M. Ullmann, *Wörterbuch zu den griechisch-arabischen Übersetzungen des neunten Jahrhunderts* (Wiesbaden 2002).
UWS 1	M. Ullmann, *Wörterbuch zu den griechisch-arabischen Übersetzungen des neunten Jahrhunderts*, suppl. 1: *A–O* (Wiesbaden 2006).
UWS 2	M. Ullmann, *Wörterbuch zu den griechisch-arabischen Übersetzungen des neunten Jahrhunderts*, suppl. 2: *Π–Ω* (Wiesbaden 2007).
UWS 3	M. Ullmann, *Wörterbuch zu den griechisch-arabischen Übersetzungen des neunten Jahrhunderts*, suppl. 3: *Zur Agronomie* (Wiesbaden 2018).
WCD	H. Wehr, *A Dictionary of Modern Written Arabic*, ed. by J. Milton Cowan, 4th ed. (Wiesbaden 1979).
WKAS	*Wörterbuch der klassischen arabischen Sprache*, ed. by Deutsche Morgenländische Gesellschaft (Wiesbaden 1957–2009).

Biblical Sources

Dan	Daniel
Deut	Deuteronomy
Ex	Exodus
Gen	Genesis
Lam	Lamentations
Lev	Leviticus
Prov	Proverbs

Abbreviations

Abl.	ablative
acc.	according(ly)
add.	added
Adj.	adjective
aka	also known as
anat.	anatomical
Arab.	Arabic

Aram.	Aramaic
attr.	attributed
Bibl.	Biblical
Cat.	Catalan
conj.	conjugation
Dat.	dative
ed.	edited/edition/editor
eds.	editors
emend. ed.	emendation editor
enl.	enlarged
esp.	especially
f.	feminine
Gr.	Greek
Hebr.	Hebrew
Inf.	infinitive
Ital.	Italian
L. Lat.	Late Latin
Lat.	Latin
M. Lat.	Middle Latin
Mod. Span.	Modern Spanish
Ms(s)	manuscript(s)
O. Cat.	Old Catalan
O. Fr.	Old French
O. Ital.	Old Italian
o.l.	other language
O. Occ.	Old Occitan
O. Sp.	Old Spanish
om.	omitted
Pass.	passive
Plur.	plural
Rabb.	Rabbinic
re	as related to
rev.	revised
resp.	respectivelly
Rom.	Romance
Sing.	singular
s.v.	*sub voce*
trans.	translated/translation(s)/translator

Introduction

The current volume[1] is part of a wider project aiming at mapping the novel[2] Hebrew[3] technical medical and general terminology as it features in medieval Hebrew medical works translated both from Arabic and Latin.[4] It is my hope that this volume, just like the earlier ones, will facilitate the consultation of medical works and the identification of translators whose identity is unknown or uncertain. One such identification is that of the author of the *Sefer ha-Mezonot*, a Hebrew translation of Abū Marwān ʿAbd al-Malik ibn Zuhr's *K. al-Aghdhiya*. In NM 6, I was able to show that the translator of this text is in all probability Nathan ha-Meʾati. In the same volume, I suggested that Nathan ha-Meʾati might also be the translator of the *Sammim Libbiyim*, i.e., a Hebrew translation of Ibn Sīnā's *K. al-Adwiya al-qalbiyya*. This translation is considered to be by an anonymous translator until now. My suggestion was based on the occurrence of the term עצלה in the unique sense of 'fatigue' (Arab. إعياء) in both Nathan's translation of the *K. al-Qānūn* and in the *Sammim Libbiyim*. This suggestion is now confirmed by a study of the terminology featuring in Nathan's translation of the *K. al-Qānūn* and the comparison with that of the *Sammim Libbiyim*. I found several unique identical terms featuring in both sources, listed below.

---

1 I thank Felix Hedderich and Fabian Käs for proofreading the manuscript.

2 With 'novel,' I mean those terms that do not feature in the current dictionaries of the Hebrew language at all or that feature in these dictionaries either without proper explanation or in a later period only. Occasionally, I include terms that have already been mentioned in the first six volumes (NM 1–6) dealing with novel Hebrew medical terminology in order to show the wider distribution of a certain term; this is especially the case with terms that appear in earlier sources than those mentioned in previous volumes.

3 In addition to the Hebrew terms, the list below also includes (common) loan words from Latin and Romance.

4 Earlier volumes published are: NM 1 = *Novel Medical and General Hebrew Terminology from the 13th Century: Translations by Hillel ben Samuel of Verona, Moses ben Samuel ibn Tibbon, Shem Tov ben Isaac of Tortosa, and Zeraḥyah ben Isaac ben Sheʾaltiel Ḥen*, = *Journal of Semitic Studies*, suppl. 27 (Oxford 2011); NM 2 = *Novel Medical and General Hebrew Terminology from the 13th Century*, vol. 2, = *Journal of Semitic Studies*, suppl. 30 (Oxford 2013); NM 3 = *Novel Medical and General Hebrew Terminology: Hippocrates'* Aphorisms *in the Hebrew Tradition*, = *Journal of Semitic Studies*, suppl. 37 (Oxford 2016); NM 4 = *Novel Medical and General Hebrew Terminology from the 13th Century*, vol. 4 (Leiden 2019); NM 5 = *Novel Medical and General Hebrew Terminology from the Middle Ages*, vol. 5 (Leiden 2022); NM 6 = *Novel Medical and General Hebrew Terminology from the Middle Ages*, vol. 6 (Leiden 2023). The terms listed in NM 1–4 feature also in an alphabetical arrangement in: BCD = *A Concise Dictionary of Novel Medical and General Hebrew Terminology from the Middle Ages* (Leiden 2020).

The main texts consulted are:

1. *Sefer Ṣedat ha-Derakhim*; Moses ben Samuel ben Judah ibn Tibbon's translation of Ibn al-Jazzār's *Zād al-musāfir wa-qūt al-ḥādir* (*Provisions for the Traveller and Nourishment for the Sedentary*), bks. 3–7.[5] The terms selected are derived from the forthcoming critical edition.[6] The basic Ms consulted for the edition is Oxford, Bodleian Libraries, Poc. 353, Uri Heb. 413 (Neubauer 2111).
2. *Sefer Ya'ir Netiv*; a translation made from Constantinus Africanus' *Viaticum*.[7] It was done by an anonymous author living in the Midi who, after his conversion to Christianity, called himself Do'eg ha-Edomi.[8] Between 1197 and 1199 he allegedly translated a corpus of twenty-four medical texts, both practical and theoretical, from Latin to Hebrew. These texts were the first complete Hebrew translations of works by non-Jewish authors on secular subjects. The terms selected are derived from the forthcoming critical edition of Ibn al-Jazzār's *Zād al-musāfir*, bks. 4–7. The basic Ms consulted for the edition is London, British Library, Add. 18969. In the case of corruptions, omissions, or variant readings, I consulted Ms Moscow, Russian State Library, Guenzburg 1481, or Parma, Biblioteca Palatina, Cod. Parm. 2474. The parallel Latin terms from Constantine's translation are also derived from the forthcoming critical edition.[9]
3. *Shinnui ha-Shemot ha-Niqra'im Synonimi*; Ms Florence, Biblioteca Medicea Laurenziana, Or. 17. The Ms consisting of 92 fols. is a medical miscellany copied by Abraham ben Moses in Anagni in the year 1464. It contains, a.o., an extensive list of 1749 entries of medical synonyms (fols. 68^{a}–92^{b})[10]

5 For this translation, possibly hailing from the year 1259, cf. the intr. in IJZ 1–2:429–437.

6 For the Arabic terms derived from bks. 6–7, I consulted G. Bos (ed. and trans.), *Ibn al-Jazzār on Sexual Diseases and Their Treatment* (London 1997) (bk. 6); G. Bos (ed. and trans.), *Ibn al-Jazzār on Fevers* (London 2000) (bk. 7, chs. 1–6); and IJZ 7 (bk. 7, chs. 7–30), which was also consulted for Moses ibn Tibbon's translation (*Sefer Ṣedat ha-Derakhim*) of bk. 7, chs. 7–30.

7 I.e., his Latin translation of Ibn al-Jazzār's *Zād al-musāfir*. The Hebrew translator attributed the text to Isaac Israeli.

8 For this translation, cf. the intr. in IJZ 1–2:595–600; see also NM 3:3 and the recent article by G. Freudenthal, M.R. McVaugh, and K. Mesler, 'Twelfth-Century Latin Medicine in Hebrew Garb: Doeg the Edomite as a Cultural Intermediary,' *Medieval Encounters* 26 (2020): 226–284.

9 For the Arabic terms derived from bks. 6–7, I consulted G. Bos (ed. and trans.), *Ibn al-Jazzār on Sexual Diseases and Their Treatment* (London 1997) (bk. 6); G. Bos (ed. and trans.), *Ibn al-Jazzār on Fevers* (London 2000) (bk. 7, chs. 1–6); and IJZ 7 (bk. 7, chs. 7–30).

10 This list is currently being edited with support of the Deutsche Forschungsgemeinschaft (DFG) by a team consisting of G. Bos, F. Hedderich, F. Käs, J. Kley, S. Lauschus, G. Mensching, L. Refrigeri, and F. Savelsberg. For a detailed description, see NM 5:6–7.

and an alphabetical list of substitute drugs, belonging to the genre of *Quid pro quo* on fols. 10^a–15^b.[11]

4. *Sefer ha-Qanun*; Nathan ha-Me'ati's translation of Ibn Sīnā's *K. al-Qānūn*, Ms Oxford, Bodleian Libraries, Can. Or. 88, copied in the fourteenth–fifteenth century in a Sephardic semi-cursive script.[12] In case of corruptions, I consulted Ms Paris, BnF, héb. 1136, which was copied in a Sephardic semi-cursive script in Villalón de Campos (Spain) in 1487.[13] Nathan's translation of the *K. al-Qānūn* is probably one of the first translations of Arabic medical works he undertook. It has several non-standard, odd, or imprecise expressions that he corrected in later translations of other medical works,[14] e.g., the *Medical Aphorisms* composed by Moses Maimonides.[15] A further indication for an early dating of the translation of the *K. al-Qānūn* can be found in its preface, in which he explicitly states that he only started his translating enterprise from Arabic into Hebrew once he had acquired sufficient knowledge of both languages to take upon himself this difficult task.[16]
5. *Sefer ha-Qanun*; Zeraḥyah Ḥen's translation of Ibn Sīnā's *K. al-Qānūn*, Ms Oxford, Bodleian Libraries, Opp. Add. Fol. 12, copied in a semi-cursive

11 For a discussion of the genre of *Quid pro quo* in medieval Hebrew medical literature, see M. Steinschneider, 'Eine medicinische hebraeische Handschrift,' *Magazin für die Wissenschaft des Judentums* 12 (1885): 182–216; G. Bos, F. Lauschus, and F. Savelsberg, 'Substitute Drugs in the Hebrew Tradition,' in: *From Formal Linguistic Theory to the Art of Historical Editions: The Multifaceted Dimensions of Romance Linguistics*, ed. by N. Pomino, E.M. Remberger, and J. Zwink, 303–316 (Göttingen 2023).

12 Cf. A. Neubauer, *Catalogue of the Hebrew Manuscripts in the Bodleian Libraries* (Repr., Oxford 1994); *Supplement of Addenda and Corrigenda*, comp. by M. Beit-Arié and ed. by R.A. May (Oxford 1994), no. 2101.

13 Cf. H. Zotenberg (ed.), *Catalogues des manuscrits hébreux et samaritains de la Bibliothèque Impériale* (Paris 1866), 212; Ktiv: The International Collection of Digitized Hebrew Manuscripts at The National Library of Israel. The Arabic edition consulted is the one printed in Būlāq 1876, repr. in 3 vols.

14 These non-standard terms are not peculiar to Ms Oxford, Bodleian Libraries, Can. Or. 88, but also feature in the same quotations in Ms Paris, BnF, héb. 1136.

15 Cf. entry סביאה.

16 Cf. BMMN 1: 'I have learned the tongues of these foreign nations among which I have dwelt. Until now I have lingered; till I have acquired distinct speech and the tongue of the learned, lovely and pleasant, Hebrew and Arabic joined together. I have kept them in my heart and they have become united in my hand.' If one accepts the supposition that the translation of the *K. al-Qānūn* is one of his earlier endeavors, if not the earliest, and was completed in 1279, it would also mean that the translation of the *Medical Aphorisms* must have been completed at some time after that date and not shortly after 1277 as supposed by Steinschneider (cf. M. Steinschneider, *Die hebräischen Übersetzungen des Mittelalters und die Juden als Dolmetscher* (Berlin 1893), 766).

Sephardic script in the fourteenth–fifteenth century.[17] The terminology featuring in this translation is that recurring in other translations from his hand, notably that of Moses Maimonides' *Medical Aphorisms*.

6. *Sefer ha-Qanun*; Anonymous I's translation of Ibn Sīnā's *K. al-Qānūn*, Ms Paris, BnF, héb. 1142. This translation is ascribed to Zeraḥyah Ḥen in Ktiv[18] and also in Benjamin Richler's list of Mss of the Hebrew translations of the *K. al-Qānūn*;[19] Zotenberg however ascribed the translation to Nathan ha-Me'ati.[20] This discrepancy hails from the technical terminology used by the translator and/or adapter, which partly agrees with Nathan and partly with Zeraḥyah, but is also partly different from that used by both translators.[21] For this reason, I have omitted the name of the translator.
7. *Sefer ha-Qanun*; Anonymous II's translation of Ibn Sīnā's *K. al-Qānūn*, Ms Parma, Biblioteca Palatina, Cod. Parm. 3045 (Richler 1505). The Ms was copied in the mid-fourteenth century in an Italian semi-cursive script. The translation is unique: The list of drugs (simplicia) is arranged according to the Arabic alphabet and not the Hebrew alphabet as in all the other translations.[22] The main entries with the names of plants and minerals are in many cases not the Arabic terms in Hebrew characters, but the parallel terms in Latin and/or Romance (Italian?).[23] Also, the sub-entries introducing the usefulness of the different plants and minerals for illnesses affecting different parts of the body,[24] such as 'wounds and ulcers' or 'organs of the head,' are generally preceded by the term: תועלתו ('its usefulness'). Some of the technical terms employed by the translator

17 Cf. Neubauer, *Catalogue* and *Supplement*, no. 2099. According to Mauro Zonta, the Ms is the archetype copied from a lost autograph (see M. Zonta, 'Zeraḥyah: Philosopher and Translator and His Role in 13th Century Rome' (paper read in Jerusalem, January 1, 2007).

18 https://www.nli.org.il/en/discover/manuscripts/hebrew-manuscripts/itempage?docId=PNX_MANUSCRIPTS990001316280205171&vid=MANUSCRIPTS&SearchTxt=paris%201142.

19 Cf. B. Richler, 'Manuscripts of Avicenna's *Kanon* in Hebrew Translation: A Revised and Up-to-Date List,' *Korot* 8, nos. 3–4 (1982): 163 (no. 77).

20 Cf. Zotenberg (ed.), *Catalogues*, 212.

21 For a more extensive discussion of this Ms, cf. NM 6:6–9.

22 Cf. B. Richler, *Hebrew Manucripts in the Biblioteca Palatina in Parma* (Jerusalem 2001); idem, 'Manuscripts of Avicenna's *Kanon*,' 165 (no. 89).

23 Some examples are: לפיז ספוגייא (Lat./Rom. LPYZ SPWGYY'), Arab. حجر الاسفنج ('sponge stone'); לפיז לטֵאֵז (Lat./Rom. LPYZ LṬe'eZ), Arab. حجر اللبن ('milk stone'); לפיז יודאיקו (Lat./Rom. LPYZ YWD'YQW), Arab. حجر اليهود ('Jews' stone'). The interpretation of these terms and specification of the Romance language is complicated and can only be done by a specialist in all medieval Romance languages. It is beyond the scope of the present study.

24 Cf. the extensive discussion in NM 6:8–9.

are uncommon, non-standard, and not to be found in any other medieval medical work or other translation as far as our current knowledge goes.[25]

8. *Glossary* of plant names in Arabic with parallel terms in Hebrew, Latin, Romance, Greek. The glossary, featuring in Ms Moscow, Russian State Library, Guenzburg 573, fols. 147ᵇ–160ᵃ, is part of an incomplete copy of Nathan ha-Me'ati's translation of Ibn Sīnā' *K. al-Qānūn* (i.e., *Sefer ha-Qanun*). The last missing leaf is possibly extant in the Genizah; according to the colophon on that leaf, it was copied in Lecce in 1441 (cf. Ktiv). The glossary is introduced on fol. 147ᵇ by the following words: ועתה אחל לכתוב הסמים בשמותם איש על דגלו לבית אבותם. At the end on fol. 160ᵃ it states: תם זכרון הסמים שהביא החכם אבן סינא בספר הקאנון ת״ל.
9. *Ma'amar ba-Haqqazah*; an anonymous Hebrew translation of Abū Bakr Muḥammad ibn Zakariyyā' al-Rāzī's *K. fī al-Faṣd*. The translation is extant in Ms Parma, Biblioteca Palatina, Cod. Parm. 2283,4, fols. 91ᵃ–97ᵇ (Richler 1535[26]). The Arabic text, extant in Ms San Lorenzo de El Escorial, Real Biblioteca, 857, has recently been edited and translated by Juhan Björn.[27]
10. Anonymous translation of Guy de Chauliac's *Inventarium sive Chirurgia Magna*,[28] Ms Paris, BnF, héb. 1189. The Ms was copied in the fifteenth century in a Sephardic script. The beginning and end are missing.[29]

---

25 A few examples are: האברים הדוחים ('the excretory organs'); האברים המגדלים ('the nutritive organs'); בשר מת ('excessive (superfluous) flesh'); זוֹב, *Plur.* זובים ('humors'); מעפץ ('astringent'); הצליח ('to be beneficial'); שפע עת הנשים ('uterine (menstrual) bleeding'); משותף ('mixed'); חבלים ('nerves'); הֶבֶל ('fomentation; hot compress'); נִפְסָל ('adulterated').

26 Cf. Richler, *Hebrew Manuscripts*.

27 Abū Bakr Muḥammad ibn Zakariyyā' al-Rāzī, *On Phlebotomy*, edition, translation, and commentary by J. Björn (PhD diss., *Studia Orientalia Lundensa*) (Lund 2023).

28 The Latin text consulted is based on the edition by M.R. McVaugh (Guigonis de Caulhiaco (Guy de Chauliac), *Inventarium sive Chirurgia Magna*, 2 vols. (Leiden 1997)). I thank Michael for his help in translating the Latin terminology.

29 Cf. Zotenberg (ed.), *Catalogues*, 218; M. Steinschneider, *Die hebräischen Übersetzungen des Mittelalters und die Juden als Dolmetscher*, 802f.

List of Terms

א

[אבן] • *Hitpaʿel* **הִתְאַבֵּן** · **to coagulate**: Arab. تحجّر · Ibn Sīnā, *K. al-Qānūn* II · trans. Nathan ha-Meʾati, *Sefer ha-Qanun* (Ms Oxford, Bodleian Libraries, Can. Or. 88, fol. 75[a]): גבסין ... יערבו אותו בלובן ביצה לבלתי יתאבן ויושם על האפר הדמיי הנקרא רמד ויועילו לו ([Arab.] *jibsīn*: Gipsum: ... When it is mixed with the white of an egg, so that it does not coagulate, and is then applied in cases of hemorrhagic conjunctivitis, called [in Arab.] *ramad*, it is beneficial). Hebr. הִתְאַבֵּן features in BM 32 in attestations from the *Sefer ha-Qanun* in the sense of 'to petrify' only. Zeraḥyah Ḥen translates Arab. تحجّر as שב כאבן. Anonymous I has התאבן, just like Nathan.

אֶבֶן • **אבן האושכפים** · **shoemaker's stone**: Arab. حجر الاساكفة (cf. IBF no. 604; Gr. λίθος ἀγηρἀτος; cf. Galen, *De simplicum medicamentorum temperamentis ac facultatibus* IX.8[1]) · Ibn Sīnā, *K. al-Qānūn* II · trans. Nathan ha-Meʾati, *Sefer ha-Qanun* (Ms Oxford, Bodleian Libraries, Can. Or. 88, fol. 88[b]): חגר אלאסאכפה כלומ׳ אבן האושכפים: איברי הנשימה והחזה: יועיל מהנגעים והמורסות הנולדים בערלת הגרון מאד ([Arab.] *ḥajar al-asākifa*; i.e., [Hebr.] *even ha-ushkafim*: Shoemaker's stone: The respiratory organs and chest: It is very beneficial for inflammations of the uvula). Hebr. אבן האושכפים is a non-attested calque from Arab. حجر الاساكفة. Zeraḥyah Ḥen transcribes the Arab. term as חגר אלאספכה (read: חגר אלאסכפה) only. Anonymous I translates the Arab. term as אבן האושכפים, just like Nathan, and Anonymous II has the mixed Hebr.-Arab. term אבן אליסיקפא (read: אבן אלאסאקפא = *even al-asākifa*).

• **אבן האספוג** · **sponge stone**: Arab. حجر الاسفنج (cf. IBF no. 611; Gr. λίθοι οἱ ἐν τοῖς σπόγγοις; cf. DW 101 (V.144); DWB 401) · Ibn Sīnā, *K. al-Qānūn* II · trans. Zeraḥyah Ḥen, *Sefer ha-Qanun* (Ms Oxford, Bodleian Libraries, Opp. Add. Fol. 12, fol. 217[b]): חגַ׳ר אַלְאַסְפַ׳נְג אבן האספוג: המהות הוא אבן הנמצא בגרם האספוג הנקיון ישבר החול שבכליות ([Arab.] *ḥajar al-isfanj*; [i.e., Hebr.] *even ha-espog*: Sponge stone. What is it? It is a stone that can be found in the body (substance) of a sponge. Excretion: It fragments bladder stones). Hebr. אבן האספוג features in a variant reading אבן הספוג in NM 5:12. Nathan ha-Meʾati transcribes Arab. حجر الاسفنج as חגר אלאספנג only, while Anonymous I renders the term, similar to Zeraḥyah, as חגר אלאספנג׳ כלומר אבן הספוג and Anonymous II has לפיז ספוגייא (Lat./Rom. LPYZ SPWGYYʾ).

• **אבן ארמיני** · **Armenian stone**: Arab. حجر أرميني (cf. SUD 76, 168 (B XIII)) · Ibn Sīnā, *K. al-Qānūn* II · trans. Anonymous I, *Sefer ha-Qanun* (Ms Paris, BnF, héb. 1142, fol. 123[a]): חגר ארמיני כלומר אבן ארמיני ובלשו׳ לפיש ארמיניק מהות יש בו מעט מראה לאזורדיות ואינה כמראה הלאזורד ולא במקשיותו ([Arab.] *ḥajar armīnī*; i.e., [Hebr.] *even armini*, and in [Lat.] LPYŠ ʾRMYNYQ [read: LPYŠ ʾRMYNWS, i.e., *lapis Armenus*]: Armenian stone: What is it? It is slightly azure in color, but its color is not like that of lapis lazuli,

1 K.G. Kühn (ed.), *Claudii Galeni Opera Omnia* (Repr., Hildesheim 1964–1965), 12:201.

nor does it have its compactness). Hebr. אבן ארמיני features as אבן ארמנית in BM 30 without any further explication or reference. Zeraḥyah Ḥen renders Arab. حجر أرمني as אבן ארמיני, just like Anonymous I.

• **אבן החלב · milk stone**: Arab. حجر اللبن (cf. IBF no. 596; Gr. γαλακτίτης; cf. DW 97 (V.132); DWB 398f.) · Ibn Sīnā, *K. al-Qānūn* II · trans. Nathan ha-Me'ati, *Sefer ha-Qanun* (Ms Oxford, Bodleian Libraries, Can. Or. 88, fol. 88[a]): חגר אללבן כלומ׳ אבן החלב המהות הוא אבן כשמחככים אותו במים יצא ממנו דבר כמו חלב הוא כגוון האפר מתוק בטעמו ושוחקים אותו במים והנתך ממנו יצניעהו בכלי עופרת ([Arab.] *ḥajar al-laban*; i.e., [Hebr.] *even he-ḥalav*: Milk stone. What is it? It is a stone that, when rubbed with water, produces a milky substance. It is ash-colored, sweet in taste. When it is rubbed in water, its solution should be kept in a lead vessel). Hebr. אבן החלב is attested in NM 5:11f. in a later attestation from *Shinnui ha-Shemot ha-Niqra'im Synonimis*, Ms Munich, Bayerische Staatsbibliothek, Cod. hebr. 8. Anonymous I and Zeraḥyah Ḥen render Arab. حجر اللبن as אבן החלב, just like Nathan. Anonymous II has לפיז לטֵאֶז (Lat./Rom. LPYZ LṬe'eZ).

• **אבן יהודית · Jews' stone**: Arab. حجر اليهود (cf. DW 99 (V.137); DWB 399f.; MIG no. 363[2]) · Ibn Sīnā, *K. al-Qānūn* II · trans. Anonymous I, *Sefer ha-Qanun* (Ms Paris, BnF, héb. 1142, fol. 121[b]): חגר אליהודי אבן[3] יהודית מהות כאגוז[4] קטן נוטה לאורך ([Arab.] *ḥajar al-Yahūdī*; [i.e., Hebr.] *even yehudit*: Jews' stone. What is it? [It looks] like a small elongated walnut[5]). Hebr. אבן יהודית features in BM 31 and is explained by Ben Yehuda as: 'olive shaped remnants of fossils' (שארית בעלי חיים מאבנים בצורת זית) in attestations, a.o., from *Sefer ha-Qanun*. Nathan ha-Me'ati and Zeraḥyah Ḥen both transcribe Arab. حجر اليهود as חגר אליהודי only. Zeraḥyah has the Hebr. term as marginal gloss: אבן יהודי. Anonymous II renders the Arab. term as לפיז יודאיקו (Lat./Rom. LPYZ YWD'YQW).

• **אבן הירח · moon stone (selenite)**: Arab. حجر القمر (cf. IBF nos. 301, 602; Gr. λίθος σεληνίτης; cf. DW 100 (V.141); DWB 400) · Ibn Sīnā, *K. al-Qānūn* II · trans. Zeraḥyah Ḥen, *Sefer ha-Qanun* (Ms Oxford, Bodleian Libraries, Opp. Add. Fol. 12, fol. 217[b]): חגַ׳ר אלקַמַר אבן הירח: המהות אמרו להו רוק הלבנה וקצף הלבנה ויוקח בתוספת הירח ([Arab.] *ḥajar al-qamar*; [i.e., Hebr.] *even ha-yare'aḥ*: Moon stone: What is it? They call it: Spittle or foam of the moon. It is taken (found) when the moon waxes). Hebr. אבן הירח is not attested in the currrent dictionaries. Nathan ha-Me'ati translates Arab. حجر القمر as אבן הלבנה (see entry below); Anonymous I renders the Arab. term as אבן הירח, just like Zeraḥyah, and in a marginal gloss as אבן הלבנה, just like Nathan. The latter term also features in Anonymous II.

---

2 'The Jews' stone (Judaic stone) (Gr. Ἰουδαϊκος λίθος) of the ancients is said to be a fossil, namely the petrified remains of a variety of 'sea urchin' (Cidaris glandaria Fraas; Cidaridae) found especially in Judaea.'

3 אבן יהודית: אבן הי יהודית Ms לאפיש יהודית Ms[1].

4 כאגוז קטן: כאלונים קטנים Ms[1].

5 'walnut': 'acorn' Ms[1].

• **אבן יכבה בשמן** · **stone quenched with oil**: Arab. حجر يطفأ بالزيت · Ibn Sīnā, *K. al-Qānūn* II · trans. Zeraḥyah Ḥen, *Sefer ha-Qanun* (Ms Oxford, Bodleian Libraries, Opp. Add. Fol. 12, fol. 218ª): אבן יכבה בשמן ... הסגולות זאת האבן יכבס בשמן ויעשה במים הסם זאת האבן ינוסו ממנו השרצים (The stone that is quenched with oil ... Properties: This stone is quenched with oil and used with water. Poisons: This stone chases vermin away). Hebr. אבן יכבה בשמן is not attested in the current dictionaries. Anonymous I renders Arab. حجر يطفأ as אבן תכובה בשמן and Anonymous II has אבן קֵיסֵי סְטֵיגְיֵי אל השמן (Hebr.-Lat./Rom. *even* QeYSeY SəṬeYGəYeY *el ha-shemen*; cf. Lat. *lapis qua extinguit in oleo*, ALC 126ᵇ).

• **אבן הכושים** · **Ethiopian stone**: Arab. حجر الحبش (cf. IBF no. 600) · Ibn Sīnā, *K. al-Qānūn* II · trans. Zeraḥyah Ḥen, *Sefer ha-Qanun* (Ms Oxford, Bodleian Libraries, Opp. Add. Fol. 12, fol. 217ᵇ): חַגַר אלחַבַּשׁ אבן הכושים המהות אבן יובא מן ארץ כוש נוטה לצִיתְרִינֵיטְצָה יחוכך ממנו חיכוך עוקצת הלשון דומה בחלב ([Arab.] *ḥajar al-ḥabash*; [Hebr.,] *even ha-Kushim*: Ethiopian stone. What is it? It is a stone that is brought from Ethiopia. It is yellowish [in color]; its powder, which is similar to that of [the milk stone], is irritant to the tongue). Hebr. אבן הכושים is not attested in the currrent dictionaries. Nathan ha-Me'ati transcribes Arab. حجر الحبش as חגר אלחבש only and Anonymous I renders it as אבן כוש.

• **אבן הלבנה** · **moon stone (selenite)**: Arab. حجر القمر (cf. IBF nos. 301, 602; Gr. λίθος σεληνίτης; cf. DW 100 (V.141); DWB 400) · Ibn Sīnā, *K. al-Qānūn* II · trans. Nathan ha-Me'ati, *Sefer ha-Qanun* (Ms Oxford, Bodleian Libraries, Can. Or. 88, fol. 88ª): חגר אלקמר כלומ׳ אבן הלבנה קוראין אותו בזאק אלקמר כלו׳ רוק הלבנה וקוראין אותו חלאת הלבונה כלומ׳ זבד אלקמר ([Arab.] *ḥajar al-qamar*; i.e., [Hebr.] *even ha-levanah*. It is called [in Arab.] *buzāq al-qamar*; i.e., 'spittle of the moon,' and it is called 'foam of the moon,' i.e., [Arab.] *zabad al-qamar*). Hebr. אבן הלבנה is not attested in the currrent dictionaries. Zeraḥyah Ḥen renders Arab. حجر القمر as אבן הירח (see entry above); Anonymous I has אבן הירח, just like Zeraḥyah, and in a marginal gloss אבן הלבנה, just like Nathan. The latter term also features in Anonymous II.

• **אבן המחצב** · **ore**: Arab. حجارة المعدن · Ibn Sīnā, *K. al-Qānūn* II · trans. Nathan ha-Me'ati, *Sefer ha-Qanun* (Ms Oxford, Bodleian Libraries, Can. Or. 88, fol. 81ª): זיבק הוא כסף חי יש שדולים אותו ממחצבו ויש ממנו שמוציאים[6] אותו מאבני מחצבו באש כמו שמוציאים הכסף והזהב ואבן מחצבו כשהוא זך לא יתערב עמו עפרורית ולא[7] אבן בגון הזנגפור ([Arab.] *zi'baq*; i.e., [Hebr.] *kesef ḥay*: Quicksilver (mercury): It is either obtained from mines or extracted from ores by means of fire as is the case with gold and silver. If the ore is pure and not contaminated with dust and stone [pieces], it looks like [Arab.] *zunjufūr* [i.e., cinnabar]). In the sense of 'ore,' Hebr. אבן המחצב is not attested in the current dictionaries. In the Bible, we find *Plur.* אבני מחצב for 'quarried, cut stones' (cf.

---

6 שמוציאים: Emend. ed. שמוצאים Ms.
7 ולא: Emend. ed. ולו Ms.

KB 571). Anonymous I renders Arab. حجارة المعدن as אבן המחצב, just like Nathan, and Zeraḥyah Ḥen translates the Arab. term as אבן המקור (see entry below). Anonymous II has מינירא (Lat./Rom. MYNYR', cf. DMLBS 2150, s.v. *minaria*: 'mine, ore').

• **אבן המקוה** · **bladder stone**: Arab. حجر المثانة (cf. IBF no. 626; SUD 90ff., 178f. (B XXI)) · Ibn Sīnā, *K. al-Qānūn* II · trans. Anonymous I, *Sefer ha-Qanun* (Ms Paris, BnF, héb. 1142, fol. 121[b]): חגר אלמתאנה כלומר אבן המקוה איברי הנפוץ מועיל שהוא מפתת חצץ הכליות והמקוה אמר גאלינוס אין מזה דבר ([Arab.] *ḥajar al-mathāna*, i.e., [Hebr.] *even ha-miqweh*: Bladder stone. Excretory organs: It is beneficial since it pulverizes kidney and bladder stones. Galen said that this is not the case (that it does not have such an effect)). Hebr. אבן המקוה is not attested in the current dictionaries. Nathan ha-Me'ati transcribes Arab. حجر المثانة as חגר אלמתאנה only; Zeraḥyah Ḥen renders it as אבן השלפוחית (see entry below) and Anonymous II has לפיז וויסיקא (Lat./Rom. LPYZ WWYSYQ'; cf. Lat. *lapis vesive*, ALC 126[a]).

• **אבן המקור** · **ore**: Arab. حجارة المعدن · Ibn Sīnā, *K. al-Qānūn* II · trans. Zeraḥyah Ḥen, *Sefer ha-Qanun* (Ms Oxford, Bodleian Libraries, Opp. Add. Fol. 12, fol. 205[a]): זיבק כסף חי המהות יש ממנו שהוא מוצא ממקורו ויש ממנו שהוא מוצא מאבן מקורו באש כמו הזהב והכסף ואבן מקורו בהיותו זך לא יתערב בו אבן ולא עפר והוא כמראה הזנגפור הצֵינַברי ([Arab.] *zi'baq*; [i.e., Hebr.] *kesef ḥay*: Quicksilver (mercury): What is it? It is either obtained from mines or extracted from ores by means of fire as is the case with gold and silver. If the ore is pure and not contaminated with stone [pieces] and dust, it looks like [Arab.] *zunjufūr*; [Lat./Rom.] ṢeYNaBRY [i.e., cinnabar]). Hebr. אבן המקור is not attested in the current dictionaries. For the term מקור on its own in the sense of 'mineral, mine,' cf. BCD 159 (NM 1:166). Nathan ha-Me'ati and Anonymous I render the Arab. term as אבן המחצב (see entry above); Anonymous II has מינירא (Lat./Rom. MYNYR', cf. DMLBS 2150, s.v. *minaria*: 'mine, ore').

• **אבן הנחש** · **snake stone (serpentine)**: Arab. حجر الحية (cf. IBF no. 614; Gr. λίθος ὀφίτης; cf. DW 101 (V.143); DWB 401) · Ibn Sīnā, *K. al-Qānūn* II · trans. Zeraḥyah Ḥen, *Sefer ha-Qanun* (Ms Oxford, Bodlein Library, Opp. Add. Fol. 12, fol. 218[a]): חג׳ר אלְחַיָּה אבן הנחש ... הנקיון: יאמרו היא תשבר החול. וגאלינוס זוכר אותו. הסם: אמרו שהוא מועיל בתלייתה מנשיכת הנחש ([Arab.] *ḥajar al-ḥayya*: [i.e., Hebr.,] *even ha-naḥash*: Snake stone ... Excretion: It is said that it pulverizes stones. It is mentioned by Galen. Poisons: It is said that it is good against snake bites when it is hung [around the neck]). Nathan ha-Me'ati transcribes Arab. حجر الحية as חגר אלחיה only and Anonymous I has אבן הנחש, just like Zeraḥyah. Anonymous II has לפיז סירפינטי (Lat./Rom. LPYZ SYRPYNṬY).

• **אבן ספירית** · **talcum (mica)**: Arab. طلق (cf. MIG no. 466) · Ibn Sīnā, *K. al-Qānūn* II · trans. Anonymous I, *Sefer ha-Qanun* (Ms Paris, BnF, héb. 1142, fol. 122[a]): טלק אבן[8] ספירית ... אמרו קצתם שיש בשתייתו סכנה למה שיש בו מהסתבכות בקפולי[9] האיסטומ׳

8 אבן ספירית: Ms[1].

9 بشظايا المعدة وخملها a.: בקפולי האיסטומ׳ ובכריכותיה

ובבריכותיה ([Arab.] *ṭalq*; [i.e., Hebr.] *even sapirit*: Talcum (mica): … According to some people, the oral intake of talcum might be dangerous because it adheres to the [musculary] fibres and hair (villi) of the stomach). Hebr. אבן ספירית is not attested in the current dictionaries.

• **אבן הפוך · antimony:** Arab. إثمد (cf. KM 205–210) · *Glossary* (Ms Moscow, Russian State Library, Guenzburg 573, fol. 148a): אתמד לטי׳ אנטמוני לעז קופולי והוא אבן הפוך ([Arab.] *ithmid*; Lat. ʾNṬMWNY [i.e., [*lapis*] *ant*[*i*]*moni*[*i*]], o.l. QWPWLY [i.e., O. Occ. *cofol*(*l*)*i*], i.e., [Hebr.] *even ha-pukh*). Hebr. אבן הפוך is possibly a non-attested calque from Arab. **ḥajar kuḥl* (cf. *kuḥl ḥajar*[10]). Cf. the parallel entry in the glossary of plant names based on Ibn Sīnā. *K. al-Qānūn* II, Ms Vatican, Biblioteca Apostolica, ebr. 550, fol. 112b: אתמד הוא לפיש אנטמוני קופולי ([Arab.] *ithmid*; i.e., LPYŠ ʾNṬMWNY [i.e., Lat. *lapis ant*[*i*]*moni*[*i*]], [i.e.,] QWPWLY [i.e., O. Occ. *cofol*(*l*)*i*]).

• **אבן הרחים · millstone:** Arab. حجر الرحى (cf. IBF no. 632) · Ibn Sīnā, *K. al-Qānūn* II · trans. Zeraḥyah Ḥen, *Sefer ha-Qanun* (Ms Oxford, Bodleian Libraries, Opp. Add. Fol. 12, fol. 217b): חַגַ׳ר אלרַחַי אבן[11] הרחים … המורסות והבתור אידי החומץ עמו ימנע הגרת הדם וימנע המורסות החמות ([Arab.] *ḥajar al-raḥā*; [i.e., Hebr.] *even ha-reḥayim*: Millstone … Swellings and growths: The fumes [emanating from it when mixed] with vinegar prevent bleedings and hot swellings). Hebr. אבן הרחים is not attested in the current dictionaries. Nathan ha-Meʾati transcribes Arab. حجر الرحى as חגר אלרחא only and Anonymous I renders it as אבן הרחים, just like Zeraḥyah. Anonymous II has לאפיז מולרא (Lat./Rom. LPYZ MWLRʾ, cf. ALC 126a: *De lapide molari*).

• **אבן השלפוחית · bladder stone:** Arab. حجر المثانة (cf. IBF no. 626; SUD 90ff., 178f. (B XXI)) · Ibn Sīnā, *K. al-Qānūn* II · trans. Zeraḥyah Ḥen, *Sefer ha-Qanun* (Ms Oxford, Bodleian Libraries, Opp. Add. Fol. 12, fol. 217b): חַגַ׳ר אלמַתַ׳אנָה אבן השלפוחית ([Arab.] *ḥajar al-mathāna*, [i.e., Hebr.] *even ha-shalpuḥit*). Hebr. אבן השלפוחית is not attested in the current dictionaries. Nathan ha-Meʾati transcribes Arab. حجر المثانة as חגר אלמתאנה only and Anonymous I renders it as אבן המקוה (see entry above). Anonymous II has לפיז וויסיקא (Lat./Rom. LPYZ WWYSYQʾ, cf. ALC 126a: *lapis vesive*).

• **אבן שן הפיל · ivory[-colored] stone:** Arab. حجر العاج · Ibn Sīnā, *K. al-Qānūn* II · trans. Anonymous I, *Sefer ha-Qanun* (Ms Paris, BnF, héb. 1142, fol. 122a): חגר[12] אלעאגי כלומר אבן שן הפיל … הפעולות והסגולות ממרק ומנגב ועוצר הדם ([Arab.] *ḥajar al-ʿājī*; i.e., [Hebr.] *even shen ha-pil*: Ivory [colored] stone: … Its effects and properties: It cleanses, dries and stops bleedings). Hebr. אבן שן הפיל is not attested in the current dictionaries. Nathan ha-Meʾati and Zeraḥyah Ḥen transcribe Arab. حجر العاج as חג׳ר אלעאג׳ resp. חגר

10 M. Meyerhof, 'Der Bazar der Drogen und Wohlgerüche in Kairo,' *Archiv für Wirtschaftsforschung im Orient* 34 (1918): 180–218.

11 אבן הרחים: Ms1.

12 חגר אלעאגי: שן הפיל ובלשונם אֵבוֹרִיש [i.e., ivory] Ms1.

אלעאג׳י only. Anonymous II renders the Arab. term as לפיז אַלַאזִים (Lat./Rom. LPYZ 'aLa'ZiYM, cf. ALC 126[a]: *lapis alagi*). See also entry שֵׁן הפיל.

אֲבַעְבֻּעָה • *Plur.* **אבעבועות** · **blisters**: Arab. تنفّط (Gr. φλύκταινα; cf. UW 737f.) · Ibn Sīnā, *K. al-Qānūn* II · trans. Zeraḥyah Ḥen, *Sefer ha-Qanun* (Ms Oxford, Bodleian Libraries, Opp. Add. Fol. 12, fols. 203[b]–204[a]): וַסְךְ שׁוּרְדִיצִיאָה לכלוך ... וליכלוך כותלי בית המרחץ לאבעבועות ([Arab.] *wasakh*; [Lat.] *sorditia*, [Hebr.] *likhlukh*: Dirt: ... The dirt of the walls of the bathhouse is [good] for blisters). Hebr. אֲבַעְבֻּעָה, *Plur.* אבעבועות, features in BM 34 in the sense of 'pustule, blister, small-pox.' In his trans. of Maimonides' *Commentary on Hippocrates'* Aphorisms (i.e., *Perush Aphorismi shel Apuqraṭ*) VII.55, Zeraḥyah uses the term אבעבועות to render Arab. نفاخات 'watery vesicles' (cf. BMCH 1:510, l. 13; BCD 15 (NM 3:21)). Nathan ha-Me'ati translates Arab. تنفّط as בועות (see entry בּוּעָה).

[אבק] • *Part. Hitpa'el* מִתְאַבֵּק • *Plur.* **מתאבקים** · **wrestlers**: Arab. مصارع, *Plur.* مصارعون · Ibn Sīnā, *K. al-Qānūn* II · trans. Zeraḥyah Ḥen, *Sefer ha-Qanun* (Ms Oxford, Bodleian Libraries, Opp. Add. Fol. 12, fol. 203[b]): וַסְךְ שׁוּרְדִיצִיאָה לכלוך ... ולכלוך[13] המתאבקים שני מינים ([Arab.] *wasakh*; [i.e., Lat.] *sorditia*, [i.e., Hebr.] *likhlukh*: Dirt: ... Dirt[14] [on the bodies] of wrestlers is of two kinds). In the sense of 'wrestler,' Hebr. מִתְאַבֵּק is not attested for medieval medical literature (cf. BM 36). Nathan ha-Me'ati translates Arab. مصارعون as עמלים (see entry עָמֵל) and Anonymous I has מתאבקים, just like Zeraḥyah. In both his trans. of Maimonides' *Medical Aphorisms* (i.e., *Sefer ha-Peraqim*) XVIII.9 and *Commentary on Hippocrates'* Aphorisms (i.e., *Perush Aphorismi shel Apuqraṭ*) I.3, Zeraḥyah translates Arab. مصارعون as מתאבקים as well (cf. BMMZ 175, l. 24; BMMG no. 2878; BMCH 1:426, l. 6). A synonymous term featuring in the anonymous trans. of Maimonides' *Commentary on Hippocrates'* Aphorisms (i.e., *Perush Aphorismi shel Apuqraṭ*) I.3 is טרחנים (cf. BCD 114 (NM 3:101f.); BMCH 1:521, l. 5).

אֵבֶר • *Plur.* **אברים** • **האברים המגדלים** · **the nutritive organs**: Arab. أعضاء الغذاء · Ibn Sīnā, *K. al-Qānūn* II · trans. Anonymous II, *Sefer ha-Qanun* (Ms Parma, Biblioteca Palatina, Cod. Parm. 3045, fol. 30[b]): תרנגלים ותרנגלות ... תועלתו לאברים המגדלים מרק תרנוגלים זכרים יצליח לכאב האצטומ׳ המולד מן הרוח (Roosters and hens (chickens): ... Their usefulness for the nutritive organs: Soup from roosters is beneficial for stomachache caused by gases). Hebr. האברים המגדלים is not attested in the current dictionaries. Zeraḥyah Ḥen translates Arab. أعضاء الغذاء as אברי המזון.

• **האברים הדוחים** · **the excretory organs**: Arab. أعضاء النفض · Ibn Sīnā, *K. al-Qānūn* II · trans. Anonymous II, *Sefer ha-Qanun* (Ms Parma, Biblioteca Palatina, Cod. Parm. 3045, fol. 48[a]): לוטוס ארמיני ... תועלתו לאברים הדוחים יועיל למורסות המעים ולשלשול ולשפע עת הנשים ([Lat.-Arab.] LWṬWS (*lutus/lutum*?) *armīnī*: Armenian bole: ... Its useful-

13 ולכלוך: וזיעה Ms[1].

14 'Dirt': 'Transpiration' Ms[1].

ness for the excretory organs: It is good for intestinal ulcers, diarrhea, and uterine (menstrual) bleeding). Hebr. האברים הדוחים is not attested in the current dictionaries. Nathan ha-Me'ati translates Arab. أعضاء النفض as איברי הנעירה (cf. NM 6:8, 14), Zeraḥyah Ḥen translates the Arab. term as איברי הנקיון (cf. NM 6:8), and Anonymous I has איברי הנפוץ (cf. NM 6:8, 14).

• **האברים המחזיקים** · **containing organs (members)**: Lat. *membra continentia* (cf. ND 665 (B 11): 'Body parts enclosing other part(s)') · Guy de Chauliac, *Inventarium sive Chirurgia Magna* (cf. CMM 1:239, ll. 12–14) · trans. Anonymous (Ms Paris, BnF, héb. 1189, fol. 131[a]): לפעמים יהיו הנגעים באברים המחזיקים ולפעמים באברים המוקפים ולפעמים באברים הנמשכים מהם כמו באמה וכיס האשכים והטבעת (Sometimes [ulcers] occur in the organs (members) that contain [other parts], sometimes in the organs that are contained [by other parts], and sometimes in the organs that can have a prolapse, such as a penis, scrotum, and anus). Hebr. האברים המחזיקים is not attested in the current dictionaries. A synonymous term used by Anonymous is האברים המקיפים (see entry below).

• **האברים הנמשכים** · **organs that can have a prolapse**: Lat. *membra procidentia* · Guy de Chauliac, *Inventarium sive Chirurgia Magna* (cf. CMM 1:239, l. 13) · trans. Anonymous (Ms Paris, BnF, héb. 1189, fol. 131[a]): ולפעמים באברים הנמשכים (Sometimes [ulcers] occur in organs that can have a prolapse). Hebr. האברים הנמשכים is not attested in the current dictionaries.

• **האברים המקיפים** · **containing organs (members)**: Lat. *membra continentia* (cf. ND 665 (B 11): 'Body parts enclosing other part(s)') · Guy de Chauliac, *Inventarium sive Chirurgia Magna* (cf. CMM 1:239, ll. 14–15) · trans. Anonymous (Ms Paris, BnF, héb. 1189, fol. 131[a]): אמנם הנעשים באברים המקיפים באותו אופן עצמו ירופא כנגעי הבטן (However, those [ulcers] that occur in the containing organs should be cured in the same way as stomach ulcers). Hebr. האברים המקיפים is not attested in the current dictionaries. A synonymous term used by Anonymous is האברים המחזיקים (see entry above).

• **האברים המוקפים** · **contained organs (members)**: Lat. *membra contenta* (cf. ND 665 (B 10): 'Body parts enclosed within larger structure') · Guy de Chauliac, *Inventarium sive Chirurgia Magna* (cf. CMM 1:239, ll. 12–14) · trans. Anonymous (Ms Paris, BnF, héb. 1189, fol. 131[a]): ולפעמים באברים המוקפים ולפעמים באברים הנמשכים מהם כמו באמה וכיס האשכים והטבעת (Sometimes ulcers occur in the organs (members) that contain [other parts], sometimes in the organs that are contained [by other parts], and sometimes in the organs that can have a prolapse, such as a penis, scrotum, and anus). Hebr. האברים המוקפים is not attested in the current dictionaries.

• **האברים המעולים** · **the vital (principal) organs**: Arab. الأعضاء النفيسة · al-Rāzī, *K. fī al-Faṣd* · trans. Anonymous, *Ma'amar ba-Haqqazah* (Ms Parma, Biblioteca Palatina, Cod. Parm. 2283,4, fol. 93[a]): וכאשר יהיה הדם הרבה בגוף ונתחמם ונרתח ונתחדשה ממנו קדחת יעשה הרקתו פתאם בעת ירידת הקפת הקדחת וקודם שיהיה נגר אל האברים המעולים

בעבור כי זאת הקדחת ואם היא דבקה יהיה לה על הרוב התחלה ותוספת ותכלית וירידה (When there is a lot of blood in the body, and it boils and causes a fever, then evacuate it all at once at the time of the decline of the paroxysm of fever before it flows towards the vital (principal) organs, because this fever, even if it was continuous, in most cases will have a beginning, rise, increase, climax, and decline). Hebr. האברים המעולים features in BCD 16 (NM 4:12) (for Arab. الأعضاء الشريفة 'the noble organs') in Zeraḥyah Ḥen's trans. of Maimonides' *Medical Aphorisms* (i.e., *Sefer ha-Peraqim*) III.79 (cf. BMMZ 44, l. 21; BMMG no. 3437). Arab. *Sing.* عضو نفيس 'principle organ, vital organ' features as אבר נכבד in Nathan's *Sefer ha-Peraqim* III.110 and XV.13 (cf. BMMN 55, l. 23; 156, l. 9; BMMG no. 3412) and in Zeraḥyah's trans. of the same aphorisms as אבר יותר מעולה ונכבד (III.110) and אבר שריי (XV.1) (cf. BMMZ 49, l. 6; 154, l. 19; BMMG no. 3412).

אֱגוֹז · **medicinal weight; dose of one walnut**: Arab. جوزة (for its varying weight; cf. HIM 12; MIG no. 217) · Ibn Sīnā, *K. al-Qānūn* II · trans. Nathan ha-Me'ati, *Sefer ha-Qanun* (Ms Oxford, Bodleian Libraries, Can. Or. 88, fol. 92[a]): כרסנה ... ויתנו ממנו אל הכחוש כמו אגוז ויסיר הרזון ([Arab.] *kirsinna*: Bitter vetch [*Vicia ervilia* (L.) Willd.]: ... When one administers a dose of one walnut to lean persons, they will gain weight). Hebr. אֱגוֹז features in the current dictionaries in the sense of 'nut' only; cf. JD 11; BM 43. Anonymous I renders Arab. جوزة as אֱגוֹז, just like Nathan, and Zeraḥyah Ḥen translates the Arab. term as אֱגוֹזָה (see next entry).

אֱגוֹזָה · **medicinal weight; dose of one walnut**: Arab. جوزة (for its varying weight; cf. HIM 12; MIG no. 217) · Ibn Sīnā, *K. al-Qānūn* II · trans. Zeraḥyah Ḥen, *Sefer ha-Qanun* (Ms Oxford, Bodleian Libraries, Opp. Add. Fol. 12, fols. 224[b]–225[a]): כַּרְסַנָּה ... ויותן לכחושים ממנו כמו האגוזה ויסיר הכחש ([Arab.] *kirsinna*: Bitter vetch [*Vicia ervilia* (L.) Willd.]: ... When one administers a dose of one walnut to lean persons, they will gain weight). Hebr. אֱגוֹזָה features in Rabb. literature in the sense of 'nut tree' only; cf. JD 11; BM 43. Nathan ha-Me'ati and Anonymous I both render Arab. جوزة as אֱגוֹז (see previous entry).

אָדוֹם • **שחין אדום** → **שְׁחִין**.

[אדם] • *Part. Pi'el* **מְאַדֵּם** • **הסם המאדם** → **סַם**.

• *Part. Hif'il* **מַאְדִים** • **הסם המאדים** → **סַם**.

• **הרפואה המאדימה** → **רְפוּאָה**.

אָדָם • **בן אדם** → **בֵּן**.

[אוה] • *Part. Pi'el* **מְאַוֶּה** • **מאוה המאכל** · **whetting the appetite**: Arab. مشهّ للطعام · Ibn Sīnā, *K. al-Qānūn* II · trans. Nathan ha-Me'ati, *Sefer ha-Qanun* (Ms Oxford, Bodleian Libraries, Can. Or. 88, fols. 84[b]–85[a]): חרף ... והוא רע לאצטומכא וידמה שיהיה זה בעד רוב נשיכתו והוא מאוה המאכל ([Arab.] *ḥurf*: Garden cress [*Lepidium sativum* L.]: ... It is bad for the stomach and this is probably due to it being intensely irritant. It whets the appetite). Hebr. אוה המאכל, *Part. Pi'el* מאוה המאכל, is not attested in the current dictionaries. Zeraḥyah Ḥen translates Arab. مشهّ للطعام as מקנה תאות המזון and Anonymous I has מאוה המאכל, just like Nathan.

אוֹזֶן → אֹזֶן.

אוֹטֵם (*Part.*) → אָטַם.

אֲוִירִיּוּת · airiness: Arab. هوائية · Ibn Sīnā, *K. al-Qānūn* II · trans. Anonymous I, *Sefer ha-Qanun* (Ms Paris, BnF, héb. 1142, fols. 99[b]–100[a]): חב[15] אלצנובר כלומר גרגרי פנייש .... ועצמיותו עפרי מימיי ויש בו מעט אויריות ([Arab.] *ḥabb al-ṣanawbar*; i.e., [Hebr.-Lat./Rom.] *gargerei* PNYYŠ: Pine nuts [*Pinus* L.]: ... Their substance is earthy, watery, and a little bit airy). Hebr. אֲוִירִיּוּת features as אֲוִירִיּוּת in BM 98 in an attestation from the *Sefer ha-Qanun*. Nathan ha-Me'ati translates Arab. هوائية as אוירי and Zeraḥyah Ḥen has אוירריית.

אוּשְׁכָּף • *Plur.* אושכפים • אבן האושכפים → אֶבֶן.

אֹזֶן • הגרת האזן → הֲגָרָה.

• זוהמת האוזן → זהמה.

• לחיצת האזן → לְחִיצָה.

• ליכלוכי האוזן → לִכְלוּךְ.

• המורסות אשר בעקר האזן → מֻרְסָה.

• רסוק האזן → רִסּוּק.

• רצוץ האזן → רִצּוּץ.

• *Dual* אזנים • טנופת האזנים → טִנּוֹפֶת.

• כאב האזנים → כְּאֵב.

• המורסות אשר בשורש האזנים → מֻרְסָה.

אָחוּ • עסיס אחו → עָסִיס.

אָטַם • *Part.* אוטם • הסם האוטם → סַם.

[איד] • *Hif'il* האיד · **to evaporate, disperse, emit vapors:** Lat. *evaporo* · Guy de Chauliac, *Inventarium sive Chirurgia Magna* (cf. CMM 1:415, ll. 36–38) · trans. Anonymous (Ms Paris, BnF, héb. 1189, fol. 122[a]): ויעץ זהרבי ועלי אביש ... הכוויה העגולה כמו הזיתים להאיד המוח ולהעתיק החמר ([Al-]Zahrāwī and 'Alī 'Abbās ... advised the application of the cautery round like an olive (olivary cautery) [to the head] to disperse vapors from the brain and to divert [superflous] matter). Hebr. *Hif'il* האיד is not attested in the current dictionaries.

אִילִיאוּשׁ · **ileus** · Arab. إيلاوس (Gr. εἰλεός; cf. UW 222) · Ibn Sīnā, *K. al-Qānūn* II · trans. Nathan ha-Me'ati, *Sefer ha-Qanun* (Ms Oxford, Bodleian Libraries, Can. Or. 88, fol. 81[a–b]): זיבק הוא כסף חי ... אמר בולש כי יש מהאנשים שמשקים הכסף חי הנמוח לחולי איליאוש ([Arab.] *zi'baq*; i.e., [Hebr.] *kesef ḥay*: Quicksilver (mercury): ... Paulus said that some people (physicians) administer 'killed'[16] quicksilver to those suffering from the illness [called] *ileus*). Hebr. איליאוש[17] is an unattested loan word from Arab. إيلاوس and features also in both Nathan's (אילאוש) and Zeraḥyah's (איליאוס) trans. of

---

15 גרגירי פינייאש והוא פינוש :חב אלצנובר Ms[1].
16 'killed': Arab. مقتول; cf. entry כֶּסֶף: כסף חי נמוח.
17 Variants: איליאוס; אליאוש.

Maimonides' *Medical Aphorisms* (i.e., *Sefer ha-Peraqim*) XXIII.93 (cf. BMMN 230, l. 23; BMMZ 229, l. 23; BMMG no. 161). Zeraḥyah Ḥen renders Arab. إيلاوس as חולי הקוליקא (see entry חֳלִי).

איסטו׳ → אִצְטוֹמְכָא.

אִישׁוֹן · **pupil of the eye**: Arab. حدقة · Ibn Sīnā, *K. al-Qānūn* II · trans. Anonymous I, *Sefer ha-Qanun* (Ms Paris, BnF, héb. 1142, fol. 201[a]): ... ערוק אלצבאג׳ין כלומר עורקי הצבעים סחיטתו מועילה מאד לחדד הראות וממרק מה שהוא לפני האישון ממים ולובן ([Arab.] *ʿurūq al-ṣabbāghīn* [lit. 'roots of the dyers']; i.e., [Hebr.] *ʿorqei ha-ṣabaʿim*: Greater celandine [*Chelidonium majus* L.] (cf. IBF no. 1525): ... Its juice is very good for sharpening the eyesight and for clearing water covering the pupil of the eye and for leucoma). Hebr. אִישׁוֹן features in MD 612 without any further reference and in BM 200f. and EM 62 without any attestation from medieval medical literature. Nathan ha-Me'ati translates Arab. حدقة as בבת העין (see entry בָּבָה) and Zeraḥyah Ḥen translates the Arab. term as בת עין (see entry בַּת).

אישפונגי • **עשה אישפונגי באף** → עָשָׂה.

אָכוּל (*Part. Pass.*) → אָכַל.

אֲכִילָה • **תאות אכילת החומר** → תַּאֲוָה.

אָכַל • *Part.* **אוֹכֵל** • **הסם האוכל** → סַם.

• **הרפואה האוכלת** → רְפוּאָה.

• *Part. Pass.* **אָכוּל** · **corrosive**: Arab. متأكّل (Gr. γαγγραινώδης; cf. UW 173f.: 'nach Art eines fressenden Geschwürs') · Ibn Sīnā, *K. al-Qānūn* II · trans. Nathan ha-Me'ati, *Sefer ha-Qanun* (Ms Oxford, Bodleian Libraries, Can. Or. 88, fols. 75[b]–76[a]): גזר ... אם ישחקו זרעו ועליו וישימו על הנגעים האכולים יועיל להם ([Arab.] *jazar* / [Hebr.] *gezer*: Carrot [*Daucus carota* L.]: ... If one pulverizes its seeds and leaves and applies them to corrosive ulcers, it is beneficial for them). Hebr. אָכוּל does not feature in this sense in the current dictionaries. Anonymous I renders Arab. متأكّل as *Part. Hitpaʿel* מִתְאַכֵּל (see entry below) and Anonymous II has *Part.* אוֹכֵל (cf. NM 6:17). Yet another variant reading is *Part. Puʿal* מְאֻכָּל (see entry below).

• *Part. Piʿel* **מְאַכֵּל** • **הסם המאכל** → סַם.

• *Part. Puʿal* **מְאֻכָּל** · **corrosive**: Lat. *corrosivus* · Guy de Chauliac, *Inventarium sive Chirurgia Magna* (cf. CMM 1:239, l. 34) · trans. Anonymous (Ms Paris, BnF, héb. 1189, fol. 131[a]): אמנם אותם הנעשים באברים הנמשכים כמו באמה וצואר הרחם הם גרידות חימומים ונגעים המימיים[18] עם מוגליות ומעופשים ומאוכלים ומסורטנים ([Ulcers] that occur in organs that can have a prolapse, such as a penis and neck of the uterus (cervix), are: excoriations, heating ulcers, virulent ulcers, putrid ulcers, corrosive ulcers, cancerous ulcers). Hebr. מְאֻכָּל is not attested in the sense of 'corrosive' in the current dictionaries.

---

18 המימיים עם מוגליות: *virulenta* L.

• *Part. Hitpa'el* מִתְאַכֵּל · **corrosive**: Arab. متأكّل (Gr. γαγγραινώδης; cf. UW 173f.: 'nach Art eines fressenden Geschwürs') · Ibn Sīnā, *K. al-Qānūn* II · trans. Nathan ha-Me'ati, *Sefer ha-Qanun* (Ms Oxford, Bodleian Libraries, Can. Or. 88, fol. 97[b]): כמאלאון ... ימשחו על הגרב ועל השחין הדק והוא קובא בערבי ויועיל ועושין ממנו תחבשת אל הנגעים המתאכלים ([Arab.] *khāmālāwun*: Chamaeleon (DT 3.8): ... It is beneficial when it is rubbed on scabies and ringworm, [called] *qūbā* in Arab. As a plaster it is used for corrosive ulcers). In the sense of 'corrosive' (for Lat. *corrosivus*), Hebr. *Part. Hitpa'el* מִתְאַכֵּל features in BCD 21 (NM 4:16) in an attestation from Abraham Avigdor's *Pirqei Arnavṭ de-Vila Nova*. For the synonymous *Part. Pass.* אָכוּל, see entry above; for *Part.* אוֹכֵל (Arab. أكّال) in the same sense, see NM 6:17. Anonymous I renders Arab. متأكّل as מִתְאַכֵּל, just like Nathan. Yet another variant reading is *Part. Pu'al* מְאֻכָּל (see previous entry).

אַמָּה • **אמת הזרוע** · **forearm**: Arab. ذراع (cf. FA no. 1150) · al-Rāzī, *K. fī al-Faṣd* · trans. Anonymous, *Ma'amar ba-Haqqazah* (Ms Parma, Biblioteca Palatina, Cod. Parm. 2283,4, fol. 93[b]): וו' גידים באמות הזרוע בכל אמת[19] הזרוע מהם ג' גידים (Six veins in the forearms, in each forearm three veins). In the sense of 'forearm,' Hebr. אמת הזרוע features as אמה in Bibl. and Rabb. literature, cf. KB 61; Low XXXVII; BM 271.

אנולוס • *Plur.* **אנולוסים** · ***oboloi***: Arab. أبولوسات (corrupted as: أنولوسات, from Gr. ὀβολός, as a weight, the sixth part of a *drachme*, i.e., 0.75 g)[20] · Ibn Sīnā, *K. al-Qānūn* II · trans. Zeraḥyah Ḥen, *Sefer ha-Qanun* (Ms Oxford, Bodleian Libraries, Opp. Add. Fol. 12, fol. 220[b]): יברוח ... ומי שירצה שיחתך ממנו אבר יושקה שלשה אנולוסים ממנו עם יין ויפיל[21] תרדמה ([Arab.] *yabrūḥ*: Mandrake [*Mandragora officinarum* L.]: ... If you want to amputate a body part of a patient, you should give him three *oboloi* (2.25 g) of mandrake [mixed] with wine so that he will fall in a deep sleep). Hebr. אנולוס, *Plur.* אנולוסים, is a non-attested Hebraization of Arab. أبولوسات (corrupted as: أنولوسات). In addition to אנולוסים, Zeraḥyah transcribes the Arab. term as אנולוסאת. Nathan ha-Me'ati renders it as אנולוסאות (see next entry) and Anonymous I has לובלוסים (read: אובלוסים?).

• *Plur.* **אנולוסאות** · ***oboloi***: Arab. أبولوسات (corrupted as: أنولوسات, from Gr. ὀβολός, as a weight, the sixth part of a *drachme*, i.e., 0.75 g) · Ibn Sīnā, *K. al-Qānūn* II · trans. Nathan ha-Me'ati, *Sefer ha-Qanun* (Ms Oxford, Bodleian Libraries, Can. Or. 88, fol. 89[b]): יברוח ... ומי שרוצים לכרות ממנו אבר ישקו לו שלש אנולוסאות ביין וירדם ([Arab.] *yabrūḥ*: Mandrake [*Mandragora officinarum* L.]: ... If you want to amputate a body part of a patient, you should give him three *oboloi* (2.25 g) of mandrake [mixed] with wine so that he will fall in a deep sleep). Hebr. אנולוס, *Plur.* אנולוסאות, is a non-

19 אמת: Emend. ed. אמות Ms.

20 The same Hebr. term features in Nathan ha-Me'ati's entry on מגנאטיס 'magnet' (Ms Oxford, Bodleian Libraries, Can. Or. 88, fol. 103[b]).

21 ויפיל תרדמה: فيسبت a.

attested Hebraization of Arab. أنولوسات (read: أبولوسات). Zeraḥyah Ḥen renders the Arab. term as אנולוסים[22] (see previous entry) and Anonymous I has לובלוסים (read: אובלוסים?)

אֲנָחָה · **anxiety**: Arab. توحّش · Ibn Sīnā, *K. al-Qānūn* II · trans. Zeraḥyah Ḥen, *Sefer ha-Qanun* (Ms Oxford, Bodleian Libraries, Opp. Add. Fol. 12, fol. 218[a]): טבאשיר אֶשְׁפּוֹדִי ... יועיל מן הקלאע ומן האנחה ([Arab.] *ṭabāshīr*; [i.e., Rom.] ʾeŠəPWoDiY [i.e., O. Occ. *espodi*]: Tabasheer (bamboo manna) [i.e., the siliceous secretions found in the internodes of bamboo stems [*Bambusa bambos* (L.) Voss]]: It is beneficial for aphthae and for anxiety). Hebr. אֲנָחָה is not attested in this sense in the current dictionaries. Nathan ha-Me'ati translates Arab. توحّش as השתוממות השכל (see entry הִשְׁתּוֹמְמוּת) and Anonymous I has הִשְׁתּוֹמְמוּת (cf. BCD 74 (NM 4:48) for an attestation from an anonymous trans. of Ibn Sīnā's *K. al-Adwiya al-qalbiyya* (i.e., *Sammim Libbiyim*)). Cf. also NM 5:196 for the variant reading שִׁמָּמוֹן, featuring in the anonymous trans. of Isḥāq ibn ʿImrān's *Treatise on Melancholy*. In addition to אֲנָחָה, Zeraḥyah translates Arab. توحّش as מַחְשָׁבָה and תּוּגָה (see entries).

אֲנָקָה · **monitor lizard [*Varanus* (Merrem, 1820)]**: Arab. ورل (cf. MIG no. 300) · i. Ibn Sīnā, *K. al-Qānūn* II · trans. Nathan ha-Me'ati, *Sefer ha-Qanun* (Ms Oxford, Bodleian Libraries, Can. Or. 88, fol. 78[b]): דם ... דם האנקה הנקרא ורל בערבי ודם הכח הנקרא חרדון בערבי יחזקו הראות (Blood: ... The blood of the monitor lizard, called *waral* in Arab., and that of the roughtail rock agama (stellion), called *ḥirdhawn* in Arab., strengthen vision). Hebr. אֲנָקָה features in the Bible (Lev 11:30) as an 'unclean animal,' perhaps: 'ferret or shrew-mouse' (BDB 60) or 'gecko' (KB 73; FAB 97), and in Rabb. literature as a 'species of lizard' (JD 87). The identification of Hebr. אֲנָקָה as Arab. ورل already features in Saʿadya's trans. of Lev 11:30[23] and subsequently in Ibn Janāḥ's *K. al-Uṣūl*: והאנקה והכח الورل وهو شيء على خلقة الضبّ[24]. Zeraḥyah Ḥen translates Arab. ورل as לוּגֵירְדְ (Ital.-Rom. LWuGeYRəDə) and Anonymous I renders the Arab. term as אֲנָקָה, just like Nathan.

· ii. *Glossary* (Ms Moscow, Russian State Library, Guenzburg 573, fol. 151[b]): ורל הוא אנקה ובלעז לוצירטון ([Arab.] *waral*; i.e., [Hebr.] *anaqah*, o.l. LWṢYRṬWN) The Rom. term is possibly South-Ital., esp. Apulean *lucertòn* (Altamura), *lucirtòn* (Taranto); for Lecce itself (where the Ms was possibly copied), we find *lucertone*.[25]

---

22 In Zeraḥyah Ḥen's entry on מַגְנֵטִס 'magnet' (Ms Oxford, Bodleian Libraries, Opp. Add. Fol. 12, fol. 239[a–b]), Arab. أبولوسات is transcribed as אנולוסאת.

23 Cf. J. Derenbourg (ed.), *Targum Ḥamishah Ḥumshei Torah be-Lashon ʿAravit le-Rabbeinu Saʿadyah Gaʾon ben Yoseph ha-Fayyumi: Version arabe du Pentateuque de R. Saadia Ben Iosef al-Fayyoûmî* (Repr., Hildesheim 1979), 158.

24 Abū l-Walīd Marwān ibn Janāḥ, *K. al-Uṣūl: The Book of Hebrew Roots*, ed. by A. Neubauer (Oxford 1875), col. 59.

25 G. Bertoni, 'Denominazioni del *ramarro* (lacerta viridis) in Italia,' *Romania* 42, no. 166 (1913): 161–173. I thank my colleague and friend Guido Mensching for this reference.

[אסף] • *Inf. Nif'al* הֵאָסֵף • **האסף פי הרחם** · **closing (narrowing) of the cervical os**. Arab. انضمام فم الرحم · Ibn Sīnā, *K. al-Qānūn* II · trans. Zeraḥyah Ḥen, *Sefer ha-Qanun* (Ms Oxford, Bodleian Libraries, Opp. Add. Fol. 12, fol. 243[b]): נַרְגַ׳ס ... יועיל מכאבי הרחם והשלפוחית וכשישתה ממנו ד׳ דראהם עם מי הדבש יפיל העובר[26] והמת והשמן שלו פותח האסף פי הרחם ויועיל מכאיביה ([Arab.] *narjis*: Narcissus [*Narcissus* L.]: ... It is useful for pain of the uterus and urinary bladder. When one drinks 4 *dirhams*[27] of it with honey water, it causes expulsion of a live[28] or dead fetus. Its oil opens a closed cervical os and is useful for pains affecting it). Hebr. האסף פי הרחם is not attested in the current dictionaries. Nathan ha-Me'ati translates Arab. انضمام فم الرحم as צרות הרחם and Anonymous I renders the Arab. term as סגירת פי הרחם.

אֶסְפּוֹג • **אבן האספוג** → אֶבֶן.

אַף • **הטפה באף** → הַטָּפָה.
• **חבש באף** → חָבַשׁ.
• **הטיף באף** → [נטף].
• **סרחון האף** → סִרְחוֹן.
• **עשה אישפונגי באף** → עָשָׂה.
• **רעיפת דם מהאף** → רְעִיפָה.

אֲפֵלָה • **מחשך באפלה** → מַחְשָׁךְ.

אצטו׳ → אִצְטוֹמְכָא.

אִצְטוֹמְכָא (*Aram.*) • **הפוך האצטו׳** → הִפּוּךְ.
• **התהפכות האיסטו׳** → הִתְהַפְּכוּת.

אַרְבֶּה · **locust**: Arab. جراد (cf. DT 222 (II.39)) · Ibn Sīnā, *K. al-Qānūn* II · trans. Zeraḥyah Ḥen, *Sefer ha-Qanun* (Ms Oxford, Bodleian Libraries, Opp. Add. Fol. 12, fol. 194[b]): גַּרָאדְ ארבה[29] ([Arab.] *jarād*; [i.e., Hebr.] *arbeh*: Locust). Hebr. אַרְבֶּה features in the current dictionaries in the sense of 'locust' in attestations from the Bible and Rabb. literature only (cf. KB 83; FAB 115; JD 114; LZ 286; BM 377 ('grasshopper')). Nathan ha-Me'ati translates Arab. جراد as חגבים and Anonymous I has חָגָב (see entry). Zeraḥyah's marginal gloss גַזַם is attested as גָּזָם in the Bible in the sense of 'locust' as well (cf. KB 187; FAB 115).

אָרוֹךְ → אָרֹךְ.

אֲרִיגָה • **אריגת העכביש** · **cobweb**: Arab. نسج · Ibn Sīnā, *K. al-Qānūn* II · trans. Zeraḥyah Ḥen, *Sefer ha-Qanun* (Ms Oxford, Bodleian Libraries, Opp. Add. Fol. 12, fol. 256[b]): עַנְכַּבוּת עכביש ... אמר קצתם כח אריגת העכביש כשתעורב עם קצת מן המשיחות ויושם על המצח ושתי הצדעים ירפא קדחת הטירצאנא ([Arab.] *ʿankabūt*; [i.e., Hebr.] *ʿakavish*]: Spider: ...

---

26 העובר: الأجنة الأحياء a.
27 '*dirhams*': The standard *dirham* is 3.125 grams; cf. HIM 3.
28 'live': Add. acc. to a.
29 ארבה: גַזַם Ms[1].

Some [physicians] said that the cobweb, when mixed with some ointments and applied to the forehead and temples, cures tertian fever). Hebr. אריגת העכביש is a non-attested calque from Arab. نسج العنكبوت. Nathan ha-Me'ati translates the Arab. term as אריגת העכביש as well. Anonymous I renders it as קורי העכביש (see entry קוּר).

אָרֹךְ · **chronic**: Arab. مزمن · Ibn Sīnā, *K. al-Qānūn* II · trans. Zeraḥyah Ḥen, *Sefer ha-Qanun* (Ms Oxford, Bodleian Libraries, Opp. Add. Fol. 12, fol. 260[b]): ... פַּ'רָאסִיּוֹן מַרוּבִּי מיצו לכאב האוזן הארוך וינקה ופותח מעברות השמיעה ויסיר הקדמון מכאבו ([Arab. *farāsiyūn* [from Gr. πράσιον]; [i.e., Rom.] MaRWuBiY [from Lat. *marrubium*]: White horehound [*Marrubium vulgare* L.]: ... Its juice is [beneficial] for chronic earache; it cleanses and opens the auditory channels and relieves chronic pain [in the ear]). Hebr. אָרֹךְ, usually meaning 'long,' is not attested in this sense in the current dictionaries. A synonym used by Zeraḥyah in the same passage is קַדְמוֹן (see entry). Nathan ha-Me'ati translates Arab. مزمن as יָשָׁן (see entry) and Anonymous I renders the Arab. term as נוֹשָׁן (see entry [ישן]).

אַרְמִינִי • אבן ארמיני → אֶבֶן.

אַרְנֶבֶת • **ארנבת הים** · **spotted sea hare [*Aplysia depilans* (Gmelin, 1791)]**: Arab. أرنب بحري (Gr. ὁ θαλάττιος λαγωός) · Ibn Sīnā, *K. al-Qānūn* II · trans. Nathan ha-Me'ati, *Sefer ha-Qanun* (Ms Oxford, Bodleian Libraries, Can. Or. 88, fol. 67[b]): ארנאב בחארי כלומר ארנבת הים המהות הוא חייוני[30] נולד בתוך קלפות ובערבי צדף ([Arab.] *arnab baḥrī*; i.e., [Hebr.] *arnevet ha-yam*: Spotted sea hare [*Aplysia depilans* (Gmelin, 1791)]. What is it? It is an animal that originates within a shell, [called] in Arab. *ṣadaf*). Hebr. ארנבת הים is not attested in the current dictionaries. A variant הארנבת הימית features in BCD 28 (NM 4:21) in an attestation from Shem Tov ben Isaac's *Sefer ha-Shimmush* XXVII. Zeraḥyah Ḥen translates Arab. أرنب بحري as ארנבת הים, just like Nathan. Anonymous I renders the Arab. term, similar to Shem Tov, as ארנבת ימיית.

אֵשׁ • **אש זר** · **carbuncle; furuncles**: Arab. النار الفارسي (Gr. ἄνθραξ; cf. UW 112) · Ibn Sīnā, *K. al-Qānūn* II · trans. Anonymous II, *Sefer ha-Qanun* (Ms Parma, Biblioteca Palatina, Cod. Parm. 3045, fols. 26[b]–27[a]): אפופונקו ... ועם דבש יצליח למורסות קדמוניות ולאש זר ([Rom.] 'PWPWNQW: Opopanax [i.e., the resin of the sweet myrrh [*Opopanax chironius* W.D.J. Koch]]: ... Together with honey, it is beneficial for chronic ulcers and for carbuncles). Hebr. אש זר is not attested in the current dictionaries. Nathan ha-Me'ati, Zeraḥyah Ḥen, and Anonymous I translate Arab. النار الفارسي as האש הפרסי (cf. NM 6:22).

אִשָּׁה • *Plur.* **נשים** • **הגרת הנשים** → הֲגָרָה.

• **עוזר עת הנשים** → [עזר].

• **שפע עת הנשים** → שֶׁפַע.

---

30 חייוני: حيوان a.

אֶשֶׁךְ • אשך המים · **hydrocele**: Arab. أدرة الماء (Gr. ὑδροκήλη; cf. UW 697) · Ibn Sīnā, *K. al-Qānūn* II · trans. Nathan ha-Me'ati, *Sefer ha-Qanun* (Ms Oxford, Bodleian Libraries, Can. Or. 88, fol. 63[b]): אקחואן ... ויועיל ממורסת העגבות החמות ויפתח הטחורים הוא ומשיחתו ויועיל מאשך המים ובער' אדרה אחר שמבקעים אותו ([Arab.] *uqḥuwān*: Feverfew [*Tanacetum parthenium* (L.) Sch. Bip.]: ... It is useful for hot swellings of the anus and opens hemorrhoids. Its oil is useful for ruptured hydrocele, [called] in Arab. *udra* [*al-mā*]). In the sense of 'hydrocele,' Hebr. אשך המים is a non-attested calque from Arab. أدرة الماء. In addition to אשך המים, Nathan translates Arab. أدرة الماء as האשך הנולד מהמים. Zeraḥyah Ḥen translates the Arab. term as המים שירדו בכיס הביצים (see entry מַיִם) and Anonymous I has הגרת המים באשך (see entry הֲגָרָה). Similarly, Nathan translates the Arab. synonym قيلة featuring in Maimonides' *Medical Aphorisms* (i.e., *Sefer ha-Peraqim*) XXIII.57 as הגרת המים (cf. BCD 62 (NM 2:38); BMMN 225, l. 23; BMMG no. 4307).

• בקיעות קרום האשך → בְּקִיעָה.

• הגרת המים באשך → הֲגָרָה.

אֶתְרוֹגִיּוּת · **yellow color (like that of the *etrog*)**: Arab. صفرة · Ibn Sīnā, *K. al-Qānūn* II · trans. Zeraḥyah Ḥen, *Sefer ha-Qanun* (Ms Oxford, Bodleian Libraries, Opp. Add. Fol. 12, fol. 230[b]): לשון השור המהות עשב רחב העלים כמו המרו ועצו[31] חלק וענפים גסים כמו רגלי החגבים ומראהו בין ירקות ואתרוגיות ([Hebr.] *leshon ha-shor* [lit. 'ox tongue']: Borage [*Borago officinalis* L.]: What is it? It is a plant with wide leaves that resemble cat thyme and[32] that are rough in touch, and the wood of its branches is like that of [Hebr.] *raglei ha-ḥagavim* [lit. 'locusts' feet,' from Arab. *rijl al-jarād*, i.e., 'Indian plum;' cf. MIG no. 923] and its color is yellowish green). Hebr. אֶתְרוֹגִיּוּת features in BM 448 in an attestation from the *Sefer ha-Qanun*. Nathan ha-Me'ati translates Arab. صفرة as כרכומות and Anonymous I has כרכמות.

---

31 ועצו חלק וענפים גסים: وخشنة الملمس وقضبان خشبه a.

32 'and that are rough in touch, and the wood of its branches': Trans. acc. to a.

ב

בְּאוּשׁ · **stench; evil smell**: Arab. نتن · al-Rāzī, *K. fī al-Faṣd* · trans. Anonymous, *Ma'amar ba-Haqqazah* (Ms Parma, Biblioteca Palatina, Cod. Parm. 2283,4, fol. 96[b]): הקזת אלאכחל ... והאות המורה על העפוש באוש השתן באוש הזיעה (Bleeding the cephalic vein: ... A symptom of the putrefaction [of the blood] is the evil smell of urine and sweat). In the sense of 'evil smell; stench,' Hebr. בְּאוּשׁ features in EM 131 in attestations from Baḥya ibn Pakuda's *Ḥovot ha-Levavot* (c. 1080) and S. Yizhar's *Yemei Ṣiqlag* (1958).

בְּאִישׁוּת • באישות הנחירים · **ozena (foul odor from the nose)**: Arab. نتن الأنف · Ibn Sīnā, *K. al-Qānūn* II · trans. Nathan ha-Me'ati, *Sefer ha-Qanun* (Ms Oxford, Bodleian Libraries, Can. Or. 88, fol. 77[a]): דארשישעאן ... יועיל לבאישות הנחירים ועושים ממנו פתילה ויועיל לזה אם ישכשכו הפה בתבשילו יועיל לנגעי הפה הנקרא קלאע בערבי וישמר השנים ([Arab.] *dārshīsha'ān*: Broom [*Genista acanthoclada* DC. or *Cytisus spinosus* Lam.] (cf. MIG no. 223): ... It is beneficial for ozena when it is used as a wick. If its decoction is used as a mouthwash, it is useful for aphthae, called *qulā'* in Arab., and for preserving the teeth). Hebr. באישות הנחירים is not attested for medieval medical literature. A synonymous באישות האף features in Nathan ben Jo'el Falaquera's *Sefer Ṣori ha-Guf* (Ms Oxford, Bodlein Library, Mich. 550 (Neubauer 2132)): .והו' באישות האף והוא פוליפוס. Zeraḥyah Ḥen translates Arab. نتن الأنف as סירחון האף (see entry סִרְחוֹן) and Anonymous I renders the Arab. term as באשת הנחירים (see entry בְּאָשָׁה), while Anonymous II has a mixture of both terms: סרחון הנחירים (see also entry סִרְחוֹן).

בְּאָשָׁה • באשת הנחירים · **ozena (foul odor from the nose)**: Arab. نتن الأنف · Ibn Sīnā, *K. al-Qānūn* II · trans. Anonymous I, *Sefer ha-Qanun* (Ms Paris, BnF, héb. 1142, fols. 79[b]–80[a]): דארשישעאן ... טוב לבאשת הנחירים וילקח ממנו פתילה וימצמץ בבשולו לשחיני הפה ושומר השנים ומועיל מאד ([Arab.] *dārshīsha'ān*: Broom [*Genista acanthoclada* DC. or *Cytisus spinosus* Lam.] (cf. MIG no. 223): ... It is beneficial for ozena when it is used as a wick. If its decoction is used as a mouthwash, it is good for aphthae. It preserves the teeth and is very beneficial). Hebr. באשת הנחירים is not attested for medieval medical literature. Hebr. בְּאָשָׁה features in BM 456 as part of the term באשת הפה in an attestation from the *Sefer ha-Qanun*. Nathan ha-Me'ati translates Arab. نتن الأنف as באישות הנחירים (see entry בְּאִישׁוּת) and Zeraḥyah Ḥen has סירחון האף (see entry סִרְחוֹן). Anonymous II has a mixture of both terms: סרחון הנחירים (see also entry סִרְחוֹן).

בָּבָה • בבת העין · **pupil of the eye**: Arab. حدقة · Ibn Sīnā, *K. al-Qānūn* II · trans. Nathan ha-Me'ati, *Sefer ha-Qanun* (Ms Oxford, Bodleian Libraries, Can. Or. 88, fol. 113[a]): ערוק אלצבאגין ... מיצו יועיל מאד בחדוד הראות וממרק מה שלפני בבת העין מהמים והלובן ([Arab.] *'urūq al-ṣabbāghīn* [lit. 'roots of the dyers']: Greater celandine [*Chelidonium majus* L.] (cf. IBF no. 1525): ... Its juice is very good for sharpening the eyesight and for clearing water covering the pupil of the eye and for leucoma). In the sense of 'pupil of the eye,' Hebr. בבת העין is not attested for medieval Hebr. medical literature (cf. BM 457 (see also 4439: בת עין כמו בבת העין); EM 132; DAN 47). Zeraḥyah Ḥen translates Arab. حدقة as בת עין (see entry בַּת) and Anonymous I renders the Arab. term as אִישׁוֹן (see entry).

בֶּגֶד • *Plur.* **בגדים** · **pieces of cloth**: Lat. *pannus*, Plur. *panni* · Guy de Chauliac, *Inventarium sive Chirurgia Magna* (cf. CMM 1:420, ll. 19–21) · trans. Anonymous (Ms Paris, BnF, héb. 1189, fol. 229[b]): ועליו יונח עלי הכרוב או האידרא תחת הבגדים או על הגדים בג׳ כפלים או בכפלים יותרא ברקוע מה מעור או מלחשת או מכסף נקשר (And on it, leaves of cabbage or ivy should be put beneath or on top of pieces of cloth, folded three times or more, and a plate (piece) of leather or copper or silver should be bound on it). In a medical context, Hebr. בֶּגֶד features in BCD 30 in the sense of 'pannus' (NM 1:18; cf. also NM 5:25)) or 'papyrus' (NM 4:24), while *Plur.* בגדים features in the sense of 'membranes' (NM 1:17f.).

[בדל] • *Part. Nif'al* **נִבְדָּל** · **superior**: Arab. فضل · Ibn Sīnā, *K. al-Qānūn* II · trans. Zeraḥyah Ḥen, *Sefer ha-Qanun* (Ms Oxford, Bodleian Libraries, Opp. Add. Fol. 12, fol. 255[b]–256[a]): עוֹד לֵין אַלוֹאֵי ... והטוב שבזה העץ הוא המנדלי ויובא מאמצע ארץ הודו לפי דעת רבים ואחריו אותו שנקרא ההודויי והוא הררי והוא נבדל מן המנדלי שהוא אינו מוליד הכנים והוא יותר[33] מעפש הבגדים ([Arab.] *'ūd*; [Rom.] LeYN 'aLWo'eY [i.e., Cat./O. Fr. *lignàloe/lignaloe* (cf. SHS 1:459 (Qof 19) and also Zeraḥyah's trans. of Maimonides' *Medical Aphorisms* (i.e., *Sefer ha-Peraqim*) XXII.56: הלין אלואי (BMMZ 213, l. 18; BMMG no. 3587)]: Agarwood [*Aquilaria malaccensis* Lam.]: ... The best variety of agarwood is *al-mandalī*. According to many people it is imported from central India. Next [in quality] comes the agarwood that is called 'Indian,' which is a mountain variety. It is [actually] superior to *al-mandalī* because it prevents lice infestation [lit. 'does not produce lice'] and makes the clothes more[34] fragrant). Hebr. נִבְדָּל does not features in this sense in the current dictionaries; cf. BM 464f.; PESHAT.[35] Nathan ha-Me'ati translates Arab. فضل as שיבח and Anonymous I has יתרון.

בַּהַק • **הבהק הלבן** · **leucoderma** [*Vitiligo alba*]: Arab. البهق الأبيض (cf. IJZ 7:108, esp. n. 195)[36] · Ibn Sīnā, *K. al-Qānūn* II · trans. Nathan ha-Me'ati, *Sefer ha-Qanun* (Ms Oxford, Bodleian Libraries, Can. Or. 88, fol. 87[a]): חב אלניל ... יועיל מהצרעת[37] והבהק הלבן ([Arab.] *ḥabb al-nīl* [lit. 'indigo-seed']: Ivy-leaved morning glory seed [*Ipomoea*

33 יותר מעפש: أعبق a.

34 'more fragrant': Trans. acc. to a.

35 https://peshat.org/display/peshat_lemmas_00003030 (accessed May 23, 2023).

36 There are three varieties of the disease called *bahaq* acc. to Ibn al-Jazzār (cf. IJZ 7:108, n. 196): white, black, and dust-colored. The white variety is perhaps identical with *Vitiligo alba*, while the black variety is possibly a sort of melanoderma. Arab. *bahaq* stands for Gr. ἀλφός, cf. UW 97: 'weiße Hautflecken.' R. Durling, *Dictionary of Medical Terms in Galen* (Leiden 1993), 34, translates the Gr. term as: 'dull-white leprosy.'

37 מהצרעת: برص a.

nil (L.) Roth] (cf. MIG no. 382): ... It is beneficial for *baraṣ*[38] and leucoderma). Hebr. הבהק הלבן is a non-attested calque from Arab. البهق الأبيض. Zeraḥyah Ḥen and Anonymous I render Arab. البهق الأبيض as הבוהק הלבן.

[בוא] • *Hifʿil* **הֵבִיא** • **הביא הוסת** · **to stimulate menstruation**: Arab. أدرّ الطمث · Ibn Sīnā, *K. al-Qānūn* II · trans. Zeraḥyah Ḥen, *Sefer ha-Qanun* (Ms Oxford, Bodleian Libraries, Opp. Add. Fol. 12, fols. 192^b–193^a): ג׳נְצִיַאנָה ... יביא הוסת ומרבה השתן ([Lat./Rom.] ǦiNəṢiY'NaH (cf. Zeraḥyah's trans. of Maimonides' *Medical Aphorisms* (i.e., *Sefer ha-Peraqim*) IX.88, XXII.29: ג(׳)נציאנה (BMMZ 111, l. 15; 210, l. 17; BMMG no. 715)): Great yellow gentian [*Gentiana lutea* L.]: ... It stimulates menstruation and micturiction). Hebr. הביא הוסת is not attested in the current dictionaries. Nathan ha-Me'ati translates Arab. أدرّ الطمث as שלשל דם הוסת (cf. NM 6:213), Anonymous I has הגיר הנדות (cf. ibid.), and Anonymous II has עורר עת הנשים (see entry [עור]).

בּוֹסֶר → בֹּסֶר.

בּוּעָה • *Plur.* **בועות** · **I. blisters**: Arab. تنفّط (Gr. φλύκταινα; cf. UW 737f.) · Ibn Sīnā, *K. al-Qānūn* II · trans. Nathan ha-Me'ati, *Sefer ha-Qanun* (Ms Oxford, Bodleian Library, Can. Or. 88, fol. 80^b): וסך ... וטנופת המרחץ טוב אל הבועה ([Arab.] *wasakh*: Dirt: ... The dirt from the bathhouse is good for blisters). Hebr. בּוּעָה is attested in the current dictionaries and secondary literature in the sense of 'abscess' (cf. BM 489; for the Aram. counterparts בועאתא or בותא, cf. SDA 128) and of 'bulla, blister' (cf. Low XXXIX). Zeraḥyah Ḥen translates Arab. تنفّط as אבעבועות (see entry אֲבַעְבֻּעָה).

· **II. pustules**: Lat. *pustulae* (cf. DMLBS 2940: 'inflamed sores, blisters, pustules, or sim.;' ND 895: 'pustule, boil, rounded inflammatory sore containing pus') · Guy de Chauliac, *Inventarium sive Chirurgia Magna* (cf. CMM 1:228, ll. 11–13) · trans. Anonymous (Ms Paris, BnF, héb. 1189, fol. 124^b): אמנם רפויו מלבד ההנהגה הכוללת מהמסעד והתבלין[39] והנקויים הנאמרים במורסות ובועות אדומות ובנגעים הוירוליוש הוא שירוחץ המקום (Beyond the general regimen consisting of a diet and frequent[40] purging that we mentioned for swellings, choleric pustules, and virulent ulcers, their cure should consist of washing the spot).

בּוּעִי • **תרופות בועיות** → תְּרוּפָה.

בּוּרְצִי • **מלח בורצי** → מֶלַח.

בּוּרְקִי • **כח בורקי** → ²כֹּחַ.

---

38 '*baraṣ*' (cf. IJZ 7:108, n. 195): This disease has two varieties, namely white and black, which are sometimes summarized under the general term *baraṣ*. The white variety is perhaps identical with *Sklerodermia circumscripta*, while the black variety may be *Psoriasis vulgaris* or *Ichthyosis vulgaris*. The Arab. term *baraṣ* stands for Gr. λέπρα ('leprosy') (cf. UW 97, 387f.). As their is no consensus on the exact meaning of the Arab. term, I have retained the Arab. term in my translation.

39 והתבלין והנקויים: *et crebra purgatione* L.

40 'frequent purging': Trans. acc. to L.

בּוֹרְקִיּוּת · **nitrous (alkaline) property**: Arab. بورقية · Ibn Sīnā, *K. al-Qānūn* II · trans. Anonymous I, *Sefer ha-Qanun* (Ms Paris, BnF, héb. 1142, fol. 189[b]): סלק ... הסלקא יש בה בורקיות מדקדקת ויש בה התכה ופתיחה יותר חזקה מהתכת ארמול ([Arab.] *silq*: Beet [*Beta vulgaris* L.]: ... Beet has a nitrous refining property; its dissolving, deobstruant property is stronger than that of ʾRMWL [i.e., O.Occ. *armol* 'orach;' cf. SHS 1:288 (Lamed 6)]. In the sense of 'nitrous (alkaline) property,' Hebr. בּוֹרְקִיּוּת is a non-attested calque from Arab. بورقية and is also used by Nathan ha-Meʾati in his trans. of Maimonides *Medical Aphorisms* (i.e., *Sefer ha-Peraqim*) XXI.59 (cf. BMMN 203, l. 11; BMMG no. 411). The Arab. term is transcribed as בורקיה in the anonymous trans. of Isḥāq ibn ʿImrān's *Treatise on Melancholy* (cf. NM 5:27). Here, Nathan translates Arab. بورقية as כח בורקי (see entry ²כֹּחַ) and Zeraḥyah Ḥen has בורקיית.

בִּטּוּל · **producing numbness**: Arab. تخدير · Ibn Sīnā, *K. al-Qānūn K. al-Qānūn* II · trans. Zeraḥyah Ḥen, *Sefer ha-Qanun* (Ms Oxford, Bodleian Libraries, Opp. Add. Fol. 12, fol. 231[a]): לשון הכבש ... שרשו יותר יבש ופחות ליחלוח וקרירותו בלתי הביטול ויבשותו בלתי נושך ועל כן הוא תכלית לנגעים ([Hebr.] *leshon ha-keves* [lit. 'lamb's tongue']: Broadleaf plantain [*Plantago major* L.]: ... Its root is very dry and contains less moisture. Its cold does not produce numbness. Its dryness does not cause irritation. This makes it the ultimate [drug] for ulcers). In the sense of 'numbness' (for Arab. خدر) Hebr. בִּטּוּל features in BCD 32 (NM 1:130) in an attestation from Zeraḥyah's trans. of Maimonides' *Medical Aphorisms* (i.e., *Sefer ha-Peraqim*) XXII.38 (cf. BMMZ 211, l. 20; BMMG no. 1297). Nathan ha-Meʾati translates Arab. تخدير as בטול ההרגש (see next entry) and Anonymous I has הרדים. Moses ibn Tibbon translates Arab. تخدير as תרדמת האברים 'numbness [of the limbs]' in his trans. of Ibn al-Jazzār's *Zād al-musāfir* (i.e., *Sefer Ṣedat ha-Derakhim*) VII.17.1 (cf. BCD 298 (NM 1:70); IJZ 7:153, l. 15). For לשון הכבש in the sense of 'broadleaf plantain [*Plantago major* L.],' see NM 6:111.

• **בטול ההרגש** · **producing numbness**: Arab. تخدير · Ibn Sīnā, *K. al-Qānūn* II · trans. Nathan ha-Meʾati, *Sefer ha-Qanun* (Ms Oxford, Bodleian Libraries, Can. Or. 88, fols. 98[b]–99[a]): לסאן אלחמל ... עקרו יבש ופחות רוטבה וקרתו פחותה בבטול ההרגש ובער׳ כדר[41] ויבשותו פחות הנשיכה ולכן הוא מופלג אל הנגעים ([Arab.] *lisān al-ḥamal* [lit. 'lamb's tongue']: Broadleaf plantain [*Plantago major* L.]: ... Its root is dry and contains less moisture. Its cold does not produce numbness, [called] *khadar* in Arab. Its dryness causes less irritation. This makes it the ultimate [drug] for ulcers). Zeraḥyah Ḥen translates Arab. تخدير as בִּטּוּל (see previous entry).

[בטל] • *Part. Piʿel* מְבַטֵּל • **הסם המבטל הרגש** → סַם.

• **הרפואה המבטלת** → רְפוּאָה.

בֶּטֶן • **הכאיב הבטן** → [כאב].

• **הניע הבטן** → [נוע].

---

41 כדר (=خدر): تخدير a.

בִּיטּוּל → **בִּטּוּל**.

בֵּיצָה • *Plur.* **בֵּיצִים** • **בֵּיצֵי הַכִּנִּים** · **nits**: Arab. صئبان · Ibn Sīnā, *K. al-Qānūn* II · trans. Nathan ha-Me'ati, *Sefer ha-Qanun* (Ms Oxford, Bodleian Libraries, Can. Or. 88, fol. 113[b]):[42] עצל ... כשמלכלכים בו ימנע הכנים וביצי הכנים ויהרג אותם ובדבש וקסט מלכלכים על הכתם הישן הנק׳ כלף בער ([Arab.] *ʿasl*: Honey: ... When it is rubbed [on the head] it prevents [infestation] with lice and nits and kills them. With costus, honey [is useful for] chronic freckles, called *kalaf* in Arab., when it is rubbed on them). Hebr. ביצי הכנים is not attested in the current dictionaries. Zeraḥyah Ḥen translates Arab. صئبان as לֵינְנֵי and, like Nathan, Anonymous I renders the Arab. term as ביצי כנים.

• **הַמַּיִם שֶׁיָּרְדוּ בְּכִיס הַבֵּיצִים** → **מַיִם**.

בַּיִת • **בֵּית הַשֶּׁחִי** · **armpit**: Arab. إبط · al-Rāzī, *K. fī al-Faṣd* · trans. Anonymous, *Maʾamar ba-Haqqazah* (Ms Parma, Biblioteca Palatina, Cod. Parm. 2283,4, fol. 93[b]): וב׳ גידים בב׳ הזרועות ונק׳ אלבטאין וימצא כל אחד מהם בין פרק הזרוע הנק׳ אלמרפק ובין בית השחי הנק׳ אלאבטא מהצד הפנימי (Two veins in the [hollows under the] arms that are called 'armpits,' both of them are located between the joint of the arm called 'elbow' and the armpit on the inner side). Hebr. בית השחי features in the current dictionaries in attestations from Rabb. literature, cf. JD 1547; BM 536; see also MD 62. Synonyms featuring in medieval medical literature are: בתי הזיעה (cf. NM 5:28f.) and תחת השחי (cf. BCD 293 (NM 1:42, 195)).

• *Plur.* **בָּתִּים** · **apiaries; beehives**: Arab. كوارة, *Plur.* كوائر · Ibn Sīnā, *K. al-Qānūn* II · trans. Zeraḥyah Ḥen, *Sefer ha-Qanun* (Ms Oxford, Bodleian Libraries, Opp. Add. Fol. 12, fol. 239[a]): מום שעוה ... הזכה שהיא מבתי הדבורים אשר יעשו ביציהם שם ואפרוחיהם ויהיה בהם הדבש והשעוה השחורה הוא ליכלוך בתיו ([Arab.-Pers.] *mūm*; [i.e., Hebr.] *sha'a-wah*: Wax: ... Pure wax is obtained from honeycombs where the bees lay and hatch eggs and store honey. The black wax is the waste product of beehives). Hebr. בַּיִת, *Plur.* בתים, is not attested in this sense in the current dictionaries. Nathan ha-Me'ati translates Arab. كوائر as בתים, just like Zeraḥyah. Anonymous I renders the Arab. term as כוורת.

בִּלְבּוּל • **בִּלְבּוּל הַיַּיִן** · **hangover**: Arab. خمار · Ibn Sīnā, *K. al-Qānūn* II · trans. Nathan ha-Me'ati, *Sefer ha-Qanun* (Ms Oxford, Bodleian Libraries, Can. Or. 88, fol. 61[a]): אפסנתין ... יועיל מכאב האוזן וכששותין ממנו קודם שתיית היין יועיל מבלבול היין ([Arab.] *afsantīn*: Absinth wormwood [*Artemisia absinthium* L.]: ... It is good for earache, also for a hangover, if one takes it before drinking wine). Hebr. בלבול היין is not attested in the current dictionaries. Zeraḥyah Ḥen translates Arab. خمار as שכרות and Anonymous I has סְבִיאָה (see entry).

---

42 Arab. صئبان features as ביצי הכנים ובער׳ ציבאן on fol. 81[a], entry זיבק '[Arab.] *ziʾbaq*: Quicksilver (mercury).'

בְּלִיטָה • בליטת העין · **abnormal protrusion of the eyeball (exophthalmos)**: Arab. جحوظ (HLA 170 (178)) · Ibn Sīnā, *K. al-Qānūn* II · trans. Nathan ha-Me'ati, *Sefer ha-Qanun* (Ms Oxford, Bodleian Libraries, Can. Or. 88, fol. 92[a]): יברוח ... אם יערבוהו בדבש ושמן זית ויושם על הנשיכות יועיל ובלבד הלבן ... ועליו קטנים באדזהר לענב השועל הממית והממית יבואו לו ממנו מקרה חניקת הרחם קודם ואודם הפנים[43] ובליטת העין והתעוררות הפנים כמו כן כאלו הוא שכור ורפואתו בחמאה ודבש ([Arab.] *yabrūḥ*: Mandrake [*Mandragora officinarum* L.]: ... Mixed with honey and olive oil, it is good for [insect] bites when it is applied to the spot, [this holds good] especially for the variety which has white [leaves]. ... But small leaves are an antidote for poisoning due to fatal black nightshade. Death [by its intake] is preceded by the symptoms of hysterical suffocation, redness of the face,[44] abnormal protrusion of the eyeball, also bloating of the face as if he is drunk. He should be treated with butter and honey). Zeraḥyah Ḥen translates Arab. جحوظ as הסתרת עין (see entry הַסְתָּרָה) and Anonymous I has בליטת עין, just like Nathan.

בְּלִיל · **fodder**: Arab. اعتلف · Ibn Sīnā, *K. al-Qānūn* II · trans. Nathan ha-Me'ati, *Sefer ha-Qanun* (Ms Oxford, Bodleian Libraries, Can. Or. 88, fol. 92[a]): כרסנה ... וטעמו ממוצע בין טעם אלמאש והעדשים והוא בליל הבקר ([Arab.] *kirsinna*: Bitter vetch [*Vicia ervilia* (L.) Willd.]: ... Its taste is intermediate between that of mung beans and lentils; it is [used as] fodder for cattle). In the sense of 'fodder,' Hebr. בְּלִיל features in the current dictionaries as a Bibl. term only (cf. KB 133; BM 549). Zeraḥyah Ḥen and Anonymous I render Arab. اعتلف as אכל.

בְּלִילָה · **moisture**: Arab. بِلّة (cf. FL 1:148) · Ibn Sīnā, *K. al-Qānūn* II · trans. Zeraḥyah Ḥen, *Sefer ha-Qanun* (Ms Oxford, Bodleian Libraries, Opp. Add. Fol. 12, fol. 212[b]): נַאנְכְּוַה[45] אַמֵיאוּשׁ ... יועיל מבלילת האצטומכא וישכך הקרבונקל והתהפך הנפש ([Arab.] *nānakhwāh*; [i.e., Lat./Rom.] ʼaMeYʼWŠ [i.e., L. Lat./O. Occ./O. Cat./O. Sp. *ameos*; cf. SHS 1:337 (Nun 3)]: Bisnaga (toothpickweed) [*Ammi visnaga* (L.) Lam.]: ... It is beneficial for [excessive] moisture in the stomach, it alleviates nausea, and it [is good for] a stomach that is upset). Hebr. בְּלִילָה features in the current dictionaries in the sense of 'mixing, mixture' only; cf. JD 172f.; BM 549. Anonymous I renders Arab. بِلّة as לחלוחית.

בֵּן • בן אדם • *Plur.* **בני אדם** • גדל בין בני האדם ← גֶּדֶל.

בֹּסֶר • בוסר הדקל · **unripe dates**: Arab. بلح · Ibn Sīnā, *K. al-Qānūn* II · trans. Zeraḥyah Ḥen, *Sefer ha-Qanun* (Ms Oxford, Bodleian Libraries, Opp. Add. Fol. 12, fol. 247[b]): סֻךְ גַאלְיַה המהות הגאליה השרשית היא הצינית הנעשית מן העפצים ובוסר הדקל על צד שנעשה האלרָאמִךְ ([Arab.] *sukk* [i.e., an astringent electuary containing musk (a.o.)];[46] [i.e.,

---

43 וحمرة وجنة وجحوظ وينتفخ أيضا :אודם הפנים ובליטת העין והתעוררות הפנים a.

44 'face': 'cheeks' a.

45 נַאנְכְּוַה: Emend. ed. נַאנְכְּהָ Ms.

46 Cf. G. Bos and G. Mensching, 'Arabic-Romance Medico-Botanical Glossaries in Hebrew Manuscripts from the Iberian Peninsula and Italy,' *Aleph* 15, no. 1 (2015), 45.

Arab.] *ghāliya* [i.e., a perfume composed of musk, ambergris, camphor, and ben oil, cf. SHS 1:413 (Pe 20)]. What is it? Real (original) *sukk* is the Chinese *sukk* that is made from gallnuts and unripe dates in the same manner as [Arab.] *al-rāmik*).[47] Hebr. בוסר הדקל is not attested in the current dictionaries. The term בֹּסֶר on its own features in BM 568 in the sense of 'unripe grapes.' Nathan ha-Me'ati transcribes Arab. بلح as בלח and Anonymous I renders the Arab. term as אמבליסיש.

בִּעְבֵּעַ (*Pi'el*) • *Part. Pi'el* **מְבַעְבֵּעַ** • *Plur.* **מבעבעים** · **vesicant[48] medicines**: Lat. *vesicancia* · Guy de Chauliac, *Inventarium sive Chirurgia Magna* (cf. CMM 1:417, ll. 16–17) · trans. Anonymous (Ms Paris, BnF, héb. 1189, fol. 228ᵃ): המבעבעים באמת מונחים במקומות שבין העור כמו תחת הזקן ואחור הצואר ובכל הפנים וביתדות הידים והרגלים כי לא ימשכו כי אם הליחה שהוא תחת העור (Vesicant medicines are really those that are put between skin [and flesh] (beneath the skin), such as [those that are put] under the chin and behind the neck, on the whole face and on the malleoli of the feet (ankles), and the bony prominence in the forearms (wrists), because they only attract the moisture that is beneath the skin. Hebr. מְבַעְבֵּעַ, *Plur.* מבעבעים, features in BM 569 in an attestation from Ibn Sīnā's *Sefer ha-Qanun*.

בַּעַל • בעל חלודה · **mouldy**: Arab. متكرّج · Ibn Sīnā, *K. al-Qānūn* II · trans. Anonymous I, *Sefer ha-Qanun* (Ms Paris, BnF, héb. 1142, fols. 182ᵇ–183ᵃ): סאדג נקרא מלבאטרום ... היותר טוב החדש הנוטה ללובן אשר לא[49] יתפתת ויהיה ריחו מתפשט במעט[50] עסוי ולא יהיה בעל חלודה ולא מליח ולא נרפה ([Arab.] *sādhaj*, called [Lat./Rom.] MLB'ṬRWM: Malabathrum [i.e., leaf of the Indian bark [*Cinnamomum tamala* (Buch.-Ham.) T. Nees & Eberm.]]: ... The best malabathrum is that which is fresh, whitish, and unbroken. Its fragrance spreads like[51] that of Indian nard and it should not be mouldy, saltish, and soft). Hebr. בעל חלודה is not attested in the current dictionaries. The term חֲלוּדָה on its own features in medieval Hebr. medical literature (cf. BCD 95) in the sense of 'filth' (NM 4:67); 'fluid, watery moisture' (NM 2:46); and 'viscous matters' (NM 3:82). Nathan ha-Me'ati translates Arab. متكرّج as סכרי (sic!).

• **בעל חנטים** · **fibrous**: Arab. ليفي · Ibn Sīnā, *K. al-Qānūn* II · trans. Zeraḥyah Ḥen, *Sefer ha-Qanun* (Ms Oxford, Bodleian Libraries, Opp. Add. Fol. 12, fol. 212ᵇ): חנטל קוֹלוֹקִינְטִידַא הקולוקינטידא יש ממנה נקבה וממנה זכר והזכר בעל חנטים והנקבה רכה ולבנה ([Arab.] *ḥanẓal*; [i.e., Rom.] QWoLWoQiYNṬYDa' [i.e., *colloquintida*, from Lat. *colocyntis*; Gr. κολοκυνθίς]: Colocynth [*Citrullus colocynthis* (L.) Schrad.]: Colocynth has a female and a male [variety]; the male one is fibrous and the female one is soft

---

47 For *rāmik*, an electuary prepared from gallnut and aromatic drugs, cf. IJZ 7:73f., n. 7.

48 'vesicant medicines': Medicines raising blisters, used to extract morbid humors from the body.

49 לא: Emend. ed. לו Ms لا a.

50 במעט עסוי: ناردانية a.

51 'like that of Indian nard': Trans. acc. to a.

and white). Hebr. בעל חנטים is not attested in the current dictionaries. The term חֲנָט features in Rabb. literature in the sense of 'formation of fruits or leaves' (JD 482; BM 1650). Nathan renders Arab. ليفي as ליפי.

• **בעל הקרן · horned viper**: Arab. مقرّنة (cf. D 2:339) · Ibn Sīnā, *K. al-Qānūn* II · trans. Anonymous I, *Sefer ha-Qanun* (Ms Paris, BnF, héb. 1142, fols. 173[a]–174[a]): מלח ... יחובש בו עם זרע פשתן לעקיצת העקרב ועם פודנג הררי ואישוף ודבש לעקיצת בעל הקרן ועם החומץ והדבש לנשיכת הולכי על ארבע וארבעים והצרעה ((Salt: ... It is plastered with linseed in cases of scorpion bite. It is applied with wild mint, hyssop, and honey for horned viper bite. It is used with vinegar and honey for [bites by] centipedes and wasps). In the sense of 'horned viper,' Hebr. בעל הקרן features as a synonymous הקרנים in BM 6198 in an attestation from Samson Bloch's, *Shevilei Olam* (1822). Nathan ha-Me'ati translates Arab. مقرّنة as ההולך על גחון (see entry הָלַךְ) and Zeraḥyah Ḥen as בעל הקרנים (see next entry).

• **בעל הקרנים · horned viper**: Arab. مقرّنة (cf. D 2:339) · Ibn Sīnā, *K. al-Qānūn* II · trans. Zeraḥyah Ḥen, *Sefer ha-Qanun* (Ms Oxford, Bodleian Libraries, Opp. Add. Fol. 12, fol. 242[a]–243[a]): מלח ... יחבוש בו עם זרע הפשתן לעקיצת העקרבים ועם המינטרשטרי ההררי והאיספו והדבש לנשיכת בעל הקרנים ועם החומץ והדבש לבעלי הארבע והארבעים והדבורים (Salt: ... It is plastered with linseed in cases of scorpion bite. It is applied with wild mint, hyssop, and honey for horned viper bite. It is used with vinegar and honey for [bites by] centipedes and wasps). Hebr. בעל הקרנים features as הקרנים in BM 6198 in an attestation from Samson Bloch's *Shevilei Olam* (1822). Nathan ha-Me'ati translates Arab. مقرّنة as ההולך על גחון (see entry הָלַךְ) and Anonymous I has בעל הקרן (see previous entry).

בָּצוּר (*Part. Pass.*) → **בָּצַר**.

בָּצָל • בצל חזיר · [lit. 'pig onion'; sea squill [*Drimia maritima* (L.) Stearn]): Arab. بصل الخنزير (cf. DT 320 (II.154); MSh no. 60) · *Shinnui ha-Shemot ha-Niqra'im Synonimi*, Ayin 5 (Ms Florence, Biblioteca Medicea Laurenziana, Or. 17, fol. 86[a]): ענצל הוא סקוילה ונק׳ בצל עכבר ובצל חזיר ([Arab.] *ʿunṣul*; i.e., [Rom.] SQWYLH [i.e., O. Occ. (*e*)*squilla*; cf. SHS 1:130f. (Bet 3)]; also called [Hebr.] *beṣal ʿakhbar* [from Arab. *baṣal al-fa'r* [lit. 'mouse (rat) onion']] and [Hebr.] *beṣal ḥazir* [lit. 'pig onion']: Sea squill [*Drimia maritima* (L.) Stearn]). In the sense of 'pig onion,' i.e., sea squill, Hebr. בצל חזיר is a non-attested calque from Arab. *baṣal al-khinzīr*. For the Arab. synonym *baṣal al-fa'r* 'mouse (rat) onion,' see NM 5:32.

בָּצַר • *Part. Pass.* **בָּצוּר · gathered; cut; picked (re: grapes)**: Arab. مقطوف · Ibn Sīnā, *K. al-Qānūn* II · trans. Nathan ha-Me'ati, *Sefer ha-Qanun* (Ms Oxford, Bodleian Libraries, Can. Or. 88, fol. 114[a]): ענב ... והענבים הבצורים באותו יום יניעו הבטן ויולידו הנפח ([Arab.] *ʿinab*/[Hebr.] *ʿenav*: Grapes: ... Freshly picked grapes trouble the belly and are flatulent). Hebr. בָּצַר features in BM 589 in attestations from the Bible and Rabb. literature only. Anonymous I renders Arab. مقطوف as *Part. Pass.* בָּצוּר, just like Nathan. Zeraḥyah Ḥen translates the Arab. term as קטוף.

בְּקוּעַ · **I. abrasion [of the skin]**: Arab. سحج · Ibn Sīnā, *K. al-Qānūn* II · trans. Nathan ha-Me'ati, *Sefer ha-Qanun* (Ms Oxford, Bodleian Libraries, Can. Or. 88, fol. 75ª): גלד[52] ... והוא תרופה לבקוע הנולד בעד המנעל הצר ([Arab.] *jild*: Skin: ... It is a remedy for abrasions caused by narrow shoes). Hebr. בְּקוּעַ is not attested in this sense in the current dictionaries. It features in Rabb. literature in the sense of 'splitting, chopping, trimming' (cf. JD 165; BM 592). In addition to בְּקוּעַ, Nathan translates Arab. سحج as קִלּוּף (see entry) and also as הֶפְשֵׁט 'abrasion [of the intestines]' in his trans. of Maimonides' *Medical Aphorisms* (i.e., *Sefer ha-Peraqim*) XXI.27 (cf. BMMN 199, l. 6; BCD 71 (NM 2:40f.)). Zeraḥyah Ḥen translates Arab. سحج as דְּחִיקָה and לְחִיצָה (see entries) and Anonymous I has הפשט העור (see entry הֶפְשֵׁט). Moses ibn Tibbon translates Arab. سحج as חמרמרות in his trans. of Maimonides' *Commentary on Hippocrates' Aphorisms* (i.e., *Perush Aphorismi shel Apuqraṭ*) IV.24 (cf. BMCH 1:363, l. 4; BCD 104 (NM 1:56)).

· **II. fissure**: Arab. شقاق · i. Ibn Sīnā, *K. al-Qānūn* II · trans. Nathan ha-Me'ati, *Sefer ha-Qanun* (Ms Oxford, Bodleian Libraries, Can. Or. 88, fol. 78ᵇ): דם אלאכוין ... ימנע נגעי המעיים ויועיל מבקוע העגבות ([Arab.] *dam al-akhawayn* [lit. 'blood of the two brothers']: The resin of the Socotra dragontree [*Dracaena cinnabari* Balf. f.] (cf. MIG no. 73): ... It prevents intestinal abrasion and is beneficial for anal fissures). Zeraḥyah Ḥen translates Arab. شقاق as נגעים.

· ii. al-Rāzī, *K. fī al-Faṣd* · trans. Anonymous, *Ma'amar ba-Haqqazah* (Ms Parma, Biblioteca Palatina, Cod. Parm. 2283,4, fol. 96ª): אלבסליק יועיל ממורסת הצלעות ... ובקוע פי הטבעת ([Bleeding] the basilic vein is beneficial for pleurisy ... and [for] anal fissures).

· **III. tear [of a muscle]**: a) Arab. وهن (Gr. ῥῆγμα; cf. UWS 2:247) · Ibn Sīnā, *K. al-Qānūn* II · trans. Nathan ha-Me'ati, *Sefer ha-Qanun* (Ms Oxford, Bodleian Libraries, Can. Or. 88, fol. 102ᵇ):[53] מגאת ... אם עושים ממנו תחבושת יועיל אל הרצוץ והשבר ובקוע העצל וההשמטה ([Arab.] *mughāth*:[54] ... It is useful when plastered in cases of contusion (bruise), fracture, muscle tear, and dislocation). Nathan translates the synonymous Arab. فسخ as בְּקוּעַ as well (see next entry) and also as בְּקִיעָה (see entry). He also translates another Arab. synonym, هتك, as חִתּוּךְ (see entry). Zeraḥyah Ḥen translates Arab. وهن as חֲלִשָׁה (see entry) and Anonymous I has רִסּוּק (see entry for his use of the term רסוק האזן 'tear (puncture) in the ear').

· b) Arab. فسخ (Gr. ῥῆγμα; cf. UWS 2:246) · Ibn Sīnā, *K. al-Qānūn* II · trans. Nathan ha-Me'ati, *Sefer ha-Qanun* (Ms Oxford, Bodleian Libraries, Can. Or. 88, fol. 102ª): מקל אליהוד ומקל אלמכי ... יועיל מבקוע העצל ומן הקווץ והוא תשנג׳ בערבי ומקושי העצבים

52 גלד: Emend. ed. גלוד Ms.

53 The same reading בקוע features in Mss Paris, BnF, héb 1136, fol. 114ᵇ, and Paris, BnF, héb 1140, fol. 113ᵇ.

54 '*mughāth*': I.e., the root of glossostemon [*Glossostemon bruguieri* Desf.]; cf. MIG no. 546.

וקשורים ([Arab.] *muql*[55] *al-Yahūd* and [Arab.] *muql Makkī*: Judean and Meccan bdellium: ... It is useful for muscle tear, spasms, i.e., Arab. *tashannuj*, and hardness and stiffness of the nerves). Synonyms featuring in Nathan's translation are בְּקוּעַ (see previous entry) and פְּתִיחָה (see entry). In his translation of Maimonides's *Medical Aphorisms* (i.e., *Sefer ha-Peraqim*) III.109, Nathan translates Arab. فسخ 'disruption' as רסוק (cf. BMMN 55, l. 17; BMMG no. 3836); about the latter term, he remarks in the glossary to his *Sefer ha-Qanun*: רסוק הוא יותר גדול מריצוץ (RSWQ (lesion). This is greater (i.e., more severe) than RYṢWṢ (contusion) (cf. NM 2:120; 159 (Resh 4)). Zeraḥyah Ḥen translates Arab. فسخ as הֶפְסֵד (see entry).

בְּקִיעַ • *Plur.* **בקיעים** • **בקיעי הקור** · **chilblains (frostbites)**: Arab. شقاق البرد (Gr. χίμεθλον; cf. UW 765) · Ibn Sīnā, *K. al-Qānūn* II · trans. Anonymous I, *Sefer ha-Qanun* (Ms Paris, BnF, héb. 1142, fol. 147[a]): לוף הוא שרפנטינה ... שרש הכווץ ממרק עדשי הפנים והבהק והנמש ... ובייחוד עם דבש ויוטח ביין על בקיעי הקור ([Arab.] *lūf*; i.e., [Rom.] ŠRPNṬYNH [i.e., O. Occ. [*herba*] *serpentina* (cf. BMZ 48f., 89 (Lamed 6))]: Arum [*Arum* sp., e.g., snakeshead [*Arum maculatum* L.]]: ... The root of the curly variety clears freckles, *bahaq*[56] (alphos), and acne ... especially [when applied] with honey. [Mixed] with wine it is put on chilblains). Hebr. בקיעי הקור does not feature in the current dictionaries. In addition to בקיעי הקור, Anonymous I renders the Arab. term as בקיעות הקור (see entry בְּקִיעָה). Nathan ha-Me'ati translates Arab. شقاق البرد as בקיעי הקור, just like Anonymous I. Zeraḥyah Ḥen translates the Arab. term as בקיעות הקרירות (see entry בְּקִיעָה).

בְּקִיעָה · **tear [of a muscle]**: Arab. فسخ (Gr. ῥῆγμα; cf. UWS 2:246) · Ibn Sīnā, *K. al-Qānūn* II · trans. Nathan ha-Me'ati, *Sefer ha-Qanun* (Ms Oxford, Bodleian Libraries, Can. Or. 88, fol. 84[a]): זראונד ... יועיל מבקיעת העצלים ([Arab.] *zarāwand*: Birthwort [*Aristolochia longa* L., *A. rotunda* L., or *A. clematis* L.]: ... It is useful for muscle tear). Hebr. בְּקִיעָה features in medieval medical literature as 'hernia' in an attestation from Moses ibn Tibbon's trans. of Ibn al-Jazzār's *Zād al-musāfir* (i.e., *Sefer Ṣedat ha-Derakhim*) (cf. BCD 38 (NM 4:28); IJZ 1–2:441). Synonyms featuring in Nathan's translation are בְּקוּעַ and פְּתִיחָה (see entries). Zeraḥyah Ḥen translates Arab. فسخ as הֶפְסֵד (see entry) and Anonymous I has פִּשּׁוּחַ (see entry).

• *Plur.* **בקיעות** • **בקיעות קרום האשך** · **hernia**: Arab. فتق (Gr. ἐντεροκήλη; cf. UW 245) · Ibn Sīnā, *K. al-Qānūn* II · trans. Anonymous I, *Sefer ha-Qanun* (Ms Paris, BnF, héb.

55 '*muql*': I.e., bdellium, i.e., the gum resin of plants from the *Burseraceae* family, esp. *Commiphora africana* (A.Rich.) Endl. and *Commiphora mukul* (Hook. ex Stocks) Engl.

56 '*bahaq* (alphos)': There are three varieties of the disease called *bahaq* acc. to Ibn al-Jazzār (cf. IJZ 7:108, n. 196): white, black, and dust-colored. The white variety is perhaps identical with *Vitiligo alba*, while the black variety is possibly a sort of melanoderma. Arab. *bahaq* stands for Gr. ἀλφός, cf. UW 97: 'weiße Hautflecken.' Durling, *Dictionary of Medical Terms*, 34, translates the Gr. term as: 'dull-white leprosy.' See entry בַּהַק: הבהק הלבן.

1142, fol. 72[a]): גוז אלסרו כלומר אגוז סיפריש ... תחבשת לבקיעות קרום האשך ([Arab.] *jawz al-sarw*; i.e., [Hebr.-Rom.] *egoz* SYPRYŠ: Nut of the Mediterranean cypress [*Cupressus sempervirens* L.]: ... [It is used as] a plaster for hernia). Hebr. בקיעות קרום האשך does not feature in the current dictionaries. Nathan ha-Me'ati translates Arab. فتق as הֶתֵּר (see entry) and Zeraḥyah Ḥen has קְרִיעָה (see entry). A synonym featuring in medieval Hebr. medical literature is Aram. פיתקא (cf. BCD 220 (NM 1:109; 2:17)).

• **בקיעות הקור** · **chilblains (frostbites)**: Arab. شقاق البرد (Gr. χίμεθλον; cf. UW 765) · Ibn Sīnā, *K. al-Qānūn* II · trans. Anonymous I, *Sefer ha-Qanun* (Ms Paris, BnF, héb. 1142, fols. 189[b]–190[a]): סלק ... תועיל סחיטתו ובשולו ועליהו מבקיעות הקור ([Arab.] *silq*: Beet [*Beta vulgaris* L.]: ... The extract or decoction [of] its leaves is beneficial for chilblains). Hebr. בקיעות הקור does not feature in the current dictionaries. In addition to בקיעות הקור, Anonymous I renders the Arab. term as בקיעי הקור (see entry בָּקִיעַ). Nathan ha-Me'ati translates Arab. شقاق البرد also as בקיעי הקור and Zeraḥyah Ḥen has בקיעות הקרירות (see next entry).

• **בקיעות הקרירות** · **chilblains (frostbites)**: Arab. شقاق البرد (Gr. χίμεθλον; cf. UW 765) · Ibn Sīnā, *K. al-Qānūn* II · trans. Zeraḥyah Ḥen, *Sefer ha-Qanun* (Ms Oxford, Bodleian Libraries, Opp. Add. Fol. 12, fol. 230[a]): לוּף שַׁרְפֵּינְטַארַא ... השרש[57] מן התלתלי יטהר הכלף והבוהק והנמש ... וכל שכן עם הדבש ויוטח עם היין על בקיעות הקרירות ([Arab.] *lūf*; [i.e., Rom.] ŠaRəPeYNəṬa'Ra': Arum [*Arum* sp., e.g., snakeshead [*Arum maculatum* L.]]: ... The root of the curly variety clears freckles, *bahaq*[58] (alphos), and acne ... especially when applied with honey. [Mixed] with wine it is put on chilblains). Hebr. בקיעות הקרירות does not feature in the current dictionaries. Nathan ha-Me'ati and Anonymous I render Arab. شقاق البرد as בקיעי הקור (see entry בָּקִיעַ).

[ברא] • *Part. Hif'il* **מַבְרִיא** • **סם המבריא** → **סַם**.

בַּרְזֶל · **cautery**: Arab. حديد · Ibn Sīnā, *K. al-Qānūn* II · trans. Nathan ha-Me'ati, *Sefer ha-Qanun* (Ms Oxford, Bodleian Libraries, Can. Or. 88, fols. 75[b]–76[a]): גנאח ... אמרו כי נוצת העוף הנקרא ורשאן כשמערבבים אותו בכמותו בנג' וישרפו וישחקו אותו ויושם בלחם כמו המלח ויתיר החזירים אשר בצואר מבלי ברזל ([Arab.] *janāḥ*: Wing [of a bird]: ... It is said that if one mixes the feathers of the wing of the bird called [in Arab.] *warashān* [i.e., wood pigeon] with an equal weight of [Arab.] *banj* [i.e., black henbane [*Hyoscyamus niger* L.]] and burns and pulverizes this and puts it into bread as salt, it dissolves the scrofula of the neck without applying cautery). Hebr. בַּרְזֶל does not feature in this sense in the current dictionaries. As a medical term, it is attested in medieval med-

---

57 a. أصل الجعد يجلو الكلف والبهق والنمش وخصوصا مع العسل :השרש מן התלתלי ... וכל שכן

58 '*bahaq* (alphos)': There are three varieties of the disease called *bahaq* acc. to Ibn al-Jazzār (cf. IJZ 7:108, n. 196): white, black, and dust-colored. The white variety is perhaps identical with *Vitiligo alba*, while the black variety is possibly a sort of melanoderma. Arab. *bahaq* stands for Gr. ἀλφός, cf. UW 97: 'weiße Hautflecken.' Durling, *Dictionary of Medical Terms*, 34, translates the Gr. term as: 'dull-white leprosy.' See entry בַּהַק: הבהק הלבן.

ical literature as 'scalpel; surgery' (cf. BCD 38 (NM 1:54; 2:33; NM 5:32)) and 'branding iron' (cf. NM 5:33). Zeraḥyah Ḥen and Anonymous I render Arab. حديد as בַּרְזֶל as well.
• קלפות הברזל → קְלִפָּה.
• רוע ברזל → רֹעַ.

בַּרְזִלִּי • מים ברזליים → מַיִם.

בְּרִיקָה • *Plur.* בריקות · **glitter; brightness; radiance**: Arab. تلميع, *Plur.* تلميعات · Ibn Sīnā, *K. al-Qānūn* II · trans. Zeraḥyah Ḥen, *Sefer ha-Qanun* (Ms Oxford, Bodleian Libraries, Opp. Add. Fol. 12, fol. 205[b]): זָאג׳ וֵיטְרִיאוֹל ... וכח הויטריאול אשר בו בריקות זהביות הוא קרוב מכח הקלקטאר ([Arab.] *zāj*; [i.e., Lat./Rom.] WeYṬRiY'WoL: Vitriol: ... The potency of vitriol that has a golden glitter is about the same as that of yellow vitriol). Hebr. בְּרִיקָה is not attested for medieval medical literature. For quotations from scientific/philosophical literature, cf. BM 626 and PESHAT.[59] Nathan ha-Me'ati translates Arab. تلميع, *Plur.* تلميعات, as בהרות and Anonymous I has ברקים.

[ברק] • *Part. Hitpa'el* מִתְבָּרֵק · **glittering; bright; radiant**: Arab. لمع · Ibn Sīnā, *K. al-Qānūn* II · trans. Zeraḥyah Ḥen, *Sefer ha-Qanun* (Ms Oxford, Bodleian Libraries, Opp. Add. Fol. 12, fol. 205[b]): וְוִיטריאול: העושים ממנו הדיו היותר טוב הוא הקשה יהיה זה בהיותו מתברק וכחו כמו הקלקטאר ([Lat./Rom.] WWeYṬRY'WL: Vitriol: The best [vitriol] for making ink has a hard [substance]; it is glittering and its potency is like that of yellow vitriol). Hebr. *Part. Hitpa'el* מִתְבָּרֵק features in BM 636 in an attestation from Isaac ibn Latif's *Iggeret ha-Teshuvot* and in EM 204 in attestations from modern Hebr. literature only. Nathan ha-Me'ati translates Arab. لمع as מזהיר and Anonymous I has [ברק], *Hif'il* הִבְרִיק.

ברקי · **nitrous**: Lat. *nitrosus* · Guy de Chauliac, *Inventarium sive Chirurgia Magna* (cf. CMM 1:230, l. 40) · trans. Anonymous (Ms Paris, BnF, héb. 1189, fol. 126[a]): ליחות חדות רעות וברקיות (Sharp, bad, and nitrous humors). Hebr. ברקי is not attested in the current dictionaries.

ברקיות · **nitrosity**: Lat. *nitrositas* · Guy de Chauliac, *Inventarium sive Chirurgia Magna* (cf. CMM 1:230, l. 33) · trans. Anonymous (Ms Paris, BnF, héb. 1189, fol. 126[a]): שהמוגלא תתהפך לברקיות (... because the pus turns nitrous). Hebr. ברקיות is not attested in the current dictionaries.

בְּשׂוּם · **fragrance; aroma**: Arab. عطرية · Ibn Sīnā, *K. al-Qānūn* II · trans. Zeraḥyah Ḥen, *Sefer ha-Qanun* (Ms Oxford, Bodleian Libraries, Opp. Add. Fol. 12, fol. 258[b]): ... פּוּ וישתעף למטה משרשו ענף ובשרשו בישום ([Arab.] *fū* [from Gr. φοῦ]: Valerian [*Valeriana officinalis* L.]: ... The lower part of its root is divided into several sub-roots, which are fragrant). Hebr. בְּשׂוּם is not attested for medieval medical literature. It features in EM 205 in an attestation from Nachmanides' commentary on Ex 25:6. In his translation of Maimonides' *Medical Aphorisms* (i.e., *Sefer ha-Peraqim*) XIII.6;

---

59 https://peshat.org/display/peshat_lemmas_00053335 (accessed June 29, 2022).

xx.74, 75; xxi.59, Zeraḥyah translates Arab. عطرية as בָּשְׂמוּת (see entry). Nathan ha-Me'ati translates Arab. عطرية as ריח בושם and Anonymous i renders the Arab. term as בשמיות.

[בשל] • *Part. Pi'el* **מְבַשֵּׁל** • **הסם המבשל** → **סַם.**

• **הרפואה המבשלת** → **רְפוּאָה.**

• *Part. Pu'al* **מְבֻשָּׁל** • **עסיס מבושל** → **עָסִיס.**

בָּשְׂמוּת · **fragrance; aroma**: Arab. عطرية · Maimonides, *K. al-Fuṣūl fī al-ṭibb* (*Medical Aphorisms*) xx.74 · trans. Zeraḥyah Ḥen, *Sefer ha-Peraqim* (*Pirqei Moshe*) (BMMN 191, ll. 4–6; BMMG no. 3450): התפוחים להריח אותם יחזקו הלב והמוח וריחו יועיל לבעלי הרישפיצי והמשועממים. אבל לאכלם אמר הם יותר מזיקים מכל שאר הפירות הנאכלים כי בשמותם יתילד ממנו רוחות בעצבים ובמושקולי בשיעור התרתם (The smell of apples strengthens the heart and the brain, and is beneficial for those suffering from marasmus and delusions. However, as to its actual consumption, he [i.e., Abū Marwān ibn Zuhr] states that it is more harmful than the consumption of any other fruit because its fragrance gives rise to gases in the nerves and in the muscles that can only be dissolved with difficulty). Hebr. בָּשְׂמוּת is not attested in the current dictionaries. Nathan ha-Me'ati translates Arab. عطرية as בשמיות (cf. BMMZ 193, l. 19; BMMG no. 3450).

בָּשָׂר · **pulp**: Arab. لحم · Ibn Sīnā, *K. al-Qānūn* ii · trans. Nathan ha-Me'ati, *Sefer ha-Qanun* (Ms Oxford, Bodleian Can. Or. 88, fol. 65[b]): אתרנג׳ ... בשרו נופח ועליו ישקיטו הנפח וציציו יותר רקיקים מזה וחומצתו קובצת ומחסרת המרה השחורה ([Arab.] *utrunj*: Lemon [*Citrus limon* (L.) Osbeck] or citron [*Citrus medica* L.]: ... The pulp is flatulent but the leaves give relief in flatulence. The buds are more tenuous; its sourness is astringent and diminishes black bile). In the sense of 'pulp,' Hebr. בָּשָׂר features in BM 645 in an attestation, a.o., from the *Sefer ha-Qanun*. The Arab. synonym لبّ is translated by Nathan as פרי פנימי (see entry פְּרִי) and the synonymous جوف is rendered by him as תָּוֶךְ (see entry).

• **בשר מת** · **[lit. 'dead flesh']; excessive (superfluous) flesh**: Arab. لحم زائد · Ibn Sīnā, *K. al-Qānūn* ii trans. Anonymous ii, *Sefer ha-Qanun* (Ms Parma, Biblioteca Palatina, Cod. Parm. 3045, fol. 38[a]): פרח נחושת ... מעפץ ואוכל הבשר ונושך תועלתו למור׳ ולחבורות אוכל בשר מת ([Hebr.] *peraḥ neḥoshet* [lit. 'flower of copper']: Copper oxide: ... It is astringent, corrodes the flesh, and irritant. Its usefulness for wounds and ulcers: It erodes excessive flesh). Hebr. בשר מת is not attested in the current dictionaries. Nathan ha-Me'ati and Anonymous ii translate Arab. لحم زائد as בשר נוסף (cf. NM 6:32).

• **הסם המצמיח הבשר** → **סַם.**

• **הרפואה המצמיחה הבשר** → **רְפוּאָה.**

בְּשָׂרִי • **חולי המים הרעים הבשריי** → **חֹלִי.**

בַּת • **בת עין** · **pupil of the eye**: Arab. حدقة · Ibn Sīnā, *K. al-Qānūn* ii · trans. Zeraḥyah Ḥen, *Sefer ha-Qanun* (Ms Oxford, Bodleian Libraries, Opp. Add. Fol. 12, fol. 256[a]): ערוק הצבעים ... מיצו מועיל מאד לחידוד הראות ויטהר מה שלפני הבת העין מן המים והלובן ([Arab.-Hebr.] *'urūq ha-ṣaba'im* [lit. 'roots of the dyers']: Greater celandine [*Chelidonium* *majus* L.] (cf. IBF no. 1525): ... Its juice is very good for sharpening the eyesight and for clearing water covering the pupil of the eye and for leucoma). In the sense of 'pupil of the eye,' Hebr. בת עין is attested in Bibl. and modern Hebr. literature (cf. BDB 123, 4439; EM 208). Zeraḥyah Ḥen uses the same Hebr. term (also for Arab. حدقة 'pupil') in his translation of Maimonides' *Medical Aphorisms* (i.e., *Sefer ha-Peraqim*) VII.69; XXIII.70; XXIV.35 (cf. BMMZ 85, ll. 24–25; 226, l. 14; 238, l. 6; BMMG no. 85), and additionally also the synonymous הרואה שלעין in XXV.17 (cf. BMMZ 246, ll. 4–5; BMMG no. 85). He also uses בת עין to render Arab. مقلة 'eyeball' (cf. BCD 41 (NM 4:30)). Nathan ha-Me'ati translates Arab. حدقة as בבת העין (see entry בָּבָה) and Anonymous I renders the Arab. term as אִישׁוֹן (see entry).

• *Plur.* **בנות • בנות הלילה** · **[lit. 'daughters of the night']; skin affection (pustules) that occurs at night**: Arab. بنات الليل (Gr. ἐπινυκτίς; cf. LSG 649; MIG no. 166; UW 258) · Ibn Sīnā, *K. al-Qānūn* II · trans. Anonymous I, *Sefer ha-Qanun* (Ms Paris, BnF, héb. 1142, fols. 79b–80a): דבק ... ומועיל מן השרי ובנות הלילה ([Arab.] *dibq*: Mistletoe (birdlime) [*Viscum album* L.]: ... It is also beneficial for *sharan*[60] [i.e.,] for the skin affection (pustules) that occurs at night). Hebr. בנות הלילה is a non-attested calque from Arab. بنات الليل. The term features in Nathan's glossary to his *Sefer ha-Qanun*, where he defines בנות הלילה as 'small growths (on the skin) that are called شرى' (cf. NM 2:110, 127 (Bet 6)). Zeraḥyah Ḥen translates Arab. بنات الليل as צמח הלילה (see entry צֶמַח).

60 Cf. MIG no. 166: بنات الليل هو الشَّرَى من الحاوي، وقال جالينوس في المقالة الثانية من كتاب حيلة البرء: سُمّي الشرى بنات الليل من قبل أنّ الشرى يعرض بالليل (*Banāt al-layl* (lit. 'daughters of the night') is a pustule (*sharan*) according to (al-Rāzī's) *Ḥāwī*. Galen said in the second chapter of his book '*On the Method of Healing*' (*Ḥīlat al-bur'*): the pustule is called 'daughters of the night', because the pustule occurs at night). For *sharan*, see also entry רְקוּעַ, *Plur.* רקועים.

ג

גַּבְשׁוּשִׁית · **gypsum**: Arab. جبسين · Ibn Sīnā, *K. al-Qānūn* II · trans. Nathan ha-Me'ati, *Sefer ha-Qanun* (Ms Oxford, Bodleian Libraries, Can. Or. 88, fol. 75ª):[61] גבסין והוא גבשושית המהות הוא אבן העושין ממנו חרסית ([Arab.] *jibsīn*; i.e., [Hebr.] *gavshushit*: Gypsum: What is it? It is a stone from which potter's clay is made). Hebr. גַּבְשׁוּשִׁית only features in the current dictionaries in the sense of 'heap of stones, pile, mound' (cf. JD 209; BM 689f.). Zeraḥyah Ḥen transcribes Arab. جبسين as גַ'בְסִין and Anonymous I renders the Arab. term as אבן החרסית.

גָּדוֹל • **זנב העין הגדול** → זָנָב.

[גדל] • *Part. Pi'el* **מְגַדֵּל** • **האברים המגדלים** → אֵבֶר.

• *Part. Pu'al* **מְגֻדָּל** · **preserved; preserve**: Arab. مربّى · Ibn Sīnā, *K. al-Qānūn* II · trans. Zeraḥyah Ḥen, *Sefer ha-Qanun* (Ms Oxford, Bodleian Libraries, Opp. Add. Fol. 12, fol. 201ᵇ): הַלִילַג' מִירַבַּלֹנִי ... מועיל לכאב הטחול ויועיל לכלי המזון כלם וכל שכן השחורים כי הם יחזקו האצטומ' וכל שכן המגודלים ויחזקו רפיון[62] האצטומ' עם העיבוד והנקיון והנישוף ([Arab.] *halīlaj* [from Pers. *halīlah*]; [Rom.] MiYRaBaLoNiY: Chebulic myrobalan: ... They are useful for pain in the spleen, and for all nutritive organs—especially the black variety—because they strengthen the stomach, above all the preserved ones. They strengthen the lining[63] of the stomach through their astringent, cleansing, and absorbing effect). In the sense of 'preserved,' Hebr. מְגֻדָּל is a non-attested semantic borrowing from Arab. مربّى. A synonym used by Zeraḥyah is *Part. Pu'al* מְרֻבָּב (see entry [רבב]). Nathan ha-Me'ati translates Arab. مربّى as מָעוֹג (cf. NM 6:121f.) and Anonymous I has מרוקח.

גָּדֵל • **גדל בין בני האדם** · **domestic**: Arab. أهلي · Ibn Sīnā, *K. al-Qānūn* II · trans. Zeraḥyah Ḥen, *Sefer ha-Qanun* (Ms Oxford, Bodleian Libraries, Opp. Add. Fol. 12, fol. 186ᵇ): בַּט אַנֶטְרַא ... חמה יותר מן כל העופות הגדלים בין בני האדם ([Arab.] *baṭṭ*; [i.e., Rom.] 'aNeṬəRa' [i.e., Ital.-Rom. *anatra*]: Duck: ... It is hotter than any other domestic fowl). Hebr. גדל בין בני האדם is not attested in the current dictionaries. Nathan ha-Me'ati and Anonymous I render Arab. أهلي as בייתי. In his trans. of Maimonides' *Medical Aphorisms* (i.e., *Sefer ha-Peraqim*) XX.69, Zeraḥyah translates the Arab. term as נגדל בבית (cf. BMMZ 190, l. 14).

גּוּמָּא (*Aram.*) · **gum**: Arab. صمغ · Ibn Sīnā, *K. al-Qānūn* II · trans. Zeraḥyah Ḥen, *Sefer ha-Qanun* (Ms Oxford, Bodleian Libraries, Opp. Add. Fol. 12, fol. 176ᵇ): אִגַ'אץ פְּרוּנְגֵי ... הגומא שלהן חותכות ומדבקות והפרונגי מדמשק יש בו עצירה וקיבוץ לפי דיאסקורידוש וזולתי ג'לינוס ([Arab.] *ijjāṣ*; [i.e., Rom.] PəRWNəGeY: Plum tree [*Prunus domestica* L.]: ... Its gum is diluting and agglutinant. According to Dioscorides, the Damascus variety is constipating and astringent, but according to Galen it is not so). Aram. גּוּמָּא is a

61 The same Hebr. term features in ed. Naples 1491, fol. 92ᵇ: גבסין הוא גיף הוא גבשושית.

62 רפיון: خمل a.

63 In the sense of 'lining' Hebr. רפיון is a non-attested semantic borrowing from Arab. خمل.

calque from Lat. *gummi* (cf. SDA 212; s.v. 2 # גּוּמָּא). Nathan ha-Me'ati and Anonymous I render Arab. صمغ as שרף.

• **גומא של הרוטא המדברית** · **[lit. 'resin of wild rue']; thapsia [*Thapsia garganica* L.]**: Arab. صمغ السذاب الجبلي ('resin of mountain rue;' a synonym of صمغ السذاب البرّي 'resin of wild rue;' cf. MIG nos. 407, 640) · Ibn Sīnā, *K. al-Qānūn* II · trans. Zeraḥyah Ḥen, *Sefer ha-Qanun* (Ms Oxford, Bodleian Libraries, Opp. Add. Fol. 12, fol. 221ᵃ): ינתון המהות הוא תאפאסיא כלומ' גומא של הרוטא המדברית ([Arab.] *yantūn*: Thapsia [*Thapsia garganica* L.]: What is it? It is [Rom.] T'P'SY' [i.e., thapsia]; i.e., resin of mountain rue [lit. 'resin of wild rue']). Aram.-Hebr. גומא של הרוטא המדברית is not attested in the current dictionaries. A synonym featuring in NM 5:200 is שרף רוטא מדברית. Nathan ha-Me'ati translates Arab. صمغ السذاب الجبلي as שרף הסדאב ההררי and Anonymous I as שרף רודא מדברית.

גּוּף • **שלשול הגוף** → שִׁלְשׁוּל.

גָּחוֹן • **ההולך על גחון** → הָלַךְ.

גִּיד • **גיד הרמון המדברי** · **root of the wild pomegranate tree**: Arab. عرق الرمان البري (cf. Ibn Sīnā, *Qānūn*, ed. Būlāq, I 364; MSh no. 219: أصل الرمان البري, now identified as: **root of glossostemon [*Glossostemon bruguieri* Desf.]**[64]) · Ibn Sīnā, *K. al-Qānūn* II · trans. Nathan ha-Me'ati, *Sefer ha-Qanun* (Ms Oxford, Bodleian Libraries, Can. Or. 88, fol. 102ᵇ): מגאת מצאתי כתוב בספר אחד: מעאד המהות אמרו קצתם שהוא גיד הרמון המדברי ולא יאות המאמר הזה למה שאמרו כי זרעו נאות לתאות המשגל ויניעהו בכח ([Arab.] *mughāth*:[65] I found in a book: What is it? Some say that it is the root of the wild pomegranate tree; however, this statement does not fit what is said that its seed is good for (strengthens) sexual lust, and that it is a strong stimulant). Hebr. גיד הרמון המדברי is a non-attested calque from Arab. عرق الرمان البري. Zeraḥyah Ḥen, mistakenly reading Arab. عرق as عَرَق, translates the Arab. term as זיעת הרמון המדברי and Anonymous I has שרש הרמון המדברי (see entry שֹׁרֶשׁ).

• *Plur.* **גידים** • **חלי פתול הגידים** → חֳלִי.

• **פתילי הגידים** → פְּתִיל.

גָּמָל • *Plur.* **גמלים** • **תבן מגמלים** → תֶּבֶן.

גַּן עֵדֶן • **גַּן** • **תפוח גן עדן** → תַּפּוּחַ.

גְּנִיחָה · **rattling sound in the throat**: Arab. حشرجة · Ibn Sīnā, *K. al-Qānūn* II · trans. Anonymous I, *Sefer ha-Qanun* (Ms Paris, BnF, héb. 1142, fols. 198ᵇ–199ᵃ): ענצל ... חומץ שלו מטיב הגרון ומקשה בשרו והוא טוב לגניחה ולקוצר הנשימה ולשעול הנושן ([Arab.] *ʿunṣul*: Sea squill [*Drimia maritima* (L.) Stearn]: ... The vinegar prepared from sea squill makes the flesh of the throat rough and hard. It is good for a rattling sound in the

---

64 Cf. El S. Amin, O. Awad, M. Abd El Samad, and M.N. Iskander, 'Isolation of Estrone from Moghat Roots and from Pollen Grains of Egyptian Date Palm,' *Phytochemistry* 8 (1969): 295ff.

65 '*mughāth*': I.e., the root of glossostemon [*Glossostemon bruguieri* Desf.]; cf. MIG no. 546.

throat, for asthma, and for chronic cough). Hebr. גְּנִיחָה features in BM 814 in the sense of 'expectoration' (s.v. גנח, ibid. 813 and JD 259: 'to groan, esp. 1) to sigh heavily under an attack of angina pectoris; 2) to cough and spit blood'). In the glossary to his *Sefer ha-Qanun*, Nathan ha-Me'ati defines the term גְּנִיחָה as follows: גניחה הוא הנקרא רבו מגזרת גונח ובלשון אזמא הנק׳ גוייש (GNYḤH (sigh, groan): This is that which is called ربو, and it is derived from GWNḤ, [in Latin it is called] 'ZM' [and in Romance it is the illness called] GWYYŚ) (cf. NM 2:111, 129 (Gimel 2)). Zeraḥyah Ḥen translates Arab. حشرجة as גַּסּוּת (see next entry) and Nathan ha-Me'ati has עלוע הגרון (see entry עִלּוּעַ).

גַּסּוּת · **rattling sound in the throat**: Arab. حشرجة · Ibn Sīnā, *K. al-Qānūn* II · trans. Zeraḥyah Ḥen, *Sefer ha-Qanun* (Ms Oxford, Bodleian Libraries, Opp. Add. Fol. 12, fol. 255[a]): עֻנְצֻל אֶשְׁקִיל ... החומץ שלו יקשה הגרון ויעבהו והוא טוב לרובו[66] ולגסות ולשעול הארוך ([Arab.] *'unṣul*; [i.e., Arab.] *ishqīl*: Sea squill [*Drimia maritima* (L.) Stearn]: ... The vinegar prepared from sea squill makes the throat hard and rough. It is good for asthma, for a rattling sound in the throat, and for chronic cough). Hebr. גַּסּוּת does not feature in the sense of 'rattling sound in the throat' in the current dictionaries. Nathan ha-Me'ati translates Arab. حشرجة as עלוע הגרון (see entry עִלּוּעַ) and Anonymous I renders the Arab. term as גְּנִיחָה (see previous entry).

• **הסם המוליד הגסות** → סַם.

גֶּפֶן • **ורד הגפן** → וֶרֶד.

גָּרָב • **הגרב הנגוע** · **ulcerating scabies**: Arab. الجرب المتقرّح · Ibn Sīnā, *K. al-Qānūn* II · trans. Zeraḥyah Ḥen, *Sefer ha-Qanun* (Ms Oxford, Bodleian Libraries, Opp. Add. Fol. 12, fol. 211[a]): חֻרְף׳ נַשְׁטוֹרצוֹ ... יועיל לגרב הנגוע ([Arab.] *ḥurf*; [i.e., Lat./Rom.] NaŠəṬ-WoRṢWo: Garden cress [*Lepidium sativum* L.]: ... It is useful for ulcerating scabies). Hebr. הגרב הנגוע is not attested in the current dictionaries. A synonym used by Zeraḥyah is הגרב כשיתנגע (cf. NM 6:37f., s.v.: גָּרָב: הגרב המנוגע). Nathan ha-Me'ati translates Arab. الجرب المتقرّح as הגרב המנוגע (cf. ibid.), and Anonymous I has הגרב המשתחן (see next entry).

• **הגרב המשתחן** · **ulcerating scabies**: Arab. الجرب المتقرّح · Ibn Sīnā, *K. al-Qānūn* II · trans. Anonymous I, *Sefer ha-Qanun* (Ms Paris, BnF, héb. 1142, fol. 90[a–b]): חרף ... מועיל מהגרב המשתחן ([Arab.] *ḥurf*: Garden cress [*Lepidium sativum* L.]: ... It is useful for ulcerating scabies). Hebr. הגרב המשתחן features in BM 7027 without further explanation in an attestation from the *Sefer ha-Qanun*. Zeraḥyah Ḥen translates Arab. الجرب المتقرّح as הגרב הנגוע (see previous entry) and Nathan ha-Me'ati has הגרב המנוגע (cf. NM 6:37f.). See also the term הסרטאן המשתחן 'the ulcerous cancer' (for Arab. السرطان المتقرّح) with the same use of *Part. Hitpa'el* מִשְׁתַּחֵן, featuring in Nathan's trans. of Maimonides' *Medical Aphorisms* (i.e., *Sefer ha-Peraqim*) XXIII.46 (cf. BMMN 224, l. 18; BMMG no. 2370).

---

66 לרובו: للربو a.

גַּרְגַּר • *Plur.* **גרגרים** • **גרגרי המלך** · **[lit. 'the seeds (berries) of the king']; caper spurge** [***Euphorbia lathyris*** L.]: Arab. حبّ الملوك (cf. MIG no. 560) · Ibn Sīnā, *K. al-Qānūn* II · trans. Anonymous I, *Sefer ha-Qanun* (Ms Paris, BnF, héb. 1142, fol. 171[a]): מאהודאנא המהות הוא אותו שיאמר לו חב אלמלוך כלומר גרגרי המלך ([Arab.] *māhūdhāna*: Caper spurge [*Euphorbia lathyris* L.]: What is it? It is [a plant] that is called [in Arab.] *ḥabb al-mulūk*, i.e., [Hebr.] *gargerei ha-melekh* [lit., 'the seeds (berries) of the king']). Hebr. גרגרי המלך is a non-attested calque from Arab. حبّ الملوك. Zeraḥyah Ḥen translates Arab. حبّ الملوك as גרעיני המלך (see entry גַּרְעִין) and Nathan ha-Me'ati transcribes the Arab. term as חב אלמלך only.

גָּרוֹן • **עלוע הגרון** → **עִלּוּעַ**.

גַּרְעִין • *Plur.* **גרעינים** • **גרעיני הדלעת** · **tapeworms**: Arab. حبّ القرع Ibn Sīnā, *K. al-Qānūn* II · trans. Zeraḥyah Ḥen, *Sefer ha-Qanun* (Ms Oxford, Bodleian Libraries, Opp. Add. Fol. 12, fol. 215[b]):[67] חַבְ אלניל[68] ... ישלשל הליחות הגסות והמרה השחורה והליחה הלבנה בכח והתולעים וגרעיני הדלעת ([Arab.] *ḥabb al-nīl* [lit. 'indigo-seed']: Ivy-leaved morning glory seed [*Ipomoea nil* (L.) Roth] (cf. MIG no. 382): ... It forcefully expels crude humors, black bile, phlegm, worms, and tapeworms). In the sense of 'tapeworms,' Hebr. גרעיני הדלעת is a non-attested calque from Arab. حبّ القرع. Nathan ha-Me'ati translates Arab. حبّ القرع as גרגרי הדלעת (cf. BCD 49 (NM 2:35) for an attestation from Nathan's trans. of Maimonides' *Medical Aphorisms* (i.e., *Sefer ha-Peraqim*) VII.31 (cf. BMMN 85, l. 15; BMMG no. 769)) and Anonymous I has התולעים הדלועיים. The latter term also features in Nathan's trans. of Maimonides' *Medical Aphorisms* (i.e., *Sefer ha-Peraqim*) XXII.9 (cf. BCD 290 (NM 2:91); BMMN 211, l. 5; BMMG no. 769). Moses ibn Tibbon translates the Arab. term as גרגיר הקרא in his trans. of Ibn al-Jazzār's *Zād al-musāfir* (i.e., *Sefer Ṣedat ha-Derakhim*) IV. 18 (cf. NM 6:38) and Shem Tov ben Isaac has גרגרי הדלועים in his trans. of al-Zahrāwī's *K. al-Taṣrīf* (i.e., *Sefer ha-Shimmush*) XXVII (cf. BCD 49 (NM 4:34)).

• **גרעיני המלך** · **[lit. 'the seeds (berries) of the king']; caper spurge [*Euphorbia lathyris* L.]**: Arab. حبّ الملوك (cf. MIG no. 560) · Ibn Sīnā, *K. al-Qānūn* II · Hebr. trans. Zeraḥyah Ḥen, *Sefer ha-Qanun* (Ms Oxford, Bodleian Libraries, Opp. Add. Fol. 12, fol. 241[b]): מְאהוּדָאנָא המהות היא אשר יאמרו לו גרעיני המלך ([Arab.] *māhūdhāna*: Caper spurge [*Euphorbia lathyris* L.]: What is it? It is [a plant] that is called [in Hebr.] *gar'inei ha-melekh* [lit. 'the seeds (berries) of the king']). Hebr. גרעיני המלך is a non-attested calque from Arab. حبّ الملوك. Nathan ha-Me'ati transcribes Arab. حبّ الملوك as חב אלמלך only and Anonymous I renders the Arab. term as גרגרי המלך (see entry גַּרְגַּר).

67 The same Hebr. term features (also for Arab. حبّ القرع) on fol. 194[a], entry גַ'עְדָה '[Arab.] *ja'da*: Germander [*Teucrium* sp.].'

68 אלניל: Emend. ed. אלתִיל Ms.

ד

דְּבוֹרָה • *Plur.* **דבורים** · **wasps**: Arab. زنبور, *Plur.* زنابير · Ibn Sīnā, *K. al-Qānūn* II · trans. Zeraḥyah Ḥen, *Sefer ha-Qanun* (Ms Oxford, Bodleian Libraries, Opp. Add. Fol. 12, fol. 194[a]): ג׳ֻמָּאר ... טוב לעקיצת הדבורים בחובש ומשיחה ([Arab.] *jummār*: Palm heart: ... It is good against stings of wasps when applied in a plaster or salve). Hebr. דְּבוֹרָה is only attested in the current dictionaries in the sense of 'bee' (cf. BM 867f.). Nathan ha-Me'ati translates Arab. زنابير as צרעות and Anonymous I has *Sing.* צרעה. Hebr. צרעות is also used by Nathan to render Arab. ذراريح 'Spanish flies (cantharides)' (see entry צִרְעָה).

[דבק] • *Part. Pi'el* **מְדַבֵּק** · **agglutinant; gluey**: Arab. مغرّ · Ibn Sīnā, *K. al-Qānūn* II · trans. Zeraḥyah Ḥen, *Sefer ha-Qanun* (Ms Oxford, Bodleian Libraries, Opp. Add. Fol. 12, fol. 193[b]): ג׳לְנַאר בְלַוְשְׁטִיאֵי ... מדבק עוצר לכל הגרה מוליד למרה השחורה ([Arab.] *jullanār*; [i.e., Lat./Rom.] BəLaWəŠəṬiY'eY]: The flower of the wild pomegranate [*Punicum granatum* L.]: ... It is agglutinant, stops the flow [of all kinds of fluids], and produces black bile). Hebr. *Part. Pi'el* מְדַבֵּק is not attested in this sense in the current dictionaries. The root דבק features as *Part. Hif'il* מַדְבִּיק in the Hebr. term הסם המדביק 'the agglutinant remedy' in an attestation from the *Sefer ha-Refu'ot ha-Libbiyot* (cf. BCD 188 (NM 4:125); see also entry below). Nathan ha-Me'ati translates Arab. مغرّ as *Part.* צוֹפֵד (see entry צָפַד) and Anonymous I has טח בדבקות (see entry טוּחַ).

• **מדבק הזהב** · **chrysocolla**: Arab. لحام الذهب (cf. MIG no. 503) · Ibn Sīnā, *K. al-Qānūn* II · trans. Zeraḥyah Ḥen, *Sefer ha-Qanun* (Ms Oxford, Bodleian Libraries, Opp. Add. Fol. 12, fol. 278[a]): תִּנְכַּאר בֹּרַשׁ יש ממנו מקורי ויש ממנו שהוא צבוע ונקרא מדבק הזהב ([Arab.] *tinkār*; [i.e., Rom.] BoRaŠ [i.e., O. Occ. *borais* (cf. SHS 1:333 (Mem 63)); from Arab. *bawraq*]: Salt, borax, salmiac, chrysocolla (cf. KM 345–349): There is [a variety] that is a mineral and another [variety] that is artificial, which is called [in Hebr.] *medabbeq ha-zahav*). Hebr. מדבק הזהב is not attested in the current dictionaries. Nathan ha-Me'ati translates Arab. لحام الذهب as חבור הזהב (see entry חִבּוּר) and Anonymous I has מתג(?) הזהב. The Arab. synonym لصاق الذهب is translated by Zeraḥyah as דבקות הזהב (cf. BCD 54 (NM 1:136) for an attestation from his trans. of Maimonides' *Medical Aphorisms* (i.e., *Sefer ha-Peraqim*) XXIII.101 (cf. BMMZ 231, l. 4; BMMG no. 4604)).

• *Hitpa'el* **הִתְדַּבֵּק** · **1. to become mouldy**: Arab. تكرّج (cf. WKAS 1:120) · Ibn Sīnā, *K. al-Qānūn* II · trans. Anonymous I, *Sefer ha-Qanun* (Ms Paris, BnF, héb. 1142, fol. 24[b]): אס הוא הדס ... והטוב שבפרחו הלבן וסחיטת פריו יותר טובה וסחיטתו אם תתישן תחלש ותתדבק ולכן ראוי שתעשה עוגות ([Arab.] *ās*; i.e., [Hebr.] *hadas*: Myrtle [*Myrtus communis* L.]: ... The flower of the white [variety] is beneficial. Better is the extract of its fruit. But if the extract becomes old, it grows weak and becomes mouldy. Therefore, one should make pastilles of them). Hebr. הִתְדַּבֵּק is not attested in the sense of 'to become mouldy' in the current dictionaries. In the sense of 'to be regenerated' (for Arab.

تجبّر) and 'to grow [together again]' (for Arab. نمى) it features in BCD 53 (NM 3:50) in attestations from Zeraḥyah Ḥen's trans. of Maimonides' *Commentary on Hippocrates' Aphorisms* (i.e., *Perush Aphorismi shel Apuqraṭ*) IV.26, VII.28 (cf. BMCH 1:460, l. 6; 1:505, l. 4). Nathan ha-Me'ati translates Arab. تكرّج as שב כדבק (see entry שׁוּב).

· II. **to close a wound and/or promote the formation of a scar:** Lat. *consolido* (cf. ND 243f.) · Guy de Chauliac, *Inventarium sive Chirurgia Magna* (cf. CMM 1:232, ll. 15–16) · trans. Anonymous (Ms Paris, BnF, héb. 1189, fol. 120[b]): ואחרי המתת הנאצור שיוכר במה שנאמר למעלה ירופא ויתדבק (Once the fistula has been subdued—which can be recognized by [the symptoms] mentioned above—, it should be healed and the wound should be closed (the formation of a scar should be promoted). See next entry.

• *Part. Hif'il* **מַדְבִּיק** • *Plur.* **מדביקים** · **medicines that close wounds and/or promote formation of scars:** Lat. *consolidantes* (cf. ND 243, s.v. *consolidativa*) · Guy de Chauliac, *Inventarium sive Chirurgia Magna* (cf. CMM 1:231, ll. 39–40) · trans. Anonymous (Ms Paris, BnF, héb. 1189, fol. 120[b]): ואחר הנקוי ירפא עם המדביקים (Once [the lacrimal fistula] is clean, it should be cured with medicines that close wounds and/or promote formation of scars). Hebr. *Part. Hif'il* מַדְבִּיק features in the sense of 'a sticking plaster' (for Arab. لصوق) in BCD 53 (NM 1:51) in an attestation from Moses ibn Tibbon's trans. of Ibn al-Jazzār's *Zād al-musāfir* (i.e., *Sefer Ṣedat ha-Derakhim*) VII.26.6 (cf. IJZ 7:168, l. 20). In the sense of 'agglutinant,' it features as הסם המדביק 'the agglutinant remedy' (for Lat. *inviscativa medicina*) in BCD 188 (NM 4:125) in an attestation from the *Sefer ha-Refu'ot ha-Libbiyot*, and as הרפואות המדביקות 'agglutinant remedies' (for Lat. *glutinantes*) in NM 6:203f. in an attestation from Abraham Avigdor's trans. of Gerard de Solo's *Practica super nono Almansoris* (i.e., *Ha-Ma'amar ha-Teshi'i le-Sefer ha-Mansuri le-Razi*)).

דָּבֵק · **continuous:** Arab. مطبق · al-Rāzī, *K. fī al-Faṣd* · trans. Anonymous, *Ma'amar ba-Haqqazah* (Ms Parma, Biblioteca Palatina, Cod. Parm. 2283,4, fol. 93[a]): וכאשר יהיה הדם הרבה בגוף ונתחמם ונרתח ונתחדשה ממנו קדחת יעשה הרקתו פתאם בעת ירידת הקפת הקדחת וקודם שיהיה נגר אל האברים המעולים בעבור כי זאת הקדחת ואם היא דבקה יהיה לה על הרוב התחלה ותוספת ותכלית וירידה (When there is a lot of blood in the body and it becomes hot and boils and causes a fever, then evacuate it all at once at the time of the decline of the paroxysm of fever before it flows towards the vital organs, because this fever, even if it was continuous, in most cases will have a beginning, increase, climax, and decline). In the sense of 'continuous fever,' Hebr. דָּבֵק features as הקדחת הדבקה in BCD 237 (NM 2:79; corr. 3:268) in an attestation from Nathan ha-Me'ati's trans. of Maimonides, *Medical Aphorisms* (i.e., *Sefer ha-Peraqim*) X.21 (cf. BMMN 125, l. 22; BMMG no. 1105).

דֶּבֶק · I. **calcification; callus:** Arab./Pers. دشبد (Gr. πῶρος; cf. UW 580f.: 'Kalkablagerung, Verkalkung, Steinbildung (in d. Gelenken), in der Blase') · Ibn Sīnā, *K. al-Qānūn* II · trans. Nathan ha-Me'ati, *Sefer ha-Qanun* (Ms Oxford, Bodleian Libraries, Can. Or.

88, fol. 102b):[69] מגאת ... והוא טוב אל הדבק הנולד בשבר העצמות הנקרא דשבד ויועיל לקושי הפרקים ([Arab.] *mughāth*:[70] ... It is good for callus resulting from a fracture of a bone, called *dushbud* [in Arab.], and for the hardening of joints). Hebr. דֶּבֶק is not attested in the sense of 'calcification; callus' in the current dictionaries. Zeraḥyah Ḥen translates Arab. دشبد as רסבוט.

· II. **resin:** Arab. علك · *Shinnui ha-Shemot ha-Niqra'im Synonimi*, Ayin 43 (Ms Florence, Biblioteca Medicea Laurenziana, Or. 17, fol. 86a): עלך[71] ה' דבק ([Arab.] *ilk*, i.e., [Hebr.] *deveq*). In the sense of 'resin,' Hebr. דֶּבֶק features in NM 6:43 in an attestation from Nathan ha-Me'ati's trans. of Ibn Sīnā's *K. al-Qānūn* (i.e., *Sefer ha-Qanun*) II.

• **דבק הדגים** · **fish glue:** Arab. غراء السمك (Gr. ἰχθυοκόλλα; cf. DT 439 (III.83) · *Shinnui ha-Shemot ha-Niqra'im Synonimi*, Gimel 42 (Ms Florence, Biblioteca Medicea Laurenziana, Or. 17, fol. 74a): גרה סמך ה' דבק הדגים ([Arab.] *ghirā' samak*; i.e., [Hebr.] *deveq ha-dagim*). Hebr. דבק הדגים is not attested in the current dictionaries. Nathan ha-Me'ati uses a similar term in his trans. of Maimonides' *Medical Aphorisms* (i.e., *Sefer ha-Peraqim*) IX.123 (cf. BMMN 121, l. 13; BMMG no. 3657): דבק של דגים הנקרא גלוט של דגים (*deveq shel dagim*, called GLWṬ *shel dagim*). GLWṬ is O. Occ. *glut* 'viscous matter; gum' (cf. BMZ 26f., 83 (Gimel 13)).

• **שב כדבק** → שׁוּב.

דְּבֵקוּת • **טח בדבקות** → טוּחַ.

• **טיחת דבקות** → טִיחָה.

• **הסם הטח בדבקות** → סַם.

דְּבֵקִי · **glutinous:** Lat. *glutinosus* · Guy de Chauliac, *Inventarium sive Chirurgia Magna* (cf. CMM 1:231, l. 2) · trans. Anonymous (Ms Paris, BnF, héb. 1189, fol. 126a): והמוגלא השעוונית והדבקיית (... and from the serous, glutinous pus). Hebr. דְּבֵקִי features in BM 873 in the sense of 'infectious' only).

דֶּבֶר · **plague boil (plague):** Arab. طاعون · Ibn Sīnā, *K. al-Qānūn* II · trans. Nathan ha-Me'ati, *Sefer ha-Qanun* (Ms Oxford, Bodleian Libraries, Can. Or. 88, fol. 123a): ריבאס ... ויועיל מהמורסא הנק' טאעון והדבר ([Arab.] *rībās*: Syrian rhubarb [*Rheum ribes* L.]: ... It is beneficial for the tumor called [in Arab.] *ṭā'ūn* and [in Hebr.] *dever*). Hebr. דֶּבֶר features in the current dictionaries in attestations from the Bible and Rabb. literature only (cf. KB 212; JD 279; BM 880f.). The Arab. *Plur.* طواعين is rendered by Nathan as טאעונים (see entry טאעון). Zeraḥyah Ḥen renders Arab. طاعون as אנדראש (cf. Rom. *antras*; Lat. *anthrax* 'maligant boil') and Anonymous I has also the Arab. term with a Hebr. trans. (הטאעון והדבר), just like Nathan.

---

69 The same Hebr. term features in Ms Paris, BnF, héb. 1140, fol. 113b.

70 '*mughāth*': I.e., the root of glossostemon [*Glossostemon bruguieri* Desf.]; cf. MIG no. 546.

71 עלך: Emend. ed. עלק Ms.

דְּבַשׁ • **הנגע הדומה לדבש** → **נֶגַע.**
דָּג • *Plur.* **דגים** • **דבק הדגים** → **דֶּבֶק.**
דּוֹחֶה (*Part.*) → **דָּחָה.**
דּוֹמֵעַ (*Part.*) → **דָּמַע.**
דָּחָה • *Part.* **דּוֹחֶה** • **האברים הדוחים** → **אֵבֶר.**
דְּחִיקָה · **abrasion:** Arab. سحج · Ibn Sīnā, *K. al-Qānūn* II · trans. Zeraḥyah Ḥen, *Sefer ha-Qanun* (Ms Oxford, Bodleian Libraries, Opp. Add. Fol. 12, fol. 238ª): מַרְדַּאסַנְג׳ לִיטַרְג׳יר ... ויועיל לדחיקת הירכים ([Arab.] *murdāsanj*; [i.e., Lat./Rom.] LiYṬaRəǦYR: Litharge: ... It is also good for abrasion of the thighs). Hebr. דְּחִיקָה is not attested in this sense in the current dictionaries. In addition to דְּחִיקָה, Zeraḥyah translates Arab. سحج as לְחִיצָה (see entry). Nathan ha-Me'ati translates the Arab. term as בקועים (see entry בְּקוּעַ for an attestation from his *Sefer ha-Qanun*) and Anonymous I has הפשט העור (see entry הֶפְשֵׁט).
דְּלַעַת • **גרעיני הדלעת** → **גַּרְעִין.**
דָּם • **הטמנת הדם תחת העין** → **הַטְמָנָה.**
• **הסתרת הדם תחת העין** → **הַסְתָּרָה.**
• **חלוף הדם** → **חִלּוּף.**
• **כמינת הדם תחת העין** → **כְּמִינָה.**
• **עצירת דם הוסת** → **עֲצִירָה.**
• **עצירות הדם** → **עֲצִירוּת.**
• **רעיפת דם מהאף** → **רְעִיפָה.**
• **רוק הדם** → **רֹק.**
• **שלשל הדם** → **שִׁלְשֵׁל.**
• **שפע הדם מן הנחירים** → **שֶׁפַע.**
דָּמַע • *Part.* דּוֹמֵעַ · **1. the inner canthus (angle) of the eye:** Arab. مأق · Ibn Sīnā, *K. al-Qānūn* II · trans. Zeraḥyah Ḥen, *Sefer ha-Qanun* (Ms Oxford, Bodleian Libraries, Opp. Add. Fol. 12, fols. 261ᵇ–262ª):[72] פֻּג׳ל צנון ... מזיק לעין אלא שהוא מטהר אותו כשיטיף בו מימיו ויעביר הסימנים אשר בעין תחת הדומע ([Arab.] *fujl*; [i.e., Hebr.] *ṣenon*: Radish [*Raphanus sativus* L.]: ... It is harmful for the eye, but dripping its juice into the eye cleanses it and removes the spots under the inner canthus). Hebr. דּוֹמֵעַ is not attested in the current dictionaries. In addition to this term, Zeraḥyah translates Arab. مأق as מדמע (see entry). The *Dual* مأقان is translated by him as הקצוות אשר הדמע יורד מהן and by Nathan ha-Me'ati as קצוות העין in their *Sefer ha-Qanun* I (cf. BCD 247f. (4:188)). Nathan translates Arab. مأق as זנב העין הגדול (see entry זָנָב) and Anonymous I renders the Arab. term as קצה העין.

---

72 The same term features as *Plur.* הדומעים in a gloss to the term הקצוות שבעינים on fol. 199ª (entry דֻּכָאן '[Arab.] *dukhān*: Smoke, fume').

· II. **lacrymal organ (duct)**: Lat. *lacrimalis* · Guy de Chauliac, *Inventarium sive Chirurgia Magna* (cf. CMM 1:416, ll. 8–9) · trans. Anonymous (Ms Paris, BnF, héb. 1189, fol. 227ᵃ): ובדומעים לחתוך[73] הבשר המותריי עם הסכניי הקטן ([Cauterization of] the lacrymal organs (ducts) in order to consume (destroy) the superfluous flesh with a small knife-shaped cautery). See previous entry.

דֶּמַע · **exudate**: Arab. دمعة (cf. FL 1:56: 'Lacryma, i.e. succus, aut gummi, resinave ex planta stillans') · Ibn Sīnā, *K. al-Qānūn* II · trans. Nathan ha-Me'ati, *Sefer ha-Qanun* (Ms Oxford, Bodleian Libraries, Can. Or. 88, fol. 89ᵇ): יברוח ... יש ממנו דמע ויש ממנו שיש לו מיץ ומיצו יותר חזק מדמעתו ([Arab.] *yabrūḥ*: Mandrake [*Mandragora officinarum* L.]: ... It has exudates [from the roots]; it also has an extract that is stronger than its exudates). In the sense of 'exudate,' Hebr. דֶּמַע is a non-attested calque from Arab. دمعة. A variant reading featuring in Nathan's trans. is דִּמְעָה. The latter term also features in Zeraḥyah's trans. (see next entry) and Anonymous I has דֶּמַע, just like Nathan.

דִּמְעָה · **exudate**: Arab. دمعة (cf. FL 1:56: 'Lacryma, i.e. succus, aut gummi, resinave ex planta stillans') · Ibn Sīnā, *K. al-Qānūn* II · trans. Zeraḥyah Ḥen, *Sefer ha-Qanun* (Ms Oxford, Bodleian Libraries, Opp. Add. Fol. 12, fol. 220ᵇ): יברוח ... מבטל ויש לו דמעה ויש לו מיץ ומיצו יותר חזק מדמעתו ([Arab.] *yabrūḥ*: Mandrake [*Mandragora officinarum* L.]: ... It is a sedative (narcotic), that has exudates [from the roots]; it also has an extract that is stronger than its exudates). In the sense of 'exudate,' Hebr. דִּמְעָה is a non-attested calque from Arab. دمعة. Nathan ha-Me'ati translates Arab. دمعة both as דֶּמַע (see previous entry) and דִּמְעָה. Anonymous I has דֶּמַע as well.

דַּעַת • רִפְיוֹן הדעת → רִפְיוֹן.

דְּפִיקָה · **[throbbing] pain**: Arab. ضربان (cf. DBK 2:18; FL 3:13) · al-Rāzī, *K. fī al-Faṣd* · trans. Anonymous, *Ma'amar ba-Haqqazah* (Ms Parma, Biblioteca Palatina, Cod. Parm. 2283,4, fol. 96ᵃ): אלבסליק יועיל ממורסת הצלעות ... ומחלי הקולנג' המתחדש מסבת[74] נפיחת המ⟨ע⟩ים או הקיא ודפיקת הבטן ([Bleeding] the basilic vein is beneficial for pleurisy ... and for the illness of a colic that occurs from a[75] swelling in the guts or for pain in the stomach). Hebr. דְּפִיקָה is attested in the sense of 'throbbing pain' in BCD 58 (NM 4:39) in an attestation from Moses ibn Tibbon's trans. of Ibn al-Jazzār's *Zād al-musāfir* (i.e., *Sefer Ṣedat ha-Derakhim*) II.1.9 (cf. IJZ 1–2:487).

• **דפיקת העין** · **a throbbing sensation in the eyes**: Arab. ضربان العين · Ibn Sīnā, *K. al-Qānūn* II · trans. Nathan ha-Me'ati, *Sefer ha-Qanun* (Ms Oxford, Bodleian Libraries, Can. Or. 88, fol. 110ᵃ): סדאב ... הוא מחדד הראות וקל וחומר מיצו עם מיץ שומר ודבש כשכוחלים בו ויש שמחבשין ממנו עם סויק לדפיקת העין ([Arab.] *sadhāb*: Common rue [*Ruta graveolens* L.]: It strengthens the eyesight especially when one uses its juice

---

73 לחתוך: ad consumendum L.

74 מסבת נפיחת המ⟨ע⟩ים או הקיא: من ورم في الأمعاء a.

75 'a swelling in the guts': Trans. acc. to a.

with fennel juice and honey as an eye salve. Moreover, it is plastered with mush[76] for a throbbing sensation in the eyes). Hebr. דפיקת העין is not attested in the current dictionaries. Zeraḥyah Ḥen translates Arab. ضربان العين as חבטת העין (see entry חֲבָטָה) and Anonymous I has דפיקת העין, just like Nathan.

דַּק • *Plur.* **דַּקִּים** · **intestines**: Arab. أحشاء · Ibn Sīnā, *K. al-Qānūn* II · trans. Zeraḥyah Ḥen, *Sefer ha-Qanun* (Ms Oxford, Bodleian Libraries, Opp. Add. Fol. 12, fol. 253[a]): סֶמְסֶם שומשמין ... רע לאצטומכא מוריש הקרבונקלי מפיל תאות המזון משביע מהרה וכשהוא נאכל עם הדבש יסור הזקו ויאחר עכולו[77] וירפה הדקים ([Arab.] *simsim*; [i.e., Hebr.] *shumshemin*: Sesame [*Sesamum indicum* L.]: ... It is bad for the stomach and causes nausea. It reduces appetite and satiates quickly. When taken with honey, its harmful effects are removed. It delays digestion and softens the intestines). In the sense of 'intestines' (for Lat. *interiora*), Hebr. דקים features in NM 5:54f. in an attestation from Isaiah's trans. of Guillaume de Congenis' *Treatise on Surgery*. In his trans. of Maimonides, *Medical Aphorisms* (i.e., *Sefer ha-Peraqim*), Zeraḥyah translates Arab. أحشاء 'internal organs; intestines; viscera' as גוף/מעים/קרב/קרבי(י)ם (cf. BMMG no. 976). Nathan ha-Me'ati translates the Arab. term as קרבים.

• **החכמות הדקות** → **חָכְמָה**.

[דקדק] • *Part. Pi'el* **מְדַקְדֵּק** • **הרפואה המדקדקת** → **רְפוּאָה**.

דֶּקֶל • **בוסר הדקל** → **בֹּסֶר**.

דֶּרֶךְ • **דרכו ל-** · **being of someone's business, property, nature to ...**: Arab. من شأنه أن (cf. Lane 1491) · Ibn Sīnā, *K. al-Qānūn* II · trans. Anonymous I, *Sefer ha-Qanun* (Ms Paris, BnF, héb. 1142, fol. 108[b]): והמבשל הוא אשר דרכו להקנות הליחה בשול כי הוא מחמם בשווי ויש בו כח קובץ שעוצר הליחה עד שתתבשל ואינו מתיך בכבדות (A ripening (coctive) [drug is a drug] that—by its nature—ripens (concocts) the humor by its moderate heat; it has an astringent property that retains the humor until it is ripe and does not dissolve it forcefully). Hebr. דרכו ל- is not attested in the current dictionaries. Nathan ha-Me'ati translates Arab. من شأنه أن as מנהגו ש- (see entry מִנְהָג) and Zeraḥyah Ḥen has מטבעו ש- (see entry טֶבַע).

[דשן] • *Hitpa'el* **הִתְדַּשֵּׁן** · **to become rancid**: Arab. زنخ · Ibn Sīnā, *K. al-Qānūn* II · trans. Nathan ha-Me'ati, *Sefer ha-Qanun* (Ms Oxford, Bodleian Libraries, Can. Or. 88, fol. 111[a]): סמסם והוא שומשמין והוא היותר מדשן שבזרעים ולכן יתדשן מהר ([Arab.] *simsim*; i.e., [Hebr.] *shumshemin*: Sesame [*Sesamum indicum* L.]: It contains more oil than other seeds and therefore the oil quickly becomes rancid). Hebr. הִתְדַּשֵּׁן features in BM 1010 in an attestation from the *Sefer ha-Qanun* in the sense of 'to become fat.' A synonym used by Nathan for Arab. زنخ is התערב בזוהמה (see entry [ערב]). Anonymous I renders Arab. زنخ as קיבל העפוש הנקרא *רנציד (see entry [קבל]).

---

76 Cf. WCD 517, s.v. *sawīq*: 'a kind of mush made of wheat or barley (also with sugar and dates);' see also entry קָלִי.

77 עכולו: Emend. ed. עקולו Ms.

דֶּשֶׁן · **ashes**: Arab. رماد · Ibn Sīnā, *K. al-Qānūn* II · trans. Zeraḥyah Ḥen, *Sefer ha-Qanun* (Ms Oxford, Bodleian Libraries, Opp. Add. Fol. 12, fol. 254[a]): סַפַ׳רְגַ׳ל ... כשירחץ דשן ענפיו ועליו יהיה כמו התותיא ומרבבו ינקה לטוב קיבוצו ומירבב התפוחים הוא חמוץ מפני שבו מן הלחות המימיית הקר ([Arab.] *safarjal*: Quince [*Cydonia oblonga* Mill.]: ... If the ashes of its branches and leaves are washed, it becomes like tutty. A rob of quince has a cleansing effect because of its sound astringency, but a rob of apples becomes sour because it contains cold watery moisture). In the sense of 'ashes,' Hebr. דֶּשֶׁן features in NM 5:56 (for Lat. *ciner*) in an earlier attestation from Do'eg ha-Edomi's trans. of Constantinus Africanus' *Viaticum* (i.e., *Sefer Ya'ir Netiv*) I.20.3 (cf. IJZ 1–2:649). Nathan ha-Me'ati and Anonymous I both render Arab. رماد as אפר.

ה

הַבְחָרָה · **choice**: Arab. اختيار · Ibn Sīnā, *K. al-Qānūn* II · trans. Zeraḥyah Ḥen, *Sefer ha-Qanun* (Ms Oxford, Bodleian Libraries, Opp. Add. Fol. 12, fol. 202ª): ... הֻנְדְּבֵא אִינְדְּבָא ההבחרה: היותר מועיל לכבד הוא היותר בו ממרירות ([Arab.] *hindibā'*; [i.e., Lat./Rom.] 'iYN-əDiBa']: Chicory [*Cichorium intybus* L.] or endive [*Cichorium endivia* L.]: ... Choice: Most effective for the liver is the variety that is most bitter). Hebr. הַבְחָרָה is not attested in the current dictionaries. A variant reading featuring in Zeraḥyah's trans. is מובחר; Nathan ha-Me'ati translates Arab. اختيار as מבחר (cf. NM 6:8).

הֶבֶל · **fomentation; hot compress**: Arab. كماد (Gr. πυρία; cf. UW 575f.; WKAS 1:354, s.v. *kimāda*) · Ibn Sīnā, *K. al-Qānūn* II · trans. Anonymous II, *Sefer ha-Qanun* (Ms Parma, Biblioteca Palatina, Cod. Parm. 3045, fol. 29ª): גווירס[78] ... מעפץ ומיבש בלא נשיכה והבלו משקיט הכאב ([Arab.] *jāwars*: Millet [*Panicum miliaceum* L.]: ... It is astringent and drying without irritation. Its use as a fomentation relieves pain). Hebr. הֶבֶל is not attested in the sense of 'fomentation; hot compress' in the current dictionaries. Nathan ha-Me'ati translates Arab. كماد as חיתל. Zeraḥyah Ḥen has חֹבֶשׁ (see entry) and Anonymous I has הנחה חמה (cf. BCD 68 (NM 2:39; corr. 4:229) for an attestation from Nathan's trans. of Maimonides' *Medical Aphorisms* (i.e., *Sefer ha-Peraqim*) XXIII.33 (cf. BMMN 222, l. 15; BMMG no. 4421)).

הַבְרָאָה · **healing over; forming a scar; cicatrization**: Arab. إدمال · Ibn Sīnā, *K. al-Qānūn* II · trans. Anonymous I, *Sefer ha-Qanun* (Ms Paris, BnF, héb. 1142, fol. 14ª): והמטנף השחינים הוא הסם המרטיב המתערב בלחויות השחינים וישימם יותר רבות וימנע הנגוב וההבראה (A [drug] that infects (contaminates) a wound is a moistening drug that mixes with the moistures (secretions) of the wound and increases them and [thus] prevents the wound from drying and from healing over (forming a scar; cicatrization)). Hebr. הַבְרָאָה does not feature in this sense in the current dictionaries. Zeraḥyah Ḥen translates Arab. إدمال as חִיּוּת (see entry).

הֲגָרָה • **הגרת האזן** · **otorrhea (ear discharge)**: Arab. سيلان الأذن · Ibn Sīnā, *K. al-Qānūn* II · trans. Zeraḥyah Ḥen, *Sefer ha-Qanun* (Ms Oxford, Bodleian Libraries, Opp. Add. Fol. 12, fols. 208ᵇ–209ª): זיתון זתים ... מיץ הזיתים המדבריים ייבש וישמור לרפואת הגרת האוזן ([Arab.] *zaytūn* [i.e., Hebr. *Plur.*] *zetim*: Olives [*Olea europaea* L.]: ... The juice of wild olives is dried and kept for treating otorrhea). Hebr. הגרת האזן does not feature in the current dictionaries. Nathan ha-Me'ati translates Arab. سيلان الأذن as הגרת האזן as well and Anonymous I has כאב האזן.

• **הגרת הזרע** · **nocturnal pollution; emission of sperm**: Arab. احتلام · al-Rāzī, *K. fī al-Faṣd* · trans. Anonymous, *Ma'amar ba-Haqqazah* (Ms Parma, Biblioteca Palatina, Cod. Parm. 2283,4, fol. 96ª): אלבסליק יועיל ממורסת הצלעות ... והגרת הזרע הנק' אלאחתלאם

78 גווירס: Emend. ed. זיגווירסי Ms.

([Bleeding] the basilic vein is beneficial for pleurisy … and [for] nocturnal pollution (emission of sperm) called [in Arab.] *al-iḥtilām*. Hebr. הגרת הזרע is not attested in the current dictionaries. Synonyms featuring in medieval medical literature are: מקרה לילה, גרישת הזרע בתוך השינה, געול (cf. NM 6:37, 39, 126f.), and חלום בראית קרי (see entry חֲלוֹם).

• **הגרת לחות הרחם · leukorrhea (aka: *Fluor albus*; a thick, whitish, yellowish, or greenish vaginal discharge)**: Arab. سيلان رطوبات الرحم · Ibn Sīnā, *K. al-Qānūn* II · trans. Zeraḥyah Ḥen, *Sefer ha-Qanun* (Ms Oxford, Bodleian Libraries, Opp. Add. Fol. 12, fols. 167b–168b: אֶס הדס … ובשול פריו מועיל מהגרת לחות הרחם ([Arab.] *ās*; [i.e., Hebr.] *hadas*: Myrtle [*Myrtus communis* L.]: … A decoction of its fruit is useful for leukorrhea). In the sense of 'leukorrhea,' Hebr. הגרת לחות הרחם is a non-attested calque from Arab. سيلان رطوبات الرحم. Nathan ha-Me'ati translates Arab. سيلان رطوبات الرحم as הגרת רוטבות הרחם (see entry below) and Anonymous I has הגרת לחויות הרחם (see next entry). The Arab. synonym سيلان الرحم is translated by Zeraḥyah as הגרת הרחם (see entry below).

• **הגרת לחויות הרחם · leukorrhea (aka: *Fluor albus*; a thick, whitish, yellowish, or greenish vaginal discharge)**: Arab. سيلان رطوبات الرحم · Ibn Sīnā, *K. al-Qānūn* II · trans. Anonymous I, *Sefer ha-Qanun* (Ms Paris, BnF, héb. 1142, fols. 24b–25b): אס הוא ההדס … ותבשיל פריו יועיל מהגרת לחויות הרחם ([Arab.] *ās*; i.e., [Hebr.] *ha-hadas*: Myrtle [*Myrtus communis* L.]: … A decoction of its fruit is useful for leukorrhea). In the sense of 'leukorrhea,' Hebr. הגרת לחויות הרחם is a non-attested calque from Arab. سيلان رطوبات الرحم. Zeraḥyah Ḥen translates Arab. سيلان رطوبات الرحم as הגרת לחות הרחם (see previous entry) and Nathan ha-Me'ati has הגרת רוטבות הרחם (see entry below).

• **הגרת המים באשך · hydrocele**: Arab. أدرة الماء (cf. UW 697, s.v. ὑδροκήλη) · Ibn Sīnā, *K. al-Qānūn* II · trans. Anonymous I, *Sefer ha-Qanun* (Ms Paris, BnF 1142, fol. 31a–b): אקחואן[79] … מועיל ממורסות הטבעת החמות ופותח הטחורים הוא ושמנו ומועיל מהגרת המים באשך אשר יבוקע ([Arab.] *uqḥuwān*: Feverfew [*Tanacetum parthenium* (L.) Sch. Bip.]: … It is useful for hot swellings of the anus and opens hemorrhoids. Its oil is useful for ruptured hydrocele). Hebr. הגרת המים באשך is not attested in the current dictionaries. Nathan ha-Me'ati translates Arab. أدرة الماء as אשך המים (see entry אֶשֶׁךְ) and Zeraḥyah Ḥen has המים שירדו בכיס הביצים (see entry מַיִם).

• **הגרת הנשים · menstrual bleeding**: Arab. نزف الحيض · Ibn Sīnā, *K. al-Qānūn* II · trans. Zeraḥyah Ḥen, *Sefer ha-Qanun* (Ms Oxford, Bodleian Libraries, Opp. Add. Fol. 12, fol. 216a): חדיד … והיין המכובה בו הברזל יעצור השלשול הארוך והדושנטאריא ויועיל מרפיון פי הטבעת ושילוח השתן והגרת הנשים ויחזק בתשמיש ([Arab.] *ḥadīd*: Iron: … Wine, in which [hot] iron is extinguished, stops chronic diarrhea and dysen-

79 אקחואן: קַמְמִילָא פֶּטִידָא Ms[1].

tery; it is good for the paralysis of the anus, enuresis (strangury), and menstrual bleeding. It also strengthens the sexual desire). Hebr. הגרת הנשים is not attested in the current dictionaries. Nathan ha-Me'ati translates Arab. نزف الحيض as יציאת דם הוסת.

• **הגרת רוטבות הרחם · leukorrhea (aka: *Fluor albus*; a thick, whitish, yellowish, or greenish vaginal discharge)**: Arab. سيلان رطوبات الرحم · Ibn Sīnā, *K. al-Qānūn* II · trans. Nathan ha-Me'ati, *Sefer ha-Qanun* (Ms Oxford, Bodleian Libraries, Can. Or. 88, fols. 61ᵇ–62ᵃ): אס והוא ההדס ... ותבשיל פריו יועיל מהגרת רוטבות הרחם ([Arab.] *ās*; i.e., [Hebr.] *ha-hadas*: Myrtle [*Myrtus communis* L.]: ... A decoction of its fruit is useful for leukorrhea). In the sense of 'leukorrhea,' Hebr. הגרת רוטבות הרחם is a non-attested calque from Arab. سيلان رطوبات الرحم. Zeraḥyah Ḥen translates the Arab. term as הגרת לחות הרחם (see entry above) and Anonymous I has הגרת לחויות הרחם (see entry above).

• **הגרת הרחם · leukorrhea (aka: *Fluor albus*; a thick, whitish, yellowish or greenish vaginal discharge)**: Arab. سيلان الرحم (cf. SN 113) · Ibn Sīnā, *K. al-Qānūn* II · trans. Zeraḥyah Ḥen, *Sefer ha-Qanun* (Ms Oxford, Bodleian Libraries, Opp. Add. Fol. 12, fol. 213ᵇ): חֻמָּאץ׳ ... וכבר אמר קצתם כי זרע האלחמאץ׳ בלתי קלוי יש בו המעדה וחלקות ושרשו הכתוש יועיל להגרת הרחם ויפוצץ החול שבכליות ([Arab.] *ḥummāḍ*: Sorrel [*Rumex acetosa* L.]: ... Some physicians state that unroasted seeds of sorrel are lubricant, while its pounded roots are useful for leukorrhea and crushes intestinal stones). In the sense of 'leukorrhea,' Hebr. הגרת הרחם is a non-attested calque from Arab. سيلان الرحم. The Arab. synonym سيلان رطوبات الرحم is translated by Zeraḥyah as הגרת לחות הרחם (see entry above).

הַדְבָּקָה · **viscosity**: Arab. لزوجة · Ibn Sīnā, *K. al-Qānūn* II · trans. Anonymous I, *Sefer ha-Qanun* (Ms Paris, BnF, héb. 1142, fol. 13ᵃ): והמבריא החבורות הוא הסם המנגב ומעבה הלחות הנופלת בין שני שטחי החבורה השכנים אל טיחת דבקות והדבקה הנקר׳ וישקושיטאט ויתדבק אחד מהם באחר כמו דם תנין ואלואן (A [drug] that heals wounds is a drug that dries up and thickens the fluid collected between the two layers of a wound that are close to each other. [It does so] to an extent that it (the fluid) becomes agglutinant and viscous, called WYŠQWŠYṬ'Ṭ, and both the ends [of the wound] adhere to each other; [examples of such a drug are] dragon's blood [i.e., the resin of *Dracaena cinnabari* Balf. f.] and aloes). Hebr. הַדְבָּקָה features in the sense of 'agglutination' (for Lat. *agglutinatio*) in BCD 62f. (NM 1:21) in an attestation from Hillel ben Samuel's trans. of Bruno Longobucco's *Cyrurgia Magna* (i.e., *Sefer Keritut*). Nathan ha-Me'ati translates Arab. لزوجة as דִּבּוּק (cf. NM 6:41).

הוֹלֵךְ (*Part.*) → הָלַךְ.

הוֹצָאָה • שמן ההוצאה → שֶׁמֶן.

הַזָּלָה • **הזלת השתן** · **enuresis; strangury**: Arab. تقطير البول (Gr. ἐνουρεω, στραγγουρία; cf. UW 244, 642) · Ibn Sīnā, *K. al-Qānūn* II · trans. Nathan ha-Me'ati, *Sefer ha-Qanun* (Ms Oxford, Bodleian Libraries, Can. Or. 88, fol. 75ᵇ): גראד ... יועיל להזלת השתן ואם יעשנו בו

יועיל מעוצר השתן ויועיל יותר אל הנשים ([Arab.] *jarād*: Locust: ... It is useful in strangury. Its fumigation is beneficial in dysuria, particularly so in women). Hebr. הזלת השתן features in the sense of 'micturition' (for Arab. إدرار البول) in BCD 65 (NM 3:63) in an attestation from the anonymous trans. of Maimonides' *Commentary on Hippocrates' Aphorisms* (i.e., *Perush Aphorismi shel Apuqraṭ*) I.2 (cf. BMCH 1:520, l. 19). Zeraḥyah Ḥen translates Arab. تقطير البول as טיפות השתן (cf. BCD 113 (NM 3:100) for an attestation from Zeraḥyah's trans. of Maimonides' *Commentary on Hippocrates' Aphorisms* (i.e., *Perush Aphorismi shel Apuqraṭ*) III.31 (cf. BMCH 1:454, ll. 8–9)) and Anonymous I has הטפת השתן (cf. BCD 66 (NM 3:64, 4:44) for attestations from Do'eg ha-Edomi's *Sefer Agur* V.58 and Shem Tov ben Isaac's *Sefer ha-Shimmush* XXVII; see also entry הַטָּפָה). Other synonyms for Hebr. הזלת השתן featuring in medieval Hebr. medical literature are הגרת טיפות השתן (cf. BCD 62 (NM 3:56)), טפטוף השתן (cf. BCD 113 (NM 3:100)), and קושי השתן (cf. BCD 252 (NM 3:211f.)).

• *Plur.* **הזלות** • **הזלות הראש** · **rheum:**[80] Arab. زُكام · al-Rāzī, *K. fī al-Faṣd* · trans. Anonymous, *Ma'amar ba-Haqqazah* (Ms Parma, Biblioteca Palatina, Cod. Parm. 2283,4, fol. 94b): הקזת הקיפאל יועיל ... מכבד התנועה הנקרא אלכדר עם אדמימות המראה ומהזלות הראש הנק' זוכאם (Bleeding the cephalic vein is beneficial ... for numbness, called [in Arab.] *al-khadar*, combined with redness of the face, and for rheum, called [in Arab.] *zukām*). Hebr. הזלות הראש is not attested in the current dictionaries. Synonyms featuring in medieval medical literature are מִלּוּי (see entry), מלוי הראש (cf. NM 6:119), סתום האף (cf. BCD 195 (NM 3:171)), and סתום הנחירים (cf. BCD 195 (NM 4:140)).

הֲטָחָה · **ointment; paste; unguent; salve:** Arab. لَطُوخ (cf. WKAS 2.2:691b–692a) · Ibn Sīnā, *K. al-Qānūn* II · trans. Zeraḥyah Ḥen, *Sefer ha-Qanun* (Ms Oxford, Bodleian Libraries, Opp. Add. Fol. 12, fols. 167b–168a): אֶס הדס ... והוא יועיל מכל הגרת דם הטחה וחובש וכן בשישתהו ([Arab.] *ās*; [i.e., Hebr.] *hadas*: Myrtle [*Myrtus communis* L.]: ... It is beneficial for all [kinds] of bleeding, whether [applied] as a salve or plaster; likewise [when used] as a drink). Hebr. הֲטָחָה is not attested in a medical sense in the current dictionaries. Arab. لُطُوخ 'to apply as a salve' is translated by Zeraḥyah (acc. to the use of the noun הֲטָחָה) as להטיח (see entry טוּחַ) or טיחה (see entry משח). In his trans. of Maimonides' *Medical Aphorisms* (i.e., *Sefer ha-Peraqim*) IX.18, Zeraḥyah translates Arab. لَطُوخ as משרה (cf. BMMZ 100, l. 17; BMMG no. 4608). Nathan ha-Me'ati translates the Arab. term as לִכְלֵךְ (see entry) and Anonymous I renders it as טיחה (cf. BCD 112 for attestations from Shem Tov ben Isaac's *Sefer ha-Shimmush* XXX.2.20 (cf. NM 1:95) and Moses ibn Tibbon's trans. of Ibn al-Jazzār's *Zād al-musāfir* (i.e., *Sefer Ṣedat ha-Derakhim*) VII.16.3 (cf. NM 1:58; IJZ 7:153, l. 1).

---

80 'rheum': Cf. F. Wallis, *Medieval Medicine: A Reader* (Toronto 2010), 550: 'a morbid discharge of phlegm in the head (e.g., a runny nose), eyes, joints, etc.'

הַטְמָנָה • הטמנת הדם תחת העין · dark blood collected beneath the tissue under the eye (ecchymosis): Arab. كهوبة الدم تحت العين · Ibn Sīnā, *K. al-Qānūn* II · trans. Nathan ha-Me'ati, *Sefer ha-Qanun* (Ms Oxford, Bodleian Libraries, Can. Or. 88, fol. 92ᵃ): ... כמון ילעסוהו ויערבוהו בשמן זית ויטיפוהו על הצפורן ובער' טפרה ועל הטמנת הדם תחת העין ([Arab.] *kammūn* / [Hebr.] *kammon*: Cumin [*Cuminum cyminum* L.]: ... Chewed and mixed with olive oil, it is applied for pterygium, in Arab. *ẓufra*, and for dark blood collected beneath the tissue under the eye (ecchymosis)). Hebr. הטמנת הדם תחת העין is not attested in the current dictionaries. Zeraḥyah Ḥen translates Arab. كهوبة الدم تحت العين as הסתרת הדם תחת העין (see entry הַסְתָּרָה) and Anonymous I has כמינת הדם תחת העין (see entry כְּמִינָה).

הַטָּפָה • הטפה באף · dripping (pouring) a medicine into the nose: Arab. سعوط · Ibn Sīnā, *K. al-Qānūn* II · trans. Anonymous I, *Sefer ha-Qanun* (Ms Paris, BnF, héb. 1142, fols. 65ᵇ–66ᵃ): בול הוא שתן ... מועיל מהכאבים העצביים וכל שכן שתן העז הבייתי וההררי וכל שכן לכויצה ולמתיחה וכן הטפה באף למתיחה ([Arab.] *bawl*; i.e., [Hebr.] *sheten*: Urine: ... Especially that of domestic and mountain goats is useful for neural pains. It is particularly useful for spasms and tetanus. For tetanus it can be dripped into the nose as well). Hebr. הטפה באף is not attested in the current dictionaries. Nathan ha-Me'ati translates Arab. سعوط as עשה סעוט (see entry עָשָׂה) and Zeraḥyah Ḥen translates the Arab. term as עשה שעיטה (see also entry עָשָׂה).

• הטפת השתן · enuresis; strangury: Arab. تقطير البول (Gr. ἐνουρεω, στραγγουρία; cf. UW 244, 642) · Ibn Sīnā, *K. al-Qānūn* II · trans. Nathan ha-Me'ati, *Sefer ha-Qanun* (Ms Oxford, Bodleian Libraries, Can. Or. 88, fol. 87ᵇ): חדיד ... ויועיל[81] מרפיון העגבות והטפת השתן ויציאת דם הוסת ויחזק תאות המשגל ([Arab.] *ḥadīd*: Iron: ... Wine, in[82] which hot iron is extinguished, stops chronic diarrhea and dysentery; it is good for the paralysis of the anus, enuresis (strangury), and menstrual bleeding. It also strengthens the sexual desire). Hebr. הטפת השתן features in BCD 66 (NM 3:64, 4:44) in the sense of 'strangury' only. Zeraḥyah Ḥen translates Arab. تقطير البول as שילוח השתן (see entry שִׁלּוּחַ).

הִין · liquid measure: Arab. قسط ('liquid measure of varying weight'[83]) · Ibn Sīnā, *K. al-Qānūn* II · trans. Nathan ha-Me'ati, *Sefer ha-Qanun* (Ms Oxford, Bodleian Libraries, Can. Or. 88, fol. 77ᵇ): דגאג ודיך ... ויבשלוהו בעשרים הין בערבי קסט ([Arab.] *dajāj* [i.e., chicken] and *dīk* [i.e., rooster]: Poultry: ... Then they [i.e, the roosters] should be cooked in twenty [Hebr.] *hin*, in Arab. *qisṭ* [of water]). Hebr. הִין is only attested as

81 ויועיל: والشراب المطفأ فيه الحديد يحبس الاسهال المزمن ودوسنطاريا وينفع a.

82 'in which hot iron is extinguished, stops chronic diarrhea and dysentery': Add. acc. to a.

83 Cf. EI² 6:119a, s.v. *makāyil* (J. Burton-Page): 'there were three measures called *qisṭ*: one containing 476 g olive oil, another 1.07 kg and yet another 2.14 kg;' Sābūr Ibn Sahl, *Dispensatorium Parvum* (*Al-Aqrābādhīn al-saghīr*), ed. by O. Kahl, 227, n. 201: '*qisṭ* is usually a regular measure of capacity, viz. 1.22–2.34 l.'

a liquid measure in the Bible (cf. KB 245) and Rabb. literature (cf. JD 348: 'a liquid measure, equal to twelve Log;' KTA 2:396f.). Zeraḥyah Ḥen transcribes Arab. قسط as *qisṭ*.

הַכְאָבָה · **causing pain**: Arab. تصديع · Ibn Sīnā, *K. al-Qānūn* II · trans. Anonymous I, *Sefer ha-Qanun* (Ms Paris, BnF, héb. 1142, fol. 31^{b}): אסטורק ... יש בו תרדמה והכבדה לראש והכאבה ([Rom.] ʾSṬWRQ [i.e., O. Occ. *estorac*; cf. SHS 1:214f. (Ḥet 10)]: Styrax: ... It causes lethargy, heaviness in the head, and pain [i.e., headache]). Hebr. הַכְאָבָה is not attested for medieval medical literature. Nathan ha-Me'ati and Zeraḥyah Ḥen translate Arab. تصديع as מכאיב.

הַכְבָּדָה · **causing heaviness**: Arab. تثقيل · Ibn Sīnā, *K. al-Qānūn* II · trans. Anonymous I, *Sefer ha-Qanun* (Ms Paris, BnF, héb. 1142, fol. 31^{b}): אסטורק ... יש בו תרדמה והכבדה לראש והכאבה ([Rom.] ʾSṬWRQ [i.e., O. Occ. *estorac*; cf. SHS 1:214f. (Ḥet 10)]: Styrax ...: It causes lethargy, heaviness in the head, and pain [i.e., headache]). Hebr. הַכְבָּדָה features in EM 368 as a modern term only. Nathan ha-Me'ati and Zeraḥyah Ḥen translate Arab. تثقيل as כובד.

הָלַךְ • *Part.* **הוֹלֵךְ** • **ההולך על גחון** · **horned viper**: Arab. مقرّنة (cf. D 2:339) · Ibn Sīnā, *K. al-Qānūn* II · trans. Nathan ha-Me'ati, *Sefer ha-Qanun* (Ms Oxford, Bodleian Libraries, Can. Or. 88, fol. 105^{a-b}): מלח ... עושין ממנו תחבשת עם זרע פשתן[84] ויועיל פודנג הררי וזופא ודבש לנשיכת ההולך על גחון ועם חומץ ודבש לנשיכת בעלי מ״ד רגלים והצרעות (Salt: ... It is used as a plaster with linseed for[85] scorpion bite. [Applied with] wild mint, hyssop, and honey, it is beneficial for horned viper bite. With vinegar and honey [it is beneficial] for bites by centipedes and wasps). Hebr. ההולך על גחון features as כל הולך על גחון in the general sense of 'snakes or reptiles [lit. 'anything that crawls on its belly']' only (cf. KB 187; BM 747). Zeraḥyah Ḥen renders Arab. مقرّنة as בעל הקרנים (see entry בַּעַל) and Anonymous I has בעל הקרן (see also entry בַּעַל).

הַמְעָדָה · **slipperiness**: Arab. زلق · Ibn Sīnā, *K. al-Qānūn* II · trans. Zeraḥyah Ḥen, *Sefer ha-Qanun* (Ms Oxford, Bodleian Libaries, Opp. Add. Fol. 12, fol. 252^{b}): סַלִיכָ'ה קָשֵׁיאָה ליגניאה ... ויועיל מכאבי הכליות והשלפוחית וכשיושב בבישולו יועיל להרחבת הרחם והמעדתה ([Arab.] *salīkha*; [i.e., Rom.] QaŠeY'aH LYGNY'H [i.e., O. Occ./O. Cat. *cassia lignea*; cf. SHS 1:466 (Qof 34)]: Chinese cinnamon [*Cinnamomum cassia* (L.) D. Don]: ... It is good for pain in the intestines and bladder. A sitz bath in the decoction is good for dilation and slipperiness of the uterus). Hebr. הַמְעָדָה features in BCD 67 (NM 1:88; corr. 2:198) for Arab. إزلاق in the sense of 'lubrication' and in BM 1117 in an attestation, a.o., from the *Sefer ha-Qanun* in the sense of 'slipping [of the foot].' Nathan ha-Me'ati translates Arab. زلق as מְעִידָה (see entry) and Anonymous I has הַמְעָדָה, just like Zeraḥyah.

---

84 פשתן: للسع العقرب add. a.

85 'for scorpion bite': Add. acc. to a.

הַמָתָה · **mortification:** Lat. *mortifico*[86] · Guy de Chauliac, *Inventarium sive Chirurgia Magna* (cf. CMM 1:231, ll. 37–42) · trans. Anonymous (Ms Paris, BnF, héb. 1189, fol. 126[b]): והעזר הג׳ הוא מגילים דשיליציט שכשמתרחב הנקב שינוקה עם אינגינט ירוק הנעשה מפרח הנחשת והאלום ודבש או עם אבק אפרודיליש ואחר הנקוי ירפא עם המדביקים ואם אלו לא יועילו אז תבא הכונה הג׳ שהוא המתת הנאצור (The third [kind of] treatment [of a lacrimal fistula] comes from Guglielmo da Saliceto: When the opening [of the fistula] has been widened, it should be cleaned with a green unguent made from copper oxide, alum, and honey, or with asphodel powder. Once it has been cleaned, it should be healed with medicines that close wounds and/or promote formation of scars. But if this is to no avail, the third intention (procedure) should be to mortify the fistula). In the sense of 'mortification,' Hebr. הַמָתָה is a non-attested calque from Lat. *mortifico*.

הֲנָחָה · I. **abandonment:** Arab. ترك · al-Rāzī, *K. fī al-Faṣd* · trans. Anonymous, *Ma'amar ba-Haqqazah* (Ms Parma, Biblioteca Palatina, Cod. Parm. 2283,4, fol. 92[a]): וכבר באר זה אבוק׳ באמרו כי החלי המגיע אל הדקות הרבה צריך שיתנהג בהנהגה הדקה הרבה ורצו׳ בזה הנחת המאכל לגמרי (This was explained by Hippocrates when he said: '[In the case of] a very subtle illness, one has to apply a very subtle regimen,' by which is meant the complete abandonment of food). Hebr. הֲנָחָה does not feature in this sense in the current dictionaries.

· II. **tepidity:** Arab. فتور · Ibn Sīnā, *K. al-Qānūn* II · trans. Nathan ha-Me'ati, *Sefer ha-Qanun* (Ms Oxford, Bodleian Libraries, Can. Or. 88, fol. 79[b]): דם ... אמר גלינוס כי זה בעד הנחת איכותו לא בעד דבר אחר (Blood: ... Galen said that this [property] is due to its tepid quality, not to anything else). Hebr. הֲנָחָה does not feature in this sense in the current dictionaries. Zeraḥyah Ḥen and Anonymous I both render Arab. فتور as פְּשִׁירָה (see entry).

הַנָּחָה • **הנחה למטה** · **application of a suppository:** Arab. حمول · Ibn Sīnā, *K. al-Qānūn* II · trans. Anonymous I, *Sefer ha-Qanun* (Ms Paris, BnF, héb. 1142, fols. 76[b]–77[a]): ג׳זר הוא פשטנגה ... ופשטינאגה מדברית אם יחשבו בכלל גזר הנה הם מעוררים תאות המשגל יותר מהגנניי ומגיר הנדות והשתן ובייחוד המדברי בשתיה והנחה למטה ([Arab.] *jazar*; i.e., [Rom.] PŠṬNGH [i.e., O. Occ./O. Cat *pastenaga*; cf. SHS1:344f (Nun 17)]: Carrot [*Daucus carota* L.]: ... Wild carrot, if it may be considered as a carrot at all, is more stimulant for sexual lust than its cultivated variety. When one consumes carrot, especially the wild variety, or applies it as a suppository, it stimulates menstruation and discharge

86 Cf. Wallis, *Medieval Medicine*, 547, s.v. *mortify*, *mortification*: 'depending on context, 'mortify' can mean either (a) to subdue or bring under control (a disease or a poison) or (b) to rot or corrupt (e.g., in cases of gangrene the flesh is 'mortified').' Here, it means that when the treatment with regular medicines is to no avail, one should apply more drastic means, such as incision or cauterization.

of urine). In the sense of 'application of a suppository,' Hebr. הנחה למטה features in a variant reading ההנחה העשויה למטה, *Plur.* ההנחות העשויות למטה, in NM 5:59 in an attestation from Do'eg ha-Edomi's trans. of Constantinus Africanus' *Viaticum* (i.e., *Sefer Ya'ir Netiv*) I.17.2 (cf. IJZ 1–2:618). Nathan ha-Me'ati and Zeraḥyah Ḥen translate Arab. حمول as סָבַל (see entry).

הַסְתָּרָה • הסתרת הדם תחת העין: dark blood collected beneath the tissue under the eye (ecchymosis): Arab. كهوبة الدم تحت العين · Ibn Sīnā, *K. al-Qānūn* II · trans. Zeraḥyah Ḥen, *Sefer ha-Qanun* (Ms Oxford, Bodleian Libaries, Opp. Add. Fol. 12, fol. 224b): כַּמּוֹן ... ילעוס ויעורב בשמן ויוטף על הציפורן ועל הסתרת הדם תחת העין (Cumin [*Cuminum cyminum* L.]: ... Chewed and mixed with olive oil, it is applied for pterygium and for dark blood collected beneath the tissue under the eye (ecchymosis)). Hebr. הסתרת הדם תחת העין is not attested in the current dictionaries. Nathan ha-Me'ati translates Arab. كهوبة الدم تحت العين as הטמנת הדם תחת העין (see entry הַטְמָנָה) and Anonymous I has כמינת הדם תחת העין (see entry כְּמִינָה).

• הסתרת עין · abnormal protrusion of the eyeball (exophthalmos): Arab. جحوظ (cf. HLA 170 (178)) · Ibn Sīnā, *K. al-Qānūn* II · trans. Zeraḥyah Ḥen, *Sefer ha-Qanun* (Ms Oxford, Bodleian Libaries, Opp. Add. Fol. 12, fol. 220b):[87] יברוח ... והממית ממנו יקדימנו מקרה חניקת הרחם ואודם פנים והסתרת עין ונפח פנים גם כן כאלו הוא שכור ([Arab.] *yabrūḥ*: Mandrake [*Mandragora officinarum* L.]: ... Death by the [intake of] the fatal variety is preceded by the symptoms of hysterical suffication, redness of the face,[88] abnormal protrusion of the eyeball, also swelling of the face as if he is drunk ...). Hebr. הסתרת עין is not attested in the current dictionaries. Nathan ha-Me'ati and Anonymous I both render Arab. جحوظ as בליטת העין (see entry בְּלִיטָה).

הִפּוּךְ • הפוך האצטו' · upset stomach (surfeit; nausea): Arab. قلب المعدة · Ibn Sīnā, *K. al-Qānūn* II · trans. Nathan ha-Me'ati, *Sefer ha-Qanun* (Ms Oxford, Bodleian Libraries, Can. Or. 88, fol. 116b: פסתק ... אמרו קצתם ולא נמצא לו באצטו' הזק מרובה ולא תועלת ואני אומר שהוא מונע האסטנסות והפוך האצטו' ויחזק פיה ([Arab.] *fustuq*: Pistachio [*Pistacia vera* L.]: ... Some said that they did not find it to be either very harmful or useful for the stomach. But I say that it prevents nausea and an upset stomach, and strengthens the cardia of the stomach). Hebr. הפוך האצטו' is not attested in the current dictionaries. Anonymous I translates Arab. as התהפכות האיסטו' (see entry הִתְהַפְּכוּת), which seems to be synonymous with התהפכות הנפש (see also entry הִתְהַפְּכוּת and next entry [הפך] for the variant התהפך הנפש). Zeraḥyah Ḥen renders Arab. قلب المعدة as הפך האצטו'.

---

87 The same term features on fol. 165b in the section לוח איברי העין 'table on the ocular organs' and on fols. 208b–209a in the entry זיתון זיתים '[Arab.] *zaytūn*; [i.e., Hebr. *Plur.*] *zetim*: Olives').

88 'face': 'cheeks' a.

[הפך] • *Inf. Hitpaʿel* **הִתְהַפֵּךְ • התהפך הנפש** · **upset stomach (surfeit; nausea)**: Arab.[89] تقلب النفس (Gr. ἀσώδης, ἄση, ναυτία; cf. UWS 1:179, 186, 717) · Ibn Sīnā, *K. al-Qānūn* II · trans. Zeraḥyah Ḥen, *Sefer ha-Qanun* (Ms Oxford, Bodleian Libaries, Opp. Add. Fol. 12, fol. 212[b]): נַאנַכְּוַה[90] אַמֵיאוּשׁ ... יועיל מבלילת האצטומכא וישכך הקרבונקלי והתהפך הנפש ([Arab.] *nānakhwāh*; [i.e., Lat./Rom.] ʾaMeYʾWŠ [i.e., L. Lat./O. Occ./O. Cat./O. Sp. *ameos*; cf. SHS 1:337 (Nun 3)]: Bisnaga (toothpickweed) [*Ammi visnaga* (L.) Lam.]: ... It is beneficial for [excessive] moisture in the stomach, it alleviates nausea, and it [is good for] an upset stomach). Hebr. התהפך הנפש is a non-attested calque from Arab. تقلب النفس. For *Part. Nifʿal* נֶהְפָּךְ and *Part. Hitpaʿel* מִתְהַפֵּךְ in the sense of 'upset (re: stomach),' see NM 5:60f. Nathan ha-Me'ati renders Arab. تقلب النفس as פוקה (i.e., the regular Hebr. term for Arab. فواق 'hiccups,' cf. BMMG no. 3977) and Anonymous I renders the Arab. term as התהפכות הנפש (see entry הִתְהַפְּכוּת).

הַפָּלָה · **causing a miscarriage; abortion**: Arab. إسقاط · Ibn Sīnā, *K. al-Qānūn* II · trans. Anonymous I, *Sefer ha-Qanun* (Ms Paris, BnF, héb. 1142, fol. 197[a–b]): ערטניתא[91] הוא סיקלמין ... תמורתו בהפלה והתועלת מן הארסים כמשקלו ארישטולוגיאה ארוכה וגרגרי אתרוג ופודנג׳ ([Arab.] *ʿarṭanīthā*; i.e., [Lat.] SYQLMYN [i.e., M. Lat. *cyclamen*]: Cyclamen [*Cyclamen* sp.]: ... An equal weight of birthwort, citron seeds, and mint acts as its substitute for causing a miscarriage and for being effective against poisons). Hebr. הַפָּלָה features in BCD 70 (NM 3:67) in the sene of 'miscarriage' (for Arab. سقط) in an attestation from Moses ibn Tibbon's trans. of Maimonides' *Commentary on Hippocrates' Aphorisms* (i.e., *Perush Aphorismi shel Apuqraṭ*) V.53 (cf. BMCH 1:387, l. 6). Nathan ha-Me'ati and Zeraḥyah Ḥen both translate Arab. إسقاط as להפיל.

הֶפְסֵד · **tear [of a muscle]**: Arab. فسخ (Gr. ῥῆγμα; cf. UW2:246) · Ibn Sīnā, *K. al-Qānūn* II · trans. Zeraḥyah Ḥen, *Sefer ha-Qanun* (Ms Oxford, Bodleian Libaries, Opp. Add. Fol. 12, fol. 237[a]): מֻקל[92] דֵילֵיאו יהודי ודֵילִיאו מכיי ... יועיל להפסד המושקלו ומן הקווץ וקושי העצבים ועיקודם ([Arab.] *muql*;[93] [Rom.-Hebr.] DeYLeYʾW *yehudi* and [Rom.-Arab.] DeYLYʾW *Makkī*: Judean and Meccan bdellium: ... It is useful for muscle tear, spasms, stiffness and twisting of the nerves). Hebr. הֶפְסֵד is not attested in the sense of 'tear' in the current dictionaries. It features also for Arab. فسخ in the sense of 'disruption' in Zeraḥyah's trans. of Maimonides' *Medical Aphorisms* (i.e., *Sefer ha-Peraqim*) III.109 (cf. BMMZ 49, l. 1; BMMG no. 3836). The Arab. synonym وهن is translated by Zeraḥyah

---

89 The Arab. term features as قلب النفس (Gr. ἀνατρέπει τὸν στόμαχον) in Maimonides' *Medical Aphorisms* IX.51, 55; the English trans. 'upset the soul' should be corrected to 'upset the stomach' (cf. BMMA 2:70, l. 19; 71, l. 21; BMMG no. 4162).

90 נַאנַכְּוַה: Emend. ed. נַאנַכְּה Ms.

91 ערטניתא: שיקלמין הוא פאן פורסי Ms[1].

92 מֻקל: Ms[1].

93 '*muql*': I.e., bdellium, i.e., the gum resin of plants from the *Burseraceae* family, esp. *Commiphora africana* (A.Rich.) Endl. and *Commiphora mukul* (Hook. ex Stocks) Engl.

as חֲלִשָׁה (see entry) and the synonymous Arab. هتك as חִתּוּךְ (see entry). Nathan ha-Me'ati translates Arab. فسخ as בְּקוּעַ (see entry).

הֶפְשֵׁט • הפשט העור · **abrasion of the skin**: Arab. سحج · Ibn Sīnā, *K. al-Qānūn* II · trans. Anonymous I, *Sefer ha-Qanun* (Ms Paris, BnF, héb. 1142, fol. 164^{a-b}): מרדסאנג ... ומועיל להפשט העור שבפחדים ([Arab.] *murdāsanj*: Litharge: ... It is also good for abrasion of the skin of the thighs). Hebr. הפשט העור is not attested in the current dictionaries. The term הֶפְשֵׁט alone features in the sense of 'abrasion' in BCD 71 (NM 2:40f.) in an attestation from Nathan ha-Me'ati's trans. of Maimonides' *Medical Aphorisms* (i.e., *Sefer ha-Peraqim*) XXI.27 (cf. BMMN 199, l. 6). Zeraḥyah Ḥen translates Arab. سحج as דְּחִיקָה (see entry) and Nathan has בקועים (see entry בְּקוּעַ for another attestation in his *Sefer ha-Qanun*).

הַצָּבָה • הצבת הנשימה · **orthopnea**: Arab. انتصاب النفس (cf. UW 471, s.v. ὀρθόπνοια: نفس (الانتصاب) · Ibn Sīnā, *K. al-Qānūn* II · trans. Nathan ha-Me'ati, *Sefer ha-Qanun* (Ms Oxford, Bodleian Libraries, Can. Or. 88, fols. 66^{b}–67^{a}): אנסאן ... אמרו כי שתן הנערים כששותין ממנו יועיל מעוצר הנשימה והצבתה[94] וימהר הרפואה ([Arab.] *insān*: Human being: ... It is said that the urine of a child, when taken orally, is good for dyspnea and orthopnea, and that it heals it more quickly). Hebr. הצבת הנשימה is not attested in the current dictionaries. Synonyms used by Nathan are הצבת הניפוש (cf. NM 6:56), מצב הנשימה (see entry מַצָּב), and הנשימה הנצבת (see entry נְשִׁימָה). Zeraḥyah Ḥen translates Arab. انتصاب النفس as הצבת הנשימה, just like Nathan. Anonymous I renders the Arab. term as התיצבות הנשימה (cf. entry הִתְיַצְּבוּת in NM 6:60 for an attestation from the anonymous trans. of Maimonides' *On Asthma* (i.e., *Sefer ha-Qaṣeret*) N.2 (cf. BMA 2:388, l. 2)).

הַקְדָּמָה • הקדמת הידיעה · **prognosis**: Lat. *pronosticon* · Guy de Chauliac, *Inventarium sive Chirurgia Magna* (cf. CMM 1:237, ll. 37–38) · trans. Anonymous (Ms Paris, BnF, héb. 1189, fol. 130^{a}): נגעי הצואר והשדרה אינם מתחלפים מן האחרים כי אם בהקדמת הידיעה שהם מסוכנים (Ulcers in the neck and back are not different from other ones except that their prognosis is that they are dangerous). In the sense of 'prognosis,' Hebr. הקדמת הידיעה features (for Arab. تقدمة المعرفة) in BCD 71 (NM 2:41) in an attestation from Nathan ha-Me'ati's trans. of Maimonides' *Medical Aphorisms* (i.e., *Sefer ha-Peraqim*) II.4 (cf. BMMN 35, l. 13).

הַקָּזָה • חזרת ההקזה → חֲזָרָה.

הֶקֵּף • הקדחות בעלי ההקף → קַדַּחַת.

הַקָּפָה · **attack; paroxysm**: Arab. نوبة · al-Rāzī, *K. fī al-Faṣd* · trans. Anonymous, *Ma'amar ba-Haqqazah* (Ms Parma, Biblioteca Palatina, Cod. Parm. 2283,4, fol. 93^{a}): וכאשר יהיה הדם הרבה בגוף ונתחמם ונרתח ונתחדשה ממנו קדחת יעשה הרקתו פתאם בעת ירידת הקפת הקדחת וקודם שיהיה נגר אל האברים המעולים בעבור כי זאת הקדחת ואם היא דבקה יהיה לה על

94 והצבתה (= Ms Paris, BnF, héb. 1136, fol. 66^{b}): ומצבתה Ms.

הרוב התחלה ותוספת ותכלית וירידה (When there is a lot of blood in the body and it gets hot and boils and causes a fever, then evacuate it all at once at the time of the decline of the paroxysm of fever before it flows towards the vital organs, because this fever, even if it was continuous, in most cases will have a beginning, increase, climax, and decline). Hebr. הַקָּפָה does not feature in this sense in the current dictionaries. Synonyms featuring in medieval medical literature are וֶסֶת (cf. BCD 79 (NM 3:75)), מִשְׁמָר (cf. NM 6:131), מִשְׁמָרָה (cf. NM 6:131f.), מִשְׁמֶרֶת (cf. NM 6:132), and עוֹנָה (cf. BCD 198 (NM 1:175; 2:70; 3:173).

• *Plur.* הקפות • הקדחות אשר להם הקפות → קַדַּחַת.

הֶרְגֵּשׁ • בטול ההרגש → בִּטּוּל.

• הסם המבטל ההרגש → סַם •

הֵרָיוֹן • חולשת קבול ההריון → חֻלְשָׁה.

• עוצר ההריון → עֹצֶר.

הֲרָרִי • הצמוקים ההרריים → צִמּוּק.

הַשְׁוָאָה · **regularity**: Arab. استواء · al-Rāzī, *K. fī al-Faṣd* · trans. Anonymous, *Ma'amar ba-Haqqazah* (Ms Parma, Biblioteca Palatina, Cod. Parm. 2283,4, fol. 93[a]): וכאשר יראה הדפק משתנה ומתחלף בגדלו או בהשואתו ויתרון[95] הכח עם חולשא צריך להפסיקו מיד (If you see the pulse changing in its magnitude or regularity aside[96] from becoming weaker, and the vehemence of the blood weakening, then end it [i.e., the bloodletting] immediately). Hebr. הַשְׁוָאָה is not attested in this sense in the current dictionaries. In their trans. of Maimonides' *Medical Aphorisms* (i.e., *Sefer ha-Peraqim*) XII.18, Nathan ha-Me'ati and Zeraḥyah Ḥen both translate Arab. استواء as שווי (cf. BMMN 141, l. 5; BMMZ 138, l. 12; BMMG no. 2573).

הַשְׁחָנָה · **ulceration**: Arab. تقريح · Ibn Sīnā, *K. al-Qānūn* II · trans. Anonymous I, *Sefer ha-Qanun* (Ms Paris, BnF, héb. 1142, fol. 13[a]): והמאכל הוא הסם שדרכו להתיך שמגיע מהתכתו או השחנתו שיחסר מעצם הבשר כמו הזנג'אר (A corrosive [drug] is a drug that—by its nature—has solvent and ulcerative properties, which are so strong that they reduce the substance of the flesh [of the organ]; an example of such a drug is verdigris). In the sense of 'ulceration,' Hebr. הַשְׁחָנָה features in BCD 73 (NM 3:71) in an attestation from Judah Shalom's trans. of Hippocrates' *Aphorisms* IV.81. Nathan ha-Me'ati translates Arab. تقريح as נְגוּעַ (see entry) and Zeraḥyah Ḥen has חַבָּלָה (see entry).

הֲשָׁרָה • השרת השער · **hair loss**: Arab. انتشار الشعر · Ibn Sīnā, *K. al-Qānūn* II · trans. Zeraḥyah Ḥen, *Sefer ha-Qanun* (Ms Oxford, Bodleian Libaries, Opp. Add. Fol. 12, fol. 248[a]): סַאדוּרַאן[97] ... ימנע השרת השער בסגולה שבו ([Arab.] *sādārawān*: A black resin or tar (cf. DT 121 (I.39), n. 5): ... It prevents loss of hair through its specific property). Hebr. השרת השער is not attested in the current dictionaries. Nathan ha-Me'ati trans-

---

95 ויתרון הכח עם חולשא: فضلا عن أن يضعف أو ضعفت حمية الدم a.

96 'aside from becoming weaker, and the vehemence of the blood weakening': Trans. acc. to a.

97 סַאדוּרַאן: سادوران a.

lates Arab. انتشار الشعر as נפילת השער (see entry נְפִילָה) and Anonymous I renders the Arab. term as השרת השער, just like Zeraḥyah.

הִשְׁתּוֹמְמוּת • השתוממות השכל · **anxiety**: Arab. توحّش · Ibn Sīnā, *K. al-Qānūn* II · trans. Nathan ha-Me'ati, *Sefer ha-Qanun* (Ms Oxford, Bodleian Libraries, Can. Or. 88, fol. 94b): טבאשיר ... יועיל מנגעי הפה הנקרא קלאע ומהשתוממות השכל ([Arab.] *ṭabāshīr*: Tabasheer (bamboo manna) [i.e., the siliceous secretions found in the internodes of bamboo stems [*Bambusa bambos* (L.) Voss]: It is beneficial for aphthae, called [in Arab.] *qulāʿ*, and for anxiety). Hebr. השתוממות השכל is not attested in the current dictionaries. Zeraḥyah Ḥen translates Arab. توحّش as אֲנָחָה (see entry) and Anonymous I has הִשְׁתּוֹמְמוּת (cf. BCD 74 (NM 4:48) for an attestation from an anonymous trans. of Ibn Sīnā's *K. al-Adwiya al-qalbiyya* (i.e., *Sammim Libbiyim*)). Cf. also NM 5:196 for the synonym שִׁמָּמוֹן, featuring in the anonymous trans. of Isḥāq ibn ʿImrān's *Treatise on Melancholy*.

הִשְׁתַּטְּחוּת · **stretching**: Arab. تمدّد · Ibn Sīnā, *K. al-Qānūn* II · trans. Nathan ha-Me'ati, *Sefer ha-Qanun* (Ms Oxford, Bodleian Libraries, Can. Or. 88, fol. 94b): כטמי ... ויועיל מגיד הנשה ומהרעישה ורצוץ אמצע העצלים והשתטחות[98] העצבים ([Arab.] *khiṭmī*: Common marshmallow [*Althaea officinalis* L.]: ... It is beneficial for sciatica, trembling, bruise of the median muscle, and stretching of the nerves). Hebr. הִשְׁתַּטְּחוּת is not attested in a medical context in the current dictionaries (cf. BM 1213). In his trans. of Maimonides' *Medical Aphorisms* (i.e., *Sefer ha-Peraqim*), Nathan translates Arab. تمدّد as המתח, המתחה, and מתיחה (cf. BMMG no. 4731). The term מְתִיחָה is used by Nathan for translating the synonymous Arab. امتداد (see entry).

הִתְהַפְּכוּת • התהפכות האיסטו' · **upset stomach (surfeit; nausea)**: Arab. قلب المعدة · Ibn Sīnā, *K. al-Qānūn* II · trans. Anonymous I, *Sefer ha-Qanun* (Ms Paris, BnF, héb. 1142, fol. 213b): פסתק[99] ... אמרו קצתם איני מוצא באיסטו' היזק רב ולא תועלת אומר אני אבל ימנע האסטנסות והתהפכות האיסטו' ומחזק פיה ([Arab.] *fustuq*: Pistachio [*Pistacia vera* L.]: ... Someone said that he did not find it to be either very harmful or useful for the stomach. But I say that it prevents nausea and an upset stomach, and strengthens the cardia of the stomach). Hebr. התהפכות האיסטו' is not attested in the current dictionaries. The Hebr. term is synonymous with התהפכות הנפש (see next entry). Nathan ha-Me'ati translates Arab. قلب المعدة as הפוך האצטו' (see entry הִפּוּךְ) and Zeraḥyah Ḥen renders it as הפך האצטו'.

• התהפכות הנפש · **upset stomach (surfeit; nausea)**: Arab.[100] تقلب النفس (Gr. ἀσώδης, ἄση, ναυτία; cf. UWS 1:179, 186, 717) · Ibn Sīnā, *K. al-Qānūn* II · trans. Anonymous I, *Sefer*

---

98 והשתטחות (= Ms Paris, BnF, héb. 1136, fol. 84b): והשטטחות Ms.

99 פסתק: פסתוק Ms1.

100 The Arab. term features as قلب النفس (Gr. ἀνατρέπει τὸν στόμαχον) in Maimonides' *Medical Aphorisms* IX.51, 55; the English trans. 'upset the soul' should be corrected as 'upset the stomach' (cf. BMMA 2:70, l. 19; 71, l. 21; BMMG no. 4162).

ha-Qanun (Ms Paris, BnF, héb. 1142, fol. 179[a]): נאנכואה[101] ... מועיל מלחלוחית האצטומ' ומשקיט אסטנסות האיסטו' והתהפכות הנפש ([Arab.] *nānakhwāh*: Bisnaga (toothpick-weed) [*Ammi visnaga* (L.) Lam.]: ... It is beneficial for [excessive] moisture in the stomach, it alleviates nausea, and it [is good for] an upset stomach). Hebr. התהפכות הנפש is a non-attested calque from Arab. تقلب النفس. The Hebr. term is synonymous with התהפכות האיסטו' (see previous entry). Zeraḥyah Ḥen renders Arab. تقلب النفس as התהפך הנפש (see entry [הפך]) and Nathan ha-Me'ati has פוקה (i.e., the regular Hebr. term for Arab. فواق 'hiccups;' cf. BMMG no. 3977).

הֶתֵּךְ · **dissolution; dissolving property**: Arab. تحليل · Ibn Sīnā, *K. al-Qānūn* II · trans. Nathan ha-Me'ati, *Sefer ha-Qanun* (Ms Oxford, Bodleian Libraries, Can. Or. 88, fol. 66[a]): אבנוס ... ואמרו שבו התך לנפח הבטן ([Arab.] *abanūs*: Ebony: ... [Some physicians] say that it dissolves flatulence in the abdomen). Hebr. הֶתֵּךְ is not attested in the current dictionaries. Zeraḥyah Ḥen translates Arab. تحليل as התרה and Anonymous I has התכה. The latter term features, in addition to להתיך, in Nathan's trans. of Maimonides' *Medical Aphorisms* (i.e., *Sefer ha-Peraqim*) (cf. BMMG no. 1051).

הִתְקַשְּׁרוּת · **stiffness**: Arab. تعقّد (Gr. ἀγκύλη; cf. UW 67) · Ibn Sīnā, *K. al-Qānūn* II · trans. Anonymous I, *Sefer ha-Qanun* (Ms Paris, BnF, héb. 1142, fol. 161[a–b]): מקל יהודי ומקל מכי ... מועיל מפשוח העצלים ומהכויצה וקושי העצבים וההתקשרות ([Arab.-Hebr.] *muql*[102] *yehudi* and [Arab.] *muql Makkī*: Judean and Meccan bdellium: ... It is useful in muscle rupture, spasms, hardness, and stiffness of the nerves). In the sense of 'stiffness,' Hebr. הִתְקַשְּׁרוּת is a non-attested calque from Arab. تعقّد. It features in medieval medical literature in the sense of 'coagulation' (for Arab. انعقاد, cf. BCD 77 (NM 2:43)), 'compactness; firmness; solidity' (for Arab. متانة; cf. BCD 77 (NM 4:51)), and 'consolidation; strengthening' (for Arab. تمتين, cf. ibid.). Nathan ha-Me'ati translates Arab. تعقّد as קִשּׁוּר (see entry) and Zeraḥyah Ḥen has עִקּוּד (see entry). A synonym of Arab. تعقّد, i.e., تحجر (featuring as تحجر المفاصل in the *K. al-Qānūn*) is rendered by Anonymous I as התאבנות (הפרקים) (cf. NM 6:59).

הֶתֵּר · **hernia**: Arab. فتق (Gr. ἐντεροκήλη; cf. UW 245) · Ibn Sīnā, *K. al-Qānūn* II · trans. Nathan ha-Me'ati, *Sefer ha-Qanun* (Ms Oxford, Bodleian Libraries, Can. Or. 88, fol. 74[b]):[103] גוז אלסרו ... עושים ממנו תחבשת אל ההתר הנקרא פתק בערבי ([Arab.] *jawz al-sarw*: Nut of the Mediterranean cypress [*Cupressus sempervirens* L.]: ... It is used as a plaster for hernia, called *fatq* in Arab.). Hebr. הֶתֵּר does not feature in this sense in the current dictionaries. Zeraḥyah Ḥen translates Arab. فتق as קְרִיעָה (see entry) and Anonymous I has בקיעות קרום האשך (see entry בְּקִיעָה). A synonym featuring in medieval Hebr. medical literature is Aram. פִּיתְקָא (cf. BCD 220 (NM 1:109; 2:17)).

---

101 נאנכואה: Emend. ed. נאנבואה Ms אמיאוש (= L. Lat./O. Occ./O. Cat./O. Sp. *ameos*) Ms[1].

102 '*muql*': I.e., bdellium, i.e., the gum resin of plants from the *Burseraceae* family, esp. *Commiphora africana* (A.Rich.) Endl. and *Commiphora mukul* (Hook. ex Stocks) Engl.

103 Hebr. הֶתֵּר features in the same sense in the entry מתיחה.

הַתָּרָה · dissolution; dissolving property: Arab. تحليل · Ibn Sīnā, *K. al-Qānūn* II · trans. Zeraḥyah Ḥen, *Sefer ha-Qanun* (Ms Oxford, Bodleian Libaries, Opp. Add. Fol. 12, fol. 202[b]): הַלְיוֹן אֶשְׁפַּארַגִ׳י ... פותח הסתימות בקרבים וכל שכן בכבד והכלייה ויש בו התרה וכל שכן הצורי ([Arab.] *hilyawn*; [i.e., Rom.] ʾeŠəPaʾRaǦY [i.e., Lat. Plur. *asparagi/esparagi* / O. Occ. *asperge/esparge/esperge* / O. Fr. *esparge*; cf. SHS1:108f. (Alef 21)]: Asparagus [*Asparagus officinalis* L.]: ... It opens intestinal obstructions, especially in the liver and kidneys; especially its rocky variety has a dissolving property). Hebr. הַתָּרָה features in BM 1248f. in the sense of 'dissolution,' but is not attested for medieval medical literature. In this genre it features in the sense of 'diarrhea' (cf. BCD 77 (NM 1:55)), 'flux (diarrhea)' (cf. BCD 77 (NM 3:74)), 'relaxation; looseness [of the bowels]' (cf. NM 6:61), and 'labor pains' (cf. NM 6:62). Nathan ha-Meʾati translates Arab. تحليل as הֶתֵּךְ (see entry) and Anonymous I has התכה.

וֶסֶת • הביא הוסת → [בוא].

• עצירת דם הוסת → עֲצִירָה.

• עצירת הוסת → עֲצִירָה.

וֶרֶד • ורד הגפן · **anagyris (bean clover)** [*Anagyris foetida* L.]: Arab. ينبوت (cf. MIG no. 427) · Ibn Sīnā, *K. al-Qānūn* II · trans. Anonymous I, *Sefer ha-Qanun* (Ms Paris, BnF, héb. 1142, fol. 87[a]): ינבות מהות הוא וורד הגפן כמו שאמרו קצת בעלי הידיעה ([Arab.] *yanbūt*: Anagyris (bean clover) [*Anagyris foetida* L.]: What is it? It is [Hebr.] *wered ha-gefen*, as stated by some experts). Hebr. ורד הגפן is not attested in the current dictionaries. Nathan ha-Me'ati and Zeraḥyah Ḥen both translate Arab. ينبوت as ורד הכרם (see next entry).

• ורד הכרם · **anagyris (bean clover)** [*Anagyris foetida* L.]: Arab. ينبوت · Ibn Sīnā, *K. al-Qānūn* II · trans. Zeraḥyah Ḥen, *Sefer ha-Qanun* (Ms Oxford, Bodleian Libraries, Opp. Add. Fol. 12, fol. 221[a]): ינבות המהות הוא ורד הכרם כמו שאמר קצת בעלי הידיעה ([Arab.] *yanbūt*: Anagyris (bean clover) [*Anagyris foetida* L.]: What is it? It is [Hebr.] *wered ha-kerem*, as stated by some experts). Hebr. ורד הכרם is not attested in the current dictionaries. Nathan ha-Me'ati translates Arab. ينبوت as ורד הכרם as well and Anonymous I renders the term as ורד הגפן (see previous entry).

זָהָב • מדבק הזהב → [דבק].
• חבור הזהב → חִבּוּר.
• קצף הזהב → קֶצֶף.

[זהם] • *Part. Puʿal* מְזֻהָם · **sordid:** Lat. *sordidus* · Guy de Chauliac, *Inventarium sive Chirurgia Magna* (cf. CMM 1:233, ll. 34–35) · trans. Anonymous (Ms. Paris, BnF, héb. 1189, fol. 127b): אמנם אם הוא מזוהם וקלפי ירוחץ המקום עם יין ודבש (But if the [ulcer/polyp in the nose] is sordid and crusted the spot should be washed with wine and honey). Hebr. *Part. Puʿal* מְזֻהָם features in BM 1297 and is explained by Ben Yehuda as 'soiled by a fat, fetid substance.'

זהמה[104] • **זוהמת האוזן** · **earwax:** Arab. أوساخ الأذن · Ibn Sīnā, *K. al-Qānūn* II · trans. Anonymous I, *Sefer ha-Qanun* (Ms Paris, BnF, héb. 1142, fols. 86b–87a): ... זראונד[105] מנקה זוהמת האוזן ומחזק השמע עם יושם בה עם דבש ([Arab.] *zarāwand*: Birthwort [*Aristolochia longa* L., *A. rotunda* L., or *A. clematis* L.]: ... It removes earwax and strengthens hearing when it is put into [the ear] with honey). Hebr. זוהמת האוזן is not attested in the current dictionaries. Nathan ha-Me'ati translates Arab. أوساخ الأذن as טנופת האזנים (see entry טִנּוֹפֶת) and Zeraḥyah Ḥen has ליכלוכי האוזן (see entry לִכְלוּךְ).

• **זוהמת השנים** · **dirty teeth (dental sordes):** Arab. أوساخ الأسنان · Ibn Sīnā, *K. al-Qānūn* II · trans. Anonymous I, *Sefer ha-Qanun* (Ms Paris, BnF, héb. 1142, fol. 86b–87a): זראונד[106] ... מועיל מן הבהק וממרק השנים ומועיל מזוהמתם ([Arab.] *zarāwand*: Birthwort [*Aristolochia longa* L., *A. rotunda* L., or *A. clematis* L.]: ... It is useful for *bahaq*[107] (alphos), it cleans the teeth, and it is useful for dirty teeth (dental sordes)). Hebr. זוהמת השנים is not attested in the current dictionaries. Nathan ha-Me'ati translates Arab. أوساخ الأسنان as טנופת השנים (see entry טִנּוֹפֶת) and Zeraḥyah Ḥen has ליכלוך השנים (see entry לִכְלוּךְ).

• **התערב בזוהמה** → [ערב].

[זוב] • *Part Hifʿil* מֵזִיב · **melting:** Arab. مذيب · Ibn Sīnā, *K. al-Qānūn* II · trans. Zeraḥyah Ḥen, *Sefer ha-Qanun* (Ms Oxford. Opp. Add. Fol. 12, fol. 201b): הַיוּפָארִיקוֹן ... מדקדק ומפתח מזיב ומתיר ([Arab.] *hayūfārīqūn* [from Gr. ὑπερικόν]: St. John's wort [*Hypericum* sp.]: ... It has a refining, opening, melting, and dissolving [effect]). Hebr. [זוב],

---

104 זהמה: זֻהֲמָה EM 459 זֻהֲמָה BM 1297 זוּהֲמָה JD 384.
105 זראונד: ארישטולוגיאה Ms1.
106 זראונד: ארישטולוגיאה Ms1.
107 '*bahaq* (alphos)': There are three varieties of the disease called *bahaq* acc. to Ibn al-Jazzār (cf. IJZ 7:108, n. 196): white, black, and dust-colored. The white variety is perhaps identical with *Vitiligo alba*, while the black variety is possibly a sort of melanoderma. Arab. *bahaq* stands for Gr. ἀλφός, cf. UW 97: 'weiße Hautflecken.' Durling, *Dictionary of Medical Terms*, 34, translates the Gr. term as: 'dull-white leprosy.' See entry הבהק הלבן: בַּהַק.

Hif'il הֵזִיב is not attested in a medical context in the current dictionaries. Nathan ha-Me'ati translates Arab. مذيب as *Part. Pi'el* מְמַסְמֵס (see entry מִסְמֵס) and Anonymous I has *Part. Hif'il* מֵמִיס (see entry [מסס]).

זוֹב • *Plur.* **זובים** · **humors**: Arab. خلط · Ibn Sīnā, *K. al-Qānūn* II · trans. Anonymous II, *Sefer ha-Qanun* (Ms Parma, Biblioteca Palatina, Cod. Parm. 3045, fol. 38[a]): פרח נחושת ... משקל ארבע אנילוזיט מתיר זובים עבים ומתיר מים הכרכומייסמ ([Hebr.] *peraḥ neḥoshet* [lit. 'flower of copper']: Copper oxide: ... A dose of four *oboloi*[108] (3 g) dissolves thick humors and [cures] jaundice). Hebr. זוֹב, *Plur.* זובים, features in the current dictionaries in the sense of 'discharge' and 'flux; gonorrhea; prolonged menstruation' in attestations from the Bible and Rabb. literature only (cf. BM 1301). Nathan ha-Me'ati translates Arab. خلط as תַּעֲרוּב (cf. NM 6:221) and Anonymous I has ליחה.

זוהמה → זהמה.

זָחַל • *Part.* **זוֹחֵל** • *Plur.* **זוחלים** • **זוחלי עפר** · **noxious insects; vermin**: Arab هوامّ · Ibn Sīnā, *K. al-Qānūn* II · trans. Anonymous II, *Sefer ha-Qanun* (Ms Parma, Biblioteca Palatina, Cod. Parm. 3045, fol. 30[b]): תרנגלים ותרנגלות ... נבקע התרנגלות על לבו ויושם על מקום[109] הניזק מזוחלי עפר יצליח ותחלפו עליו בכל שעה ושעה ומונעים היזק הארס (Roosters and hens (chickens): ... If one takes the heart from a hen and puts it on the spot of the bite of vermin and replaces it every hour (regularly), it prevents the poison from causing harm). Hebr. זוחלי עפר is attested in the sense of 'snakes,' in the Bible (Deut 32:24; cf. KB 267). Nathan ha-Me'ati translates Arab. هوامّ as שרצים (cf. entry עָרֹב), Zeraḥyah Ḥen has עָרֹב (see ibid.), and Anonymous I has אפעה.

זַיִת • **שמן זית המסתפקים ממנו** → שֶׁמֶן.

זְכוּכִית • **מלח זכוכית** → מֶלַח.

[זמן] • *Part Pu'al* **מְזֻמָּן** · **susceptible**: Arab مستعدّ · al-Rāzī, *K. fī al-Faṣd* · trans. Anonymous, *Ma'amar ba-Haqqazah* (Ms Parma, Biblioteca Palatina, Cod. Parm. 2283,4, fol. 92[b]): ואם יקיזו אותם אשר כזה ענינם יקרה להם רפיון וחולשה וקרירות המזג ויהיו מזומנים אל החליים הקרים עד שא״א להם לשוב אל ענינם הראשון (Whenever one bleeds someone with this condition [i.e., of overfilling], he becomes feeble and weak, his temperament becomes cold, and he becomes susceptible to cold illnesses so that he cannot return to his former condition). Hebr. *Part Pu'al* מְזֻמָּן does not feature in a medical context in the current dictionaries. In medieval philosophical literature it features in the sense of 'prepared, disposed.'[110]

זְמַן • **הזמן הנמצא** · **the current time**: Arab. الوقت الحاضر · al-Rāzī, *K. fī al-Faṣd* · trans. Anonymous, *Ma'amar ba-Haqqazah* (Ms Parma, Biblioteca Palatina, Cod. Parm. 2283,4, fol. 92[b]): אמנם הזמן הנמצא כבר זכרתי אותו למעלה בזה הספר במקום ההקזה כמו

---

108 See entry אנולוס, *Plur.* אנולוסים.

109 מקום הניזק: نهش a.

110 https://peshat.org/display/peshat_lemmas_00044103 (accessed December 6, 2022).

שזכרו חנין בן אסחק (As to the current time, I already mentioned it in this treatise [when treating the topic] of bloodletting, as it was mentioned by Ḥunayn ibn Isḥāq). Hebr. הזמן הנמצא is not attested in the current dictionaries.

זֶמֶר • זמר הרועה · **European water plantain [*Alisma plantago-aquatica* L.]**: Arab مزمار الراعي · Ibn Sīnā, *K. al-Qānūn* II · trans. Zeraḥyah Ḥen, *Sefer ha-Qanun* (Ms Oxford. Opp. Add. Fol. 12, fol. 238[a]): מזמאר הרועה זמר הרועה ([Arab.-Hebr.] *mizmār ha-ro'eh*; [i.e., Hebr.] *zemer ha-ro'eh*). Hebr. זמר הרועה is a non-attested calque from Arab. مزمار الراعي. Nathan ha-Me'ati transcribes the Arab. term as מזמאר אלראע only and Anonymous I renders it as מזמר הרועה (see entry מִזְמֹר).

זָנָב • זנב הסוס · **[lit. 'horsetail']; field/common horsetail [*Equisetum arvense* L.]**: Arab. ذنب الخيل (cf. MIG no. 501) · *Glossary* (Ms Moscow, Russian State Library, Guenzburg 573, fol. 151[a]): דנב אלכיל כלומ' זנב הסוס ([Arab.] *dhanab al-khayl*; i.e., [Hebr.] *zenav ha-sus*). Hebr. זנב הסוס features in BM 1366 in the sense of 'Equisetum, shave-grass' in an attestation from the *Sefer Asaph ha-Rofe*. The term is also attested in Shem Tov ben Isaac's *Sefer Almansur* (cf. BMZ 28f. (Dalet 10)).

• זנב העין · **the inner canthus (angle) of the eye**: Arab. مأق · Ibn Sīnā, *K. al-Qānūn* II · trans. Nathan ha-Me'ati, *Sefer ha-Qanun* (Ms Oxford, Bodleian Libraries, Can. Or. 88, fol. 117[b]): צבר ... יועיל מנגעי העין ומורסותיה ומכאוביה הנולדים מחדוד זנב העין ([Arab.] *ṣabir*: Aloe [*Aloe vera* L.]: ... It is useful for ocular ulcers, swellings, pain, and irritation of the inner canthus (angle) of the eye). Hebr. זנב העין is not attested in the current dictionaries. The term, actually meaning 'the *outer* corner of the eye,' features in BCD 85 (NM 1:90) (for Arab. ذنب العين in an attestation from Shem Tov ben Isaac's *Sefer ha-Shimmush* XXX.1.13). In addition to זנב העין, Nathan translates Arab. مأق as זנב העין הגדול (see next entry). Zeraḥyah Ḥen translates Arab. مأق as מדמע (see entry) and Anonymous I renders the Arab. term as קצות העין (cf. Nathan's use of the term קצוות העין for Arab. *Dual* مأقان in his *Sefer ha-Qanun* I (cf. BCD 248 (NM 4:188)).

• זנב העין הגדול · **the inner canthus (angle) of the eye**: Arab. مأق · Ibn Sīnā, *K. al-Qānūn* II · trans. Nathan ha-Me'ati, *Sefer ha-Qanun* (Ms Oxford, Bodleian Libraries, Can. Or. 88, fol. 116[a]): פגל הוא צנון ... הוא מזיק אל העין אלא שהוא ממרק אותה כשמטיפים ממנו בה ויסיר הסמנים אשר בזנב[111] העין הגדול ובערבי אמאק ([Arab.] *fujl*; i.e., [Hebr.] *ṣenon*: Radish [*Raphanus sativus* L.]: ... It is harmful for the eye, but dripping its juice into [the eye] cleanses it and removes the spots under the inner canthus of the eye). Hebr. זנב העין הגדול, which is a synonym for זנב העין (see previous entry), actually meaning 'the *outer* corner of the eye' (cf. BCD 85 (NM 1:90)), is not attested in the current dictionaries. Arab. *Dual* مأقان is translated by Nathan as s קצוות העין (cf. BCD 248 (NM 4:188)). Zeraḥyah Ḥen translates Arab. مأق as *Part.* דּוֹמֵעַ (see entry) and Anonymous I renders the Arab. term as קצה העין הנק' אמאק.

111 בזנב: Emend. ed. בעין זנב Ms.

זַנְגָּבִיל • זנגביל הכלבים · [lit. 'ginger of the dogs']; **marshpepper knotweed [*Persicaria hydropiper* (L.) Delabre]**: Arab. زنجبيل الكلب (cf. IBF no. 1126) · Ibn Sīnā, *K. al-Qānūn* II · trans. Zeraḥyah Ḥen, *Sefer ha-Qanun* (Ms Oxford, Bodleian Libaries, Opp. Add. Fol. 12, fol. 204[b]): זַנְגְּבִיל הכלבים המהות הוא עשב ידוע ([Hebr.] *zangavil ha-kelavim* [lit. 'ginger of the dogs']: Marshpepper knotweed [*Persicaria hydropiper* (L.) Delabre]: What is it? It is a well-known herb). In the sense of 'marshpepper knotweed,' Hebr. זנגביל הכלבים is a non-attested calque from Arab. زنجبيل الكلب and features in Anonymus I's trans. as זנגביל אלכלאב כלומ׳ זנגביל הכלבים ([Arab.] *zanjabīl al-kalb*; i.e., [Hebr.] *zangavil ha-kelavim*). The latter term features almost exactly so in *Shinnui ha-Shemot ha-Niqra'im Synonimi*, Zayin 3 (Ms Florence, Biblioteca Medicea Laurenziana, Or. 17, fol. 77[a]): זנגביל אלכלב כלומ׳ זנגביל הכלבים. Nathan ha-Me'ati transcribes Arab. زنجبيل الكلب as זנגביל אלכלאב only.

זֵעָה · **gum**: Arab. صمغ · Ibn Sīnā, *K. al-Qānūn* II · trans. Anonymous II, *Sefer ha-Qanun* (Ms Parma, Biblioteca Palatina, Cod. Parm. 3045, fol. 26[b]): אפופונקו ... וחותכין שרשו ומוציאין ממנו הזיעה שלו כשיראה[112] ([Rom.] ʾPWPWNQW: Opopanax [i.e., the resin of the sweet myrrh [*Opopanax chironius* W.D.J. Koch]]: ... The gum is taken out by incising its root after the[113] first stem appears). In the sense of 'gum,' Hebr. זֵעָה features in BM 1371 in an attestation from *Sefer Asaph ha-Rofe*: זיעת הבוטנים היא תרבינטינא (The gum (resin) from pine trees is turpentine). Nathan ha-Me'ati and Anonymous I both translate Arab. صمغ as שרף and Zeraḥyah Ḥen has Aram. גּוּמָא (see entry).

זְעִיפָה · **wrinkles**: Arab. تغضّن · Ibn Sīnā, *K. al-Qānūn* II · trans. Zeraḥyah Ḥen, *Sefer ha-Qanun* (Ms Oxford, Bodleian Libaries, Opp. Add. Fol. 12, fol. 200[a–b]): דהן ... ושורש השושן והשעוה הניתכת יועיל מן זעיפת הפנים והספחת והרושם ודומיהם ([Arab.] *duhn*: Oil: ... Root of the blue lily and melted wax is beneficial for facial wrinkles, freckles and other spots and the like). Hebr. זְעִיפָה is only attested as a modern term in EM 480 in the sense of 'anger.' The term was possibly coined on the basis of Dan 1:10: אֲשֶׁר לָמָּה יִרְאֶה אֶת-פְּנֵיכֶם זֹעֲפִים, מִן-הַיְלָדִים אֲשֶׁר כְּגִילְכֶם (For why should he see your faces sad in comparison with the youths that are of your own age?). Nathan ha-Me'ati and Anonymous I both translate Arab. تغضّن as קמטים.

זָקָן · **chin**: Arab. ذقن · al-Rāzī, *K. fī al-Faṣd* · trans. Anonymous, *Ma'amar ba-Haqqazah* (Ms Parma, Biblioteca Palatina, Cod. Parm. 2283,4, fol. 93[b]): וב׳ גידים בתוך הזקן לפנים ואם יגביה הלשון יראה הא׳ אל הימין והאחר אל השמאל (Two veins inside the chin; if the tongue is lifted, you see one on the right and one on the left). In the sense of 'chin,' Hebr. זָקָן features in BCD 85 (NM 4:59) in an attestation from Nathan ha-Me'ati's trans. of Ibn Sīnā's *K. al-Qānūn* (i.e., *Sefer ha-Qanun*) I.

---

112 כשיראה: في أول ظهور الساق a.

113 'the first stem': Trans. acc. to a.

זָר • אש זר → אֵשׁ.
זְרוֹעַ • אמת הזרוע → אַמָּה.
• יתרי הזרוע → יֶתֶר.
זֶרַע • הגרת הזרע → הֲגָרָה.

ח

[חבא] • *Part. Nif'al* נֶחְבָּא • הלחויות הנחבאות תחת העור → לַחוּת.

חִבּוּר • חבור הזהב · **chrysocolla**: Arab. لحام الذهب (cf. MIG no. 503) · Ibn Sīnā, *K. al-Qānūn* II · trans. Nathan ha-Me'ati, *Sefer ha-Qanun* (Ms Oxford, Bodleian Libraries, Can. Or. 88, fol. 126[a]): תנכאר המהות יש ממנו יוצא מהמחצב וממנו שעושים אותו ונק' חבור הזהב ובערבי לחאם אלדהב ([Arab.] *tinkār*: Salt, borax, salmiac, chrysocolla (cf. KM 345–349): What is it? There is [a kind] that is a mineral and another [kind] that is artificial. [In Hebr.] it is called *ḥibbur ha-zahav* and in Arab. *liḥām al-dhahab*). Hebr. חבור הזהב is not attested in the current dictionaries. Zeraḥyah Ḥen translates Arab. لحام الذهب as מדבק הזהב (see entry [דבק]) and Anonymous I has מתג(?) הזהב. The Arab. synonym لصاق الذهب is translated by Nathan as מדביק הזהב (cf. BCD 54 (NM 2:57) for an attestation from his trans. of Maimonides' *Medical Aphorisms* (i.e., *Sefer ha-Peraqim*) XXIII.101 (cf. BMMN 232, l. 1; BMMG no. 4604).

חֲבָטָה • חבטת העין · **a throbbing sensation in the eyes**: Arab. ضربان العين · Ibn Sīnā, *K. al-Qānūn* II · trans. Zeraḥyah Ḥen, *Sefer ha-Qanun* (Ms Oxford, Bodleian Libaries, Opp. Add. Fol. 12, fol. 251[a]): סַדֶאבְּ ... יחדד הראות וכל שכן מיצו עם מיץ השומר והדבש לכחול בו וגם לאכלו וגם יחובש בו עם הקלי על חבטת העין ([Arab.] *sadhāb*: Common rue [*Ruta graveolens* L.]: ... It strengthens the eyesight especially when its juice is used with fennel juice and honey for an eye salve, or when it is taken orally. Moreover it is plastered with mush[114] for a throbbing sensation in the eyes). Hebr. חבטת העין is not attested in the current dictionaries. Hebr. חֲבָטָה on its own features in Rabb. literature in the sense of 'beating; striking' (cf. BM 1420). Nathan ha-Me'ati and Anonymous I both render Arab. ضربان العين as דפיקת העין (see entry דְּפִיקָה).

[חבל] • *Part. Pi'el* מְחַבֵּל • הרפואה המחבלת → רְפוּאָה.

חֶבֶל • *Plur.* חבלים · **nerves**: Arab. عصب Ibn Sīnā, *K. al-Qānūn* II · trans. Anonymous II, *Sefer ha-Qanun* (Ms Parma, Biblioteca Palatina, Cod. Parm. 3045, fol. 30[a]): דַרְסִיסִיאַם ... יצליח לרכוך החבלים ([Arab.] *dārshīsha'ān*: Broom [*Genista acanthoclada* DC. or *Cytisus spinosus* Lam.] (cf. MIG no. 223): ... It is beneficial for relaxation (slackening) of the nerves). Hebr. חֶבֶל is not attested as an anat. term in the current dictionaries (cf. BM 1423f.) Nathan ha-Me'ati, Zeraḥyah Ḥen, and Anonymous I translate Arab. عصب as עצבים.

חֲבָלָה · **ulceration**: Arab. تقريح · Ibn Sīnā, *K. al-Qānūn* II · trans. Zeraḥyah Ḥen, *Sefer ha-Qanun* (Ms Oxford, Bodleian Libaries, Opp. Add. Fol. 12, fol. 160[a]): והאוכלת היא שטבעה להפליג בהתרתו וחבלתו שתפחות מעצם הבשר כמו הזינגאר (A corrosive [drug] is—by its nature—[a drug] with strong solvent and ulcerative properties, which reduce the

114 Cf. WCD 517, s.v. *sawīq*: 'a kind of mush made of wheat or barley (also with sugar and dates);' see also entry קָלִי.

substance of the flesh [of the organ]; [an example of such a drug is verdigris). Hebr. חֲבָלָה is not attested in this sense in the current dictionaries. As 'ulcer' or 'wound' it is attested in medieval Hebr. medical literature (cf. BCD 88 (NM 1:146)). Nathan ha-Me'ati translates Arab. تقريح as נְגוּעַ (see entry) and Anonymous I has הַשְׁחָנָה (see entry).

[חבר] • *Piʿel* חִבֵּר · **to add**: Lat. *addo* · Guy de Chauliac, *Inventarium sive Chirurgia Magna* (cf. CMM 1:236, ll. 18–19) · trans. Anonymous (Ms Paris, BnF, héb. 1189, fol. 129[a]): אמנם ביותר גדולים אני מחבר קלקנטוס ויין עפיץ (But in those who are older [than children], I add chalcanthum and astringent wine). In the sense of 'to add,' Hebr. *Piʿel* חִבֵּר features in NM 5:71 (also for Lat. *addo*) in an earlier attestation from Do'eg ha-Edomi's trans. of Constantinus Africanus' *Viaticum* (i.e., *Sefer Ya'ir Netiv*) III.6.

• *Part. Hitpaʿel f.* מִתְחַבֶּרֶת · **conjunctiva**: Lat. *coniunctiva* · Guy de Chauliac, *Inventarium sive Chirurgia Magna* (cf. CMM 1:229, ll. 2–3) · trans. Anonymous (Ms Paris, BnF, héb. 1189, fol. 125[a]): וכשיפתח העין אם היה במתחברת יראה נקודה אדומה (When the eye is opened and [the ulcer] is in the coniunctiva then a red spot can be seen). In the sense of 'conjunctiva,' Hebr. *Part. Hitpaʿel f.* מִתְחַבֶּרֶת features in NM 6:70 in an attestation from Abraham Avigdor's trans. of Gerard de Solo's *Practica super nono Almansoris* (i.e., *Ha-Ma'amar ha-Teshiʿi le-Sefer ha-Mansuri le-Razi*).

חָבַשׁ • **חבש באף** · **to drip (pour) a medicine into the nose**: Arab. سعط في الأنف · Ibn Sīnā, *K. al-Qānūn* II · trans. Zeraḥyah Ḥen, *Sefer ha-Qanun* (Ms Oxford, Bodleian Libaries, Opp. Add. Fol. 12, fol. 251[a]): סַדַאבְּ רוּטאָ ... יעביר ריח השומים והבצלים ויחבוש בו עם החומץ באף להגרת הדם ממנו ויעצרנו ([Arab.] *sadhāb*; [i.e., Lat.] RWuṬ'a [i.e., *ruta*]: Common rue [*Ruta graveolens* L.]: ... It removes the smell of garlic and onion. Dripping it into the nose with vinegar stops a nosebleed). Hebr. חבש באף does not feature in the current dictionaries. The Arab. synonym سعط is translated by Zeraḥyah as עשה שעיטה and as עשה אישפונגי באף (for both terms, see entry עָשָׂה), and שָׁעַט (see entry). Nathan ha-Me'ati translates Arab. سعط في الأنف as עשה תחבשת בחוטם (see also entry עָשָׂה) and Anonymous I has חבש באף, just like Zeraḥyah.

חֹבֶשׁ · I. **plaster; poultice**: Arab. ضماد · Ibn Sīnā, *K. al-Qānūn* II · trans. Zeraḥyah Ḥen, *Sefer ha-Qanun* (Ms Oxford, Bodleian Libaries, Opp. Add. Fol. 12, fol. 216[a]): חַבּ אַלְצָנַוְבַּר גרעִינֵי פִּינְיִי ... וימנעו מנגעי השלפוחית ומן החול וירבו השתן ויועיל החובש ממנו עם האינשינצו ([Arab.] *ḥabb al-ṣanawbar*; i.e., [Hebr.-Lat./Rom.] *garʿinei* PiYNəYiY: Pine nuts [*Pinus* L.]: ... They prevent the formation of ulcers and stones in the bladder, and increase the urine; their plaster with absinth wormwood is also beneficial). In the sense of 'plaster; poultice,' Hebr. חֹבֶשׁ features in NM 5:71 in the sense of 'plaster, poultice' in attestations from Abraham ben Isaac's trans. Ibn al-Jazzār's *Zād al-musāfir* (i.e., *Sefer Ṣedah la-Oreḥim*) and an adaptation thereof. Nathan ha-Me'ati and Anonymous I both render Arab. ضماد as תחבשת.

· II. **fomentation; hot compress**: Arab. كماد (Gr. πυρία; cf. UW 575f.; WKAS 1:354, s.v. *kimāda*) · Ibn Sīnā, *K. al-Qānūn* II · trans. Zeraḥyah Ḥen, *Sefer ha-Qanun* (Ms

Oxford, Bodleian Libaries, Opp. Add. Fol. 12, fol. 195[b]): ג׳אוֹרס דוחן ... יש בו קיבוץ וניגוב בלא נשיכה והוא חובש מדכך הכאב ([Arab.] *jāwars*; [i.e., Hebr.] *doḥan*: Millet [*Panicum miliaceum* L.]: ... It is astringent and drying without irritation. Its use as a fomentation relieves pain). Anonymous I renders Arab. كماد as הנחה חמה (cf. BCD 68 (NM 2:39f.; corr. 4:229) for an attestation from Nathan ha-Me'ati's trans. of Maimonides' *Medical Aphorisms* (i.e., *Sefer ha-Peraqim*) XXIII.33 (cf. BMMN 222, l. 15)) and Anonymous II has הֶבֶל (see entry).

חָגָב · **locust**: Arab. جراد (cf. DT 222 (II.39)) · Ibn Sīnā, *K. al-Qānūn* II · trans. Anonymous I, *Sefer ha-Qanun* (Ms Paris, BnF, héb. 1142, fol. 75[a]): גראד הוא חגב ([Arab. *jarād*; i.e., [Hebr.] *ḥagav*). Hebr. חָגָב does not feature in a medical context in the current dictionaries (cf. BM 1441; EM 501). Nathan ha-Me'ati translates Arab. جراد as *Plur.* חגבים and Zeraḥyah Ḥen has אַרְבֶּה (see entry).

• *Plur.* **חגבים** • **רגלי החגבים** → רֶגֶל.

חִדּוּשׁ • **חדוש הנפש** · **anxiety**: Arab. حديث النفس (cf. D 1:259: 'crainte, inquiétude, mélancolie') · Ibn al-Jazzār, *Zād al-musāfir wa-qūt al-ḥādir* · trans. Moses ibn Tibbon, *Sefer Ṣedat ha-Derakhim* III.14: תאר אבק מצליח ממהר בתועלת הדפיקה והגעש[115] וחדוש הנפש והחום הקיים[116] בלב (Recipe of a powder quickly successful in curing cardialgia, trepidation,[117] anxiety, and the heat firmly[118] settled in the heart). In the sense of 'anxiety,' Hebr. חדוש הנפש is a non-attested calque from Arab. حديث النفس.

חוֹבֵשׁ → חָבַשׁ.

חוּט • *Plur.* **חוטים** · **lines**: Arab. خطوط · Ibn Sīnā, *K. al-Qānūn* II · trans. Zeraḥyah Ḥen, *Sefer ha-Qanun* (Ms Oxford, Bodleian Libaries, Opp. Add. Fol. 12, fol. 217[b]): חג׳ר אליהודי המהות הוא כמו האגוז הקטון נוטה לאורך מעט חוטים בקצה וחוטים אחרים באלכסונה וזה חותך בזה ([Arab.] *ḥajar al-Yahūdī*: Jews' stone:[119] What is it? It resembles a small acorn; it is somewhat elongated; [it has] lines coming from [different] ends and diagonal lines that intersect with them). Hebr. חוט, *Plur.* חוטים, does not feature in this sense in the current dictionaries (cf. JD 431: 'thread, cord, strap, sinew;' BM 1461f.: 'thread'). Nathan ha-Me'ati and Anonymous I both render Arab. خطوط as קוים.

• **כרך מחוטים** → כָּרַךְ.

חוֹטֶם • **עשה תחבשת בחוטם** → עָשָׂה.

חוֹל • **פוצץ החול** → [פצץ].

---

115 והגעש: والرجف a.

116 הקיים: المستحكم a.

117 'trepidation': Trans. acc. to a.

118 'firmly settled': Trans. acc. to a.

119 Cf. MIG no. 363: 'The Jews' stone (Judaic stone) (Gr. Ἰουδαϊκὸς λίθος) of the ancients is said to be a fossil, namely the petrified remains of a variety of 'sea urchin' (Cidaris glandaria Fraas; Cidaridae) found especially in Judaea.'

חוּלְדָּה · **weasel:** Arab. ابن عرس · Ibn Sīnā, *K. al-Qānūn* II · trans. Anonymous II, *Sefer ha-Qanun* (Ms Parma, Biblioteca Palatina, Cod. Parm. 3045, fol. 29[a]): רוקא ... אם יאכל וישתה אחריו יין טוב[120] וריחני הוא כעין צרי לנשיכת חולדה ([Lat.] RWQ' [i.e., (*e*)*ruca*]: Rocket [*Eruca sativa* Mill.]: ... If one eats it and then drinks some fragrant wine, it acts as an antidote for the bite of a weasel). Hebr. חוּלְדָּה is attested in Rabb. literature in the sense of 1) 'mole,' 2) 'weasel' (cf. JD 433). Nathan ha-Me'ati renders Arab. ابن عرس as החיה הנקרא בן ערס, Zeraḥyah Ḥen has בעל חיים הנקרא בן ערוס, and Anonymous I transcribes the Arab. term as אבן ערס only. In his trans. of Maimonides' *Medical Aphorisms* (i.e., *Sefer ha-Peraqim*) XXI.54, Nathan renders the Arab. term as אבן ערס הוא עכבר פרעה (cf. BCD 201 (NM 2:71), s.v. עַכְבַּר; BMMN 202, l. 17).

חוּלִי¹ → חֹלִי.

חוּלִי² · **sandy:** Arab. رملي · Ibn Sīnā, *K. al-Qānūn* II · trans. Anonymous I, *Sefer ha-Qanun* (Ms Paris, BnF, héb. 1142, fol. 195[a]): סמך הוא דג ... ואמנם כפי מעון הדגים הנה אותו אשר ישכון המקומות הסלעיים טוב ואחריו החוליים ([Arab.] *samak*; i.e., [Hebr.] *dag*: Fish: ... According to the place where they live: Fish that live in rocky water [are the best]; then fish that live in sandy water). Hebr. חוּלִי is a non-attested Adj. coined from חול 'sand.' Zeraḥyah Ḥen translates Arab. رملي as חוּלִי, just like Anonymous I and Nathan ha-Me'ati translates the Arab. term الأماكن الرملية as חול.

חוּלְיָה → חֻלְיָה.

חוּלְשָׁה → חֻלְשָׁה.

חוּמֶט → חֹמֶט.

חוּמְצָה → חֻמְצָה.

חוּמֶר → חֹמֶר.

חוּרְפָּה → חֻרְפָּה.

חוּשׁ • **הסם המרדים החוש** → סַם.

חוֹתֵם (*Part.*) → חָתַם.

חָזֶה • **מרחב החזה** → מֶרְחָב.

חֲזִיר • **בעל חזיר** → בַּעַל.

[חזק] • *Pi'el* חִזֵּק · **to contain:** Lat. *contineo* · Guy de Chauliac, *Inventarium sive Chirurgia Magna* (cf. CMM 1:413, l. 33) · trans. Anonymous (Ms Paris, BnF, héb. 1189, fol. 124[a]): הנה הפנים אחר שהם מחזקים אברים רבים ומתחלפים ויש להם מינים ברקותיהם מהנגעים (Since the face contains many different organs and [different] kinds of ulcers in the cheeks). Hebr. *Pi'el* חִזֵּק does not feature in the sense of 'to contain' in the current dictionaries.

- *Part. Pi'el* מְחַזֵּק • **הסם המחזק** → סַם.
- **הרפואה המחזקת** → רְפוּאָה.
- *Part. Hif'il* מַחְזִיק • **האברים המחזיקים** → אֵבָר.

---

120 טוב וריחני: ريحاني a.

חֲזָרָה • חזרת ההקזה · **epaphairesis (repeated evacuation of blood)**: Arab. تثنية (Gr. ἐπαφαίρεσις; cf. LSG 612) · al-Rāzī, *K. fī al-Faṣd* · trans. Anonymous, *Ma'amar ba-Haqqazah* (Ms Parma, Biblioteca Palatina, Cod. Parm. 2283,4, fol. 95[a]): השער הט' בחזרת ההקזה הנק' אלתתניה (Ch. 9: On epaphairesis (repeated evacuation of blood), called [in Arab.] *al-tathnīyah*). Hebr. חזרת ההקזה is not attested in the current dictionaries.

חַי • כסף חי → כֶּסֶף.

[חיה] • *Pi'el* חִיָּה · **to heal; to promote cicatrization**: Arab. أدمل (Gr. ἐπουλόω, ἰάομαι; κολλάω; cf. UW 264, 303f., 354f.) · Ibn Sīnā, *K. al-Qānūn* II · trans. Zeraḥyah Ḥen, *Sefer ha-Qanun* (Ms Oxford, Bodleian Libaries, Opp. Add. Fol. 12, fol. 217[b]): נחשת ... יחייה הנגעים הפירדולינט המתפשטים וימנעם מן ההתפשט ויאכל הבשר הנוסף והרחוץ יחייה החבלות (Copper: ... It heals malignant spreading ulcers and prevents their further expansion. It corrodes the excessive flesh. Washed [copper] heals the wounds). Hebr. *Pi'el* חִיָּה does not feature in this sense in the current dictionaries. Nathan ha-Me'ati translates Arab. أدمل as סָגַר (see entry) and Anonymous I has *Hif'il* הִבְרִיא. Moses ibn Tibbon translates Arab. أدمل as סָתַם in his trans. of Ibn al-Jazzār's *Zād al-musāfir* (i.e., *Sefer Ṣedat ha-Derakhim*) III.8 (cf. NM 5:142). The synonymous Arab. term ختم is translated as חָתַם by both Zeraḥyah and Nathan in their translation of Maimonides' *Medical Aphorisms* (i.e., *Sefer ha-Peraqim*) XV.56 (cf. BMMZ 162, l. 22; BMMN 163, l. 10; BMMG no. 1288).

• *Part. Pi'el* מְחַיֶּה • הרפואה המחיה → רְפוּאָה.

חַיּוּת · **healing over; forming a scar; cicatrization**: Arab. إدمال · Ibn Sīnā, *K. al-Qānūn* II · trans. Zeraḥyah Ḥen, *Sefer ha-Qanun* (Ms Oxford, Bodleian Libaries, Opp. Add. Fol. 12, fol. 161[a]): והמלכלכת הנגעים היא הרפואה הלחה אשר תתערב עם לחות הנגעים וישימה הרבה וימנע הניגוב והחיות (A [drug] that infects (contaminates) a wound is a moist drug whose moisture mixes with that of the wound and increases it and [thus] prevents the wound from drying and from forming a scar (cicatrization)). Hebr. חַיּוּת does not feature in this sense in the current dictionaries. Anonymous I renders Arab. إدمال as הַבְרָאָה (see entry).

חִילּוּף → חִלּוּף.

חִכּוּךְ · **twisting; cramp; spasm**: Arab. تشبّك (cf. D 722) · Ibn Sīnā, *K. al-Qānūn* II · trans. Nathan ha-Me'ati, *Sefer ha-Qanun* (Ms Oxford, Bodleian Libraries, Can. Or. 88, fol. 98[a]): לבני ... יחזק האיברים ויועיל לחכוך הפרקים כששותין אותו או אם מושחין בו ומערבין אותו ויכנס במשיחות העיפות ([Arab.] *lubnā*: Styrax: ... It strengthens the organs and is useful in twisting of joints both when taken orally or applied as a salve. It is mixed in oils [used] in fatigue). Hebr. חִכּוּךְ does not feature in this sense in the current dictionaries. Zeraḥyah Ḥen translates Arab. تشبّك as שִׁבּוּךְ (see entry) and Anonymous I has הִסְתַּבְּכוּת (cf. BCD 68 (NM 4:45) for an attestation from Shem Tov ben Isaac's *Sefer ha-Shimmush* XXVII).

[חכך] • *Part Pi'el* מְחַכֵּךְ • הסם המחכך → סַם.

• הרפואה המחככת → רְפוּאָה.

חָכְמָה • *Plur.* **חכמות** • **החכמות הדקות** · **the sciences that require concentration; the exacting sciences:**[121] Arab. العلوم الدقيقة · al-Rāzī, *K. fī al-Faṣd* · trans. Anonymous, *Ma'amar ba-Haqqazah* (Ms Parma, Biblioteca Palatina, Cod. Parm. 2283,4, fol. 92[a]): ואמנם האומנות מי שיהיה רופא[122] ברב העמל והמשגל והתנועה והיגיעה והאנחות והתעורה ורוב המחשבות בחכמות הדקות צריך שימעט[123] הדם וההפך בהפך (As to the occupation, when someone is a physician,[124] [or someone has] a lot of fatigue, coitus, movement, exertion, worries, insomnia and thought on the sciences that require concentration (the exacting sciences), one should reduce the[125] evacuation of blood, and the opposite in the opposite case).

חֶלְאָה · **foam:** Arab. زبد · Ibn Sīnā, *K. al-Qānūn* II · trans. Nathan ha-Me'ati, *Sefer ha-Qanun* (Ms Oxford, Bodleian Libraries, Can. Or. 88, fol. 88[a]): חגר אלקמר כלומ' אבן הלבנה קוראין אותו בזאק אלקמר כלו' רוק הלבנה וקוראין אותו חלאת הלבונה כלומ' זבד אלקמר ([Arab.] *ḥajar al-qamar*; i.e., [Hebr.] *even ha-levanah*: Moonstone. It is called [in Arab.] *buzāq al-qamar*; i.e., 'spittle of the moon,' and it is called 'foam of the moon,' i.e., [Arab.] *zabad al-qamar*). In the sense of 'foam,' Hebr. חֶלְאָה features (for Arab. رغوة) in BCD 94 (NM 4:66) in an attestation from Shem Tov ben Isaac's *Sefer ha-Shimmush* XXVII. Zeraḥyah Ḥen and Anonymous I both render Arab. زبد as קצף.

חָלָב · **latex (milky liquid from plants):** Pers. شير ديودار (cf. D 1:810: 'le suc laiteux du pin indien') · Ibn Sīnā, *K. al-Qānūn* II · trans. Zeraḥyah Ḥen, *Sefer ha-Qanun* (Ms Oxford, Bodleian Libaries, Opp. Add. Fol. 12, fols. 198[b]–199[a]): דִּיוּדָאר ... יש[126] בו חדוד מועט ושיר דיודאר הוא החלב שלו ([Arab.] *diyūdār*: Deodar cedar (or Himalayan cedar) [*Cedrus deodara* (Roxb. ex Lamb.) G.Don] (cf. MIG no. 235): ... The latex of deodar cedar is somewhat pungent). Hebr. חָלָב is not attested in this sense in the current dictionaries. Nathan ha-Me'ati and Anonymous I both render Pers. شير ديودار as חָלָב as well.

• **אבן החלב** → אֶבֶן.

• **המיץ היוצא מן החלב** → מִיץ.

חֲלוּדָה • **בעל חלודה** → בַּעַל.

חֲלוֹם • **החלום בראית קרי** · **nocturnal pollution; emission of sperm:** Arab. احتلام · Ibn Sīnā, *K. al-Qānūn* II · trans. Zeraḥyah Ḥen, *Sefer ha-Qanun* (Ms Oxford, Bodleian Libaries, Opp. Add. Fol. 12, fol. 187[v]: בַּנְגַנְגּ׳סְת אַיְנוּ קַשְׁטוֹ ... וכשיפרשנו תחת גבו ימנע החלום בראית קרי ([Arab.] *banjankusht*; [i.e., Rom.] 'aYəNWu QaŠəṬW [from Lat. *agnus castus*]: Chaste tree [*Vitex agnus-castus* L.]: ... When one spreads [its branches] under

---

121 I thank Tzvi Langermann for this translation.
122 רופא: مباطشا a.
123 שימעט הדם: إخراج الدم a.
124 'physician': 'hard-working' a.
125 'the evacuation of blood': Trans. acc. to a.
126 יש בו חדוד מועט ושיר דיודאר הוא החלב שלו: وشير ديودار وهو لبنه حار حريف a.

one's back, it prevents nocturnal pollution). Hebr. החלום בראית קרי is not attested in the current dicitonaries. Nathan ha-Me'ati and Anonymous I both render Arab. احتلام as קרי. In the anonymous trans. of al-Rāzī's *K. fī al-Faṣd* (i.e., *Ma'amar ba-Haqqazah*), Arab. احتلام is translated as הגרת הזרע (see entry הֲגָרָה). For other synonyms see ibid.

חִלּוּף · **diarrhea**: Arab. اختلاف · Ibn Sīnā, *K. al-Qānūn* II · trans. Zeraḥyah Ḥen, *Sefer ha-Qanun* (Ms Oxford, Bodleian Libaries, Opp. Add. Fol. 12, fol. 245[a]): נַשֵׂא אָמִידוֹ ... האמידו לבדו עם העדשים יעצור הטבע וימנע חילוף המרירות ([Arab.] *nashā*; [i.e., Rom.] 'aMiYDWo [i.e., M. Lat. *amido* / O. Occ. *amido(n)* / O. Cat. *amidó* [from Lat. *amidum*]; cf. SHS 1:217 (Ḥet 14)]: Starch: ... [Its application] alone [or] with lentils stops constipation and prevents bilious diarrhea). In the sense of 'diarrhea,' Hebr. חִלּוּף is a non-attested semantic borrowing from Arab. اختلاف. Nathan ha-Me'ati and Anonymous I both render the Arab. term as שִׁלְשׁוּל. Synonymous terms featuring in medieval medical literature are בִּשּׁוּל (cf. NM 6:30), הגרת הבטן (cf. BCD 62 (NM 3:55f.)), הַזָּלָה (cf. BCD 64 (NM 3:60)), התרת הבטן (BCD 77 (NM 1:143)), חֲלָקוּת/חַלְקוּת (cf. NM 6:76f.), and שִׁלּוּחַ (cf. NM 6:212).

• **חלוּף הדם** · **bloody diarrhea (dysentery)**: Arab. اختلاف الدم · Ibn Sīnā, *K. al-Qānūn* II · trans. Nathan ha-Me'ati, *Sefer ha-Qanun* (Ms Oxford, Bodleian Libraries, Can. Or. 88, fols. 88[b]–89[a]): טראתית ... הוא מעכב ועוצר יציאת[127] הדם וחלוף הדם והעקיצה[128] אם שותין בחלב עזין נבושל ([Arab.] *ṭarāthīth*: Maltese fungus [*Cynomorium coccineum* L.]: ... It constipates and stops the flow of menstrual blood, bloody diarrhea (dysentery), and post-coital[129] bleeding (?)). Hebr. חלוף הדם is not attested in the current dictionaries. Anonymous I renders Arab. اختلاف الدم as שלשול הדם (cf. BCD 276 (NM 3:228) for an attestation from Moses ibn Tibbon's trans. of Maimonides' *Commentary on Hippocrates' Aphorisms* (i.e., *Perush Aphorismi shel Apuqraṭ*) III.11 (cf. BMCH 1:352, l. 2). For more synonymous Hebr. terms, cf. NM 6:163, s.v. עִצּוּר.

חֹלִי · **affliction; defect**: Arab. آفة · Ibn Sīnā, *K. al-Qānūn* II · trans. Zeraḥyah Ḥen, *Sefer ha-Qanun* (Ms Oxford, Bodleian Libaries, Opp. Add. Fol. 12, fol. 259[a]): פוּאַת הצבעים ... ישתה אותה עם מי הקראטין ויועיל מגיד הנשה והפלג אשר עם חולי בהרגשה ([Arab.-Hebr.] *fuwwat ha-ṣabba'im* [lit. 'dyers' madder']: Common madder [*Rubia tinctorum* L.]: ... When taken with honey water (*melikraton*), it is beneficial for sciatica and hemiplegia with a sensory defect). Hebr. חלי does not feature in this sense in the current dic-

---

127 יציאת הדם: نزف الدم a.

128 והעקיצה: والاعراس a.

129 'post-coital bleeding (?)': The meaning of Arab. اعراس is uncertain. Acc. to Lane 1998, *i'rās* can also refer to 'coitus' and in our context possibly to 'bleeding resulting from coitus.' The Engl. online trans. published by The Department of Islamic Studies (Hamdard University, New Delhi, India), 2:306, has 'post parturition mucous discharge from the womb.' The Hebr. trans. *aqiṣah* ('biting; burning; pricking pain') is unclear.

tionaries. The same Hebr. term features in Zeraḥyah's trans. of Maimonides' *Medical Aphorisms* (i.e., *Sefer ha-Peraqim*), next to Hebr. מחלה (cf. BMMG no. 140). Nathan ha-Me'ati translates Arab. آفة as מְאֹרָע (see entry) and Anonymous I renders the Arab. term as פגע.

• **חולי המים הרעים הבשריי** · **dropsy of the flesh**: Arab. الاستسقاء اللحمي · al-Rāzī, *K. fī al-Faṣd* · trans. Anonymous, *Ma'amar ba-Haqqazah* (Ms Parma, Biblioteca Palatina, Cod. Parm. 2283,4, fol. 96[a]): אלבסליק יועיל ממורסת הצלעות ... ומחלי המים הרעים הבשריי ([Bleeding] the basilic vein is beneficial for pleurisy ... and for dropsy of the flesh). Hebr. חולי המים הרעים הבשריי is not attested in the current dictionaries. In the sense of 'dropsy,' the term חולי המים הרעים features in BCD 97 (NM 3:84) in an attestation from Do'eg ha-Edomi's trans. of Hippocrates' *Aphorisms* (i.e., *Sefer Agur*) VI.43.

• **חלי פתול הגידים** · **varicose veins**: Arab. دالية, *Plur.* دوال · al-Rāzī, *K. fī al-Faṣd* · trans. Anonymous, *Ma'amar ba-Haqqazah* (Ms Parma, Biblioteca Palatina, Cod. Parm. 2283,4, fol. 94[a]): וב' גידים נמצאים במקום הנק' מאבד אלרכבתאן והם עבים ומלאים מהגידים אשר בשוקים ותועיל הקזתם מנפיחת השוקים ומחלי פתול הגידים הנק' אלדולי ולהוריד דם הוסת (Two veins are in the places called [in Arab.] *ma'biḍ al-rukbatayn* (popliteal fossa); they are thicker and fuller than the other veins that are in the legs; bleeding them is beneficial for swellings in the legs, for varicose veins called [in Arab.] *al-dawālī*, and to induce the menses). Hebr. חולי פתול הגידים is not attested in the current dictionaries. A variant featuring in the *Ma'amar ba-Haqqazah* is פתילי הגידים (see entry פְּתִיל). Synonyms featuring in medieval medical literature are דליות (cf. BCD 57 (NM 4:38f.)) and חולי הנקרא גפנים (cf. BCD 48 (NM 1:134), s.v. גֶּפֶן).

• **חולי הצלעות** · **pleurisy** · Arab. ذات الجنب · Ibn Sīnā, *K. al-Qānūn* II · trans. Nathan ha-Me'ati, *Sefer ha-Qanun* (Ms Oxford, Bodleian Libraries, Can. Or. 88, fol. 65[a–b]): אנגרה ... כשמשקים אותו עם השעורים ינקה החזה וכשמבשלים עליו במי השעור יוציא מה שיש בחזה מתערובים הגסים וזרעו יותר חזק ויסיר עוצר[130] הנשימה ויניח הנשימה הנצבת ומחולי[131] הקר אשר מחולי הצלעות ([Arab.] *anjura*: Roman nettle [*Urtica pilulifera* L.]: ... When one takes it with barley water, it cleanses the chest, and when one takes its leaves boiled with barley water, it expels the thick humors in the chest. The seeds are more potent and cure asthma, orthopnea, and cold[132] pleurisy). Hebr. חולי הצלעות is not attested in the current dictionaries. Anonymous I renders Arab. ذات الجنب as בעלת הצד. The latter term also features in Nathan's trans. of Maimonides' *Medical Aphorisms* (i.e., *Sefer ha-Peraqim*) (cf. BMMG no. 1999). Zeraḥyah Ḥen translates the Arab.

---

130 עוצר הנשימה ויניח הנשימה הנצבת (= Ms Paris, BnF, héb. 1136, fol. 65[b]): עוצר הנשימה הנצבת Ms الربو ونفس الانتصاب a.

131 ומחולי הקר אשר מחולי הצלעות والبارد من ذات الجنب a.

132 'cold pleurisy': Trans. acc. to a.

term as חולי הצד (cf. BCD 98 (NM 1:148) for an attestation from his *Sefer ha-Peraqim* IV.42 (cf. BMMZ 55, l. 23; BMMG no. 1999)). The synonymous Arab. شوصة is translated by Nathan as מורסת הצלעות (see entry מֻרְסָה).

• **חולי הקוליקא** · **ileus:** Arab. إيلاوس (Gr. εἰλεός; cf. UW 222) · Ibn Sīnā, *K. al-Qānūn* II · trans. Zeraḥyah Ḥen, *Sefer ha-Qanun* (Ms Oxford, Bodleian Libaries, Opp. Add. Fol. 12, fol. 205a): זיבק כסף חי ... זכר בולש כי יש מבני אדם שישקו המומת ממנו בחולי הקוליקא הנק׳ איליאוס ([Arab.] *zi'baq*; [i.e., Hebr.] *kesef ḥay*: Quicksilver (mercury): ... Paulus said that some people (physicians) administered calcinated quicksilver in the case of [Hebr.-Rom.] *ḥoli ha-colica*, called *ileus*). Hebr.-Rom. חולי הקוליקא is a non-attested combined term consisting of Hebr. *ḥoli* and M. Lat./Rom. *colica/colice* (cf. ND 223: 'a painful affliction in the lower abdomen; in some texts said to originate in the colon and involve pain, constipation, flatulence, nausea'). In addition to חולי הקוליקא, Zeraḥyah translates Arab. إيلاوس as קוליקא (see entry). Nathan ha-Me'ati renders إيلاوس as אילִיאוש (see entry). The latter term is also used by Anonymous I and features in both Nathan's (אילאוש) and Zeraḥyah's (איליאוס) trans. of Maimonides' *Medical Aphorisms* (i.e., *Sefer ha-Peraqim*) XXIII.93 (cf. BMMN 230, l. 23; BMMZ 229, l. 23; BMMG no. 161).

חֲלִיָה • **חולית הצואר** · **the hollow of the neck:** Arab. نقرة (cf. FA no. 2256) · Maimonides, *Medical Aphorisms* XII.43 · trans. Zeraḥyah Ḥen, *Sefer ha-Peraqim* (cf. BMMZ 142, l. 13; BMMG no. 5256): תתלה הכוסות על חולית הצואר ותמשוך החומר אשר ירוץ אל העינים (Apply cupping glasses to the hollow of the neck to attract the matter that streams to the eyes). Hebr. חולית הצואר is not attested in the current dictionaries. Nathan ha-Me'ati translates Arab. نقرة as הנקרה בעורף (see entry נְקָרָה). Additionaly, Anonymous translates the Arab. term as נקב העורף in his trans. of al-Rāzī's *K. fī al-Faṣd* (i.e., *Ma'amar ba-Haqqazah*) (see entry נֶקֶב).

חָלָל • *Plur.* **חללים** · **vessels (anat.):** Arab. وعاء, *Plur.* أوعية · al-Rāzī, *K. fī al-Faṣd* · trans. Anonymous, *Ma'amar ba-Haqqazah* (Ms Parma, Biblioteca Palatina, Cod. Parm. 2283,4, fol. 92b): השער הג׳ בסבות המחייבות ההקזה מהסבות לזה הוא המלוי ונחלק לב׳ חלקים הא׳ מהם החללים והם הגידים והם שיהיו הגידים והשרינים מלאי דם (Chapter 3: On the causes (circumstances) that make bloodletting necessary. One of them is overfilling, which is divided into two parts, one of which is relating to vessels, i.e., the veins, and that is when the veins and arteries are full with blood). Hebr. חָלָל, *Plur.* חללים, does not feature as an anat. term in the sense of 'vessel' in the current dictionaries. *Sing.* חָלָל features in BCD 99 in the sense of 'cavity' (cf. NM 3:87), 'concave (part)' (cf. NM 1:148f.), and 'ventricle' (cf. NM 2:48). *Plur.* חללים features ibid. in the sense of 'intestines' only (cf. NM 4:69). In their trans. of Maimonides' *Medical Aphorisms* (i.e., *Sefer ha-Peraqim*), Nathan ha-Me'ati translates Arab. أوعية as כלים, while Zeraḥyah Ḥen has כיסים or גידים (cf. BMMG no. 5589). For כיסים see also BCD 127 (NM 1:97, 158) for attestations from Shem Tov ben Isaac's *Sefer ha-Shimmush* XXX.2.4 and Zeraḥyah's *Sefer ha-Peraqim* XVIII.8.

חֲלָלִיּוּת · **cavity; hollow part:** Lat. *concavitas* · Guy de Chauliac, *Inventarium sive Chirurgia Magna* (cf. CMM 1:230, ll. 2–3) · trans. Anonymous (Ms Paris, BnF, héb. 1189, fol. 125[b]): ואחר הנקוי ימלא החלליות מאותם שיצמיחו בשר (Once [the ulcer in the case of ophthalmia] is clean, the cavity (hollow part) should be filled with those [medicines] that make the flesh grow). Hebr. חֲלָלִיּוּת is not attested in the current dictionaries.

[חלק] • *Hifʿil* **הֶחֱלִיק** · **to soften, relieve:** Arab. ليّن · Ibn Sīnā, *K. al-Qānūn* II · trans. Zeraḥyah Ḥen, *Sefer ha-Qanun* (Ms Oxford, Bodleian Libaries, Opp. Add. Fol. 12, fol. 277[b]): תַּרוּנְגְּבִין מַנְנָא ... יועיל מן השעול ויחליק החזה ([Arab.] *taranjubīn* [from Pers. *tarangubīn*]; [Aram.] *manna*ʾ: Manna:[133] It is beneficial for cough and for relieving a [congested] chest). Hebr. *Hifʿil* הֶחֱלִיק features as part of the terms החליק הטבע 'to soften the stools' and החליק הבטן 'to prescribe laxatives' in BCD 101 (NM 1:149f.) and also as *Part. Hifʿil* as part of the term הרפואה המחליקה 'the softening remedy' in NM 5:190 in an attestation from Zeraḥyah's trans. of Maimonides' *Medical Aphorisms* (i.e., *Sefer ha-Peraqim*) XXI.64 (cf. BMMZ 201, l. 24; BMMG no. 1873; see also entry רְפוּאָה). Nathan ha-Meʾati and Anonymous I both render Arab. ليّن as *Piʿel* רִכֵּךְ (see entry).

• *Part. Hifʿil* **מַחְלִיק** • **הסם המחליק** → **סַם**.

• **הרפואה המחליקה** → **רְפוּאָה**.

חֲלִשָׁה · **tear [of a muscle]:** Arab. وهن (Gr. ῥῆγμα; cf. UWS 2:247) · Ibn Sīnā, *K. al-Qānūn* II · trans. Zeraḥyah Ḥen, *Sefer ha-Qanun* (Ms Oxford, Bodleian Libaries, Opp. Add. Fol. 12, fol. 238[a]): מֻגַאתְ ... הוא מועיל כשיחובש בו הרסבוט והשבירה וחולשת המושקלו וההשמטה ([Arab.] *mughāth*:[134] ... It is useful when plastered in cases of contusion (bruise), fracture, muscle tear, and dislocation). In the sense of 'tear,' Hebr. חֲלִשָׁה is a non-attested semantic borrowing from Arab. وهن. Nathan translates Arab. وهن as בְּקוּעַ (see entry) and Anonymous I has רִסּוּק (see entry for his use of the term רסוק האזן 'tear (puncture) in the ear'). The synonymous Arab. term فسخ is translated by Zeraḥyah as הֶפְסֵד (see entry) and the synonymous هتك as חִתּוּךְ (see entry).

• **חולשת קבול ההריון** · **infertility:** Arab. عسر الحبل · Ibn Sīnā, *K. al-Qānūn* II · trans. Anonymous II, *Sefer ha-Qanun* (Ms Parma, Biblioteca Palatina, Cod. Parm. 3045, fol. 29[a]): ייזאר ... ויצליח זרעו ושרשיו לחולשת קבול ההריון ([Arab.] *jazar*: Carrot [*Daucus carota* L.]: ... Its seed and roots are beneficial for [women suffering from] infertility). Hebr. חולשת קבול ההריון is not attested in the current dictionaries. Nathan ha-Meʾati and Anonymous I both translate Arab. عسر الحبل as קושי ההריון and Zeraḥyah Ḥen has עוצר ההריון (see entry עֹצֶר).

---

133 'Manna': I.e., the crystallized honeydew of certain scale insects, in particular the manna mealybug [*Trabutina mannipara* (Hemprich & Ehrenberg, 1829)] that feeds on the tamarisk [*Tamarix* L.]; cf. Lane 306; MSh no. 386.

134 '*mughāth*': I.e., the root of glossostemon [*Glossostemon bruguieri* Desf.]; cf. MIG no. 546.

• **חולשת הראות** · **night blindness (nyctalopia)**: Arab. عشاوة (cf. MMT 195 (253);[135] D 2:132) · al-Rāzī, *K. fī al-Faṣd* · trans. Anonymous, *Ma'amar ba-Haqqazah* (Ms Parma, Biblioteca Palatina, Cod. Parm. 2283,4, fol. 93[b]): וב׳ גידים בקצוי העורקים הנק׳ אלמאקין ותועיל הקזתם משארית חלי העינים הנק׳ אלרמאד והדמעות וחולשת הראות הנק׳ אלעשוא (Two veins in the canthi, called [in Arab.] *al-ma'qayn*; bleeding them is beneficial for remains of ophthalmia, called [in Arab.] *al-ramad*, for rhyas, and for nyctalopia, called [in Arab.] *al-'ashāwa*). Hebr. חולשת הראות does not feature in the current dictionaries. Ben Yehuda mentions a reading חולשת כח הראות featuring in the treatise *Minchat Kenaot* by Yechiel ben Samuel of Pisa (cf. BM 1605). Synonyms featuring in medieval Hebr. medical literature are: אֹפֶל, featuring in Abraham Avigdor's trans. of Gerard de Solo's *Practica super nono Almansoris* (i.e., *Ha-Ma'amar ha-Teshi'i le-Sefer ha-Mansuri le-Razi* (cf. NM 6:20f.); לִילִית, featuring in Moses ibn Tibbon's trans. of Ibn al-Jazzār's *Zād al-musāfir* (i.e., *Sefer Ṣedat ha-Derakhim*) II.5.0–1 (cf. BCD 137 (NM 4:91); IJZ 1–2:491); and סַנְוֵר, featuring in Shem Tov ben Isaac's trans. of al-Rāzī's *K. al-Manṣūrī* (i.e., *Sefer Almansur*) (cf. NM 6:152).

• **חולשת השתן** · **dysuria**: Arab. عسر البول · Ibn Sīnā, *K. al-Qānūn* II · trans. Anonymous II, *Sefer ha-Qanun* (Ms Parma, Biblioteca Palatina, Cod. Parm. 3045, fol. 30[a]): דַּרְסֵיסִיאַם ... מי בשולו עוצר הבטן ויצליח אל הנפח[136] לחולשת[137] השתן ([Arab.] *dārshīsha'ān*: Broom [*Genista acanthoclada* DC. or *Cytisus spinosus* Lam.] (cf. MIG no. 223): ... Its decoction causes constipation. It is beneficial for the flatulence of[138] intestines and for dysuria). Hebr. חולשת השתן is not attested in the current dictionaries. Nathan ha-Me'ati translates Arab. عسر البول as עוצר השתן (cf. BCD 212 (NM 3:181) for an attestation from Moses ibn Tibbon's trans. of Maimonides' *Commentary on Hippocrates' Aphorisms* (i.e., *Perush Aphorismi shel Apuqraṭ*) VI.36 (cf. BMCH 1:400, l. 6)) and Anonymous I has קשי יציאת השתן (cf. BCD 252 (NM 3:211) for an attestation from Nathan's trans. of Hippocrates' *Aphorisms* (i.e., *Pirqei Abuqraṭ*) VI.36). For other synonyms featuring in medieval medical literature, see NM 6:126, s.v. מצוקת השתן.

חַם • **כוית המים החמים** → כְּוִיָּה.

• **שרפת המים החמים** → שְׂרֵפָה.

חֹמֶט · **chameleon**: Arab. حرباء (cf. JAD 1:519) · *Glossary* (Ms Moscow, Russian State Library, Guenzburg 573, fol. 152[b]): חרבא הוא החומט ([Arab.] *ḥirbā'*; i.e., [Hebr.] *ha-ḥomeṭ*). Hebr. חֹמֶט is attested in the Bible as an unclean animal of unknown identity (cf. KB 328), 'a kind of lizard' (cf. BDB 328), or 'skink' (cf. FAB 98); and in Rabb. literature

---

135 The Arab. term can also refer to the opposite of night blindness, i.e., hemeralopia (cf. IJZ 1–2:273, n. 429).

136 הנפח: في الأمعاء add a.

137 לחולשת: ومن عسر a.

138 'of intestines and': Trans. acc. to a.

as 'lizard (chamaeleon)' (cf. JD 435, s.v. חומטא). Ben Yehuda (cf. BM 1619) translates חֹמֶט as 'chamaeleon,' a.o., following Sa'adya's trans. of Lev 11:30[139] and Ibn Janāḥ's *K. al-Uṣūl*.[140]

חֲמְצָה · **sourness**: Arab. حموضة · Ibn Sīnā, *K. al-Qānūn* II · trans. Nathan ha-Me'ati, *Sefer ha-Qanun* (Ms Oxford, Bodleian Libraries, Can. Or. 88, fol. 77[b]): דאדי[141] ... הוא עוצר ויעצר הבטן ובמה שיש בו מהקבוץ ישמור שכר התמרים מהחומצה ([Arab.] *dādī*:[142] ... It is astringent and constipative. Its astringency prevents the date wine from becoming sour). Hebr. חֲמְצָה features in EM 555 (s.v. חֲמְצָה) as a modern term in the sense of 'acid.' Zeraḥyah Ḥen translates Arab. حموضة as חמץ and Anonymous I has חמיצות.

חֹמֶר • **תאות אכילת החומר** → תַּאֲוָה.

חָנוּק (*Part. Pass.*) → חָנַק.

חֲנֶט • *Plur.* **חנטים** • **בעל חנטים** → בַּעַל.

חֲנִיקָה • *Plur.* **חניקות** · **sore throat; quinsy**: Arab. خوانيق (Gr. συνάγχη; cf. UW 654) · i. Ibn Sīnā, *K. al-Qānūn* II · trans. Nathan ha-Me'ati, *Sefer ha-Qanun* (Ms Oxford, Bodleian Libraries, Can. Or. 88, bk. 2, fols. 99[b]–100[a]): לבן ... חלב הרחלים יותר מועיל לרקיקת הדם וכן החלב הוא מתרופות נגעי הריאה והכליון והוא סל בערבי ואם ישכשך בו או עם יעשה ממנו גרגור ובערבי גרגרה יועיל מהחניקות והאסכרה ובער׳ דבאח ומורסת ערלת הגרון והוא לאהה בערבי ([Arab.] *laban*: Milk: ... Ewe's milk is more beneficial in hemoptysis; milk is a [good] drug in pulmonary ulcers and phthisis, i.e., *sill* in Arab. Rinsing the mouth and gargling, [i.e.,] in Arab *gharghara*, with milk is useful in quinsy, angina, [i.e.,] in Arab. *dhibḥa*, and swollen uvula, i.e., *lahāt* in Arab.). Hebr. *Plur.* חניקות is not attested in this sense in the current dictionaries. *Sing.* חֲנִיקָה (for Arab. خوانيق) features in BCD 104 (NM 1:94) in an attestation from Shem Tov ben Isaac's *Sefer ha-Shimmush* XXX.2.95. Zeraḥyah Ḥen translates Arab. خوانيق as חֶנֶק (cf. BCD 104f. (NM 1:150f.; corr. 4:229) for an attestation from Zeraḥyah's trans. of Maimonides' *Medical Aphorisms* (i.e., *Sefer ha-Peraqim*) XXV.11 (cf. BMMZ 245, l. 1; BMMG no. 1599) and NM 6:79f. for an attestation from Shem Tov ben Isaac's *Sefer Almansur*) and Anonymous I has מחנקים (see entry מַחֲנַק).

· ii. al-Rāzī, *K. fī al-Faṣd* · trans. Anonymous, *Ma'amar ba-Haqqazah* (Ms Parma, Biblioteca Palatina, Cod. Parm. 2283,4, fol. 93[b]): וב׳ גידים בפנימי הלשון ותועיל הקזתם מנפיחת הלשון ומהחניקות אשר מסבת הדם (Two veins inside the tongue, bleeding them is beneficial for swelling of the tongue and sanguine quinsy).

---

139 Cf. Derenbourg (ed.), *Targum Ḥamishah Ḥumshei Torah be-Lashon 'Aravit le-Rabbeinu Sa'adyah Ga'on ben Yoseph ha-Fayyumi*, 158.

140 Col. 233.

141 דאדי: Emend. ed. דארי Ms.

142 *'Dādī'*: A term that can refer to a sort of lichen, to St John's wort, and to tar made of plant resins; cf. MIG no. 242.

חָנַק • *Part. Pass.* חָנוּק • הרחם החנוק → רֶחֶם.
• *Part. Nif'al* נֶחְנָק • הרחם הנחנק → רֶחֶם.

חֶנֶק • חנק הרחם · **hysterical suffocation**: Arab. احتناق الرحم · Ibn Sīnā, *K. al-Qānūn* II · trans. Zeraḥyah Ḥen, *Sefer ha-Qanun* (Ms Oxford, Bodleian Libraries, Opp. Add. Fol. 12, fol. 262ᵇ): פ׳סֶאפ׳סְן ... כשישתה[143] תועיל מחנק הרחם ([Arab.] P̄Se'P̄YSiN [read: P̄S'P̄YS, i.e., *fasāfis*] Bed bugs: ... When a woman inhales them, they are beneficial for hysterical suffocation). Hebr. חנק הרחם features in BM 1661 in a later attestation from Meir Aldabi's *Shevilei Emunah*. In addition to this term, Zeraḥyah translates Arab. احتناق الرحم as חניקת הרחם (cf. BCD 104 (NM 3:94) for an attestation from Zeraḥyah's trans. of Maimonides' *Commentary on Hippocrates' Aphorisms* (i.e., *Perush Aphorismi shel Apuqraṭ*) V.35 (cf. BMCH 1:479, l. 14); cf. also NM 6:79). The latter term (חניקת הרחם) is also used by Nathan ha-Me'ati and Anonymous I renders Arab. احتناق الرحم as מחנק הרחם (cf. BCD 146 (NM 2:58) for an attestation from Nathan's trans. of Maimonides' *Medical Aphorisms* (i.e., *Sefer ha-Peraqim*) XXIV.58 (cf. BMMN 242, l. 7; BMMG no. 1598)).

חסו · **sip; broth**: Arab. حسو · Ibn Sīnā, *K. al-Qānūn* II · trans. Zeraḥyah Ḥen, *Sefer ha-Qanun* (Ms Oxford, Bodleian Libaries, Opp. Add. Fol. 12, fol. 251ᵇ): ... סַקַנְקוּר אֶשְׁטִינְק יעורר התשמיש עד שלא ינוח אלא אם חסו ממרק העדשים והחסות ([Arab.] *saqanqūr*; [i.e., Rom.] 'eŠəṬiYNəQ [from Lat. *stincus*]: Skink: ... It arouses sexual lust that can only be reduced by sipping lentil soup and [eating] lettuce). In the sense of 'sip; broth,' Hebr. חסו is a non-attested calque from Arab. حسو. Zeraḥyah employs the same term in the sense of 'broth' (for Arab. حسو) in his trans. of Maimonides' *Medical Aphorisms* (i.e., *Sefer ha-Peraqim*) XVII.21 (cf. BMMZ 171, l. 18; BMMG no. 966). Anonymous I renders Arab. حسو as גמיעה. In the glossary to his *Sefer ha-Qanun*, Nathan ha-Me'ati defines חסו as: חסו הוא שם לחביץ קדרה כלומר איזה קמח או פתיתות מבושל בקדרה (ḤSW. This is the name for a type of broth (corr.) (ḤBYṢ QDRH); i.e., flour or breadcrumbs boiled in a pot) (cf. NM 2:114, 139 (Ḥet 17)). A synonym used by Shem Tov ben Isaac in his *Sefer ha-Shimmush* XXVII is Hebr. שֶׁרֶף (cf. BCD 286 (NM 4:213)).

חִפּוּשִׁית · **beetle**: Arab. خنفس (cf. Lane 817f.: 'black beetle or a species thereof;' D 1:409: 'bupreste' (*buprestis*); FL 1:533: 'Scarabaeus niger')[144] · *Glossary* (Ms Moscow, Russian State Library, Guenzburg 573, fol. 154ᵇ): כנאפש הוא חפושית ([Arab.] *khanāfis* (*Plur.* of *khunfus*); i.e., [Hebr.] *ḥippushit*). Hebr. חִפּוּשִׁית features in Rabb. literature in the sense of 'scarabee; beetle' (cf. JD 459; BM 1683; LZ 305).

חֲפִירָה · **dental erosion; caries; cavity**: Arab. حفر (cf. VL 1:401: 'Erosio dentium circa radices, vel flavedo, qua dentes corrumpuntur') · Ibn Sīnā, *K. al-Qānūn* II · trans.

143 כשישתנה: شمت a.
144 Cf. also A. Malouf, *Mu'jam al-ḥayawān* (*An Arabic Zoological Dictionary*) (Cairo 1932), 33: 'beetle.'

Zeraḥyah Ḥen, *Sefer ha-Qanun* (Ms Oxford, Bodleian Libaries, Opp. Add. Fol. 12, fol. 242[a–b]): מלח ... המלח השרוף ינקה השנים מן החפירה (Salt: ... Burnt salt cleanses the teeth [so that they are not affected by] dental erosion (caries)). Hebr. חֲפִירָה is attested in BCD 106 (NM 4:71) in the sense of 'cavity' in an attestation from Jacob ibn Tibbon's trans. of Ibn Zuhr's *Regimen of Health* (i.e., *Hanhagat ha-Beri'ut le-Abu 'Ali Ben Zuhr*) XXVIII. Nathan ha-Me'ati and Anonymous I both render Arab. حفر as חפירה as well.

חֵפֶץ • **התנועה מאין חפץ** → תְּנוּעָה.

חֲצִי • **כאב חצי הראש** → כְּאֵב.

חֶרֶס • *Plur.* **חרסים** · **shells**: Arab. أصداف · Ibn Sīnā, *K. al-Qānūn* II · trans. Zeraḥyah Ḥen, *Sefer ha-Qanun* (Ms Oxford, Bodleian Libaries, Opp. Add. Fol. 12, fol. 214[b]): חַלָּזוֹן המהות הוא מכלל החרסים קוֹנְקוֹלִי ([Arab.] *ḥalazūn* / [Hebr.] *ḥilazon*: Snail: What is it? It is a kind of [mollusc] that has a shell [called in Rom.] QWoNəQWoLiY). In the sense of 'shell,' Hebr. חֶרֶס, *Plur.* חרסים, features in BM 1772 in an attestation from Simeon ben Zemah Duran's *Magen Avot*. Nathan ha-Me'ati translates Arab. أصداف as קליפות (הנק׳ צרף (*צדף and Anonymous I has מגן הנק׳ צדף (see entry מָגֵן).

חַרְסִית · **potter's clay**: Arab. جبسين · Ibn Sīnā, *K. al-Qānūn* II · trans. Nathan ha-Me'ati, *Sefer ha-Qanun* (Ms Oxford, Bodleian Libraries, Can. Or. 88, fol. 75[a]):[145] גבסין והוא גבשושית המהות הוא אבן העושין ממנו חרסית ([Arab.] *jibsīn*; i.e., [Hebr.] *gavshushit*: Gypsum: What is it? It is a stone from which potter's clay is made). Hebr. חַרְסִית is attested in Rabb. literature (cf. JD 504; BM 1773). In his commentary on *Mishnah Shabbat* 8:4 (ed. Kafih, 49), Maimonides explains the term חַרְסִית as טיט אלחכמה (i.e., Arab. *ṭiṭ al-ḥakama*: 'plaster that is put around vessels so that they do not break when heated')[146] and in his commentary on *Mishnah Ma'aser Sheni* 5:1 he explains the Hebr. term as אלטין אלמטבוך (i.e., Arab. *al-ṭīn al-maṭbūkh* [lit. 'cooked clay']) (cf. SHS 1:230 (Ḥet 37)). Anonymous I renders Arab. جبسين as חַרְסִית as well.

חֲרִפָּה · **pungency**: Arab. حرافة · Ibn Sīnā, *K. al-Qānūn* II · trans. Anonymous II, *Sefer ha-Qanun* (Ms Parma, Biblioteca Palatina, Cod. Parm. 3045, fol. 41[b]): אניסו הוא זרע פינוקלו רומנו וחורפתו תהיה פחות מחורפת נַאבַּתִי ('NYSW [i.e., Ital.-Rom. *aniso*]; i.e., seed of PYNWQLW RWMNW [i.e., Ital.-Rom. from M. Lat. *foeniculum romanum*, 'Roman fennel']: Anise [*Pimpinella anisum* L.]: Its pungency is less than that of Nabataean [fennel]). Hebr. חֲרִפָּה is attested as synonymous with חריפות in BM 1778 in an attestation from Eliah Misrachi's *Ḥokhmat* (= *Sefer*?) *ha-Mispar*. Nathan ha-Me'ati and Zeraḥyah Ḥen both translate Arab. حرافة as חריפות and Anonymous I renders the Arab. term as חריף.

חֲשֵׁכָה · **dimness [of sight]**: Arab. ظلمة (البصر) (Gr. ἀμβλυωπία; cf. UW 99f.) · Ibn Sīnā, *K. al-Qānūn* II · trans. Nathan ha-Me'ati, *Sefer ha-Qanun* (Ms Oxford, Bodleian Lib-

145 The same Hebr. term features in ed. Naples 1491, fol. 92[bii]: גבסין הוא גיף הוא גבשושית.

146 J. Blau, *A Dictionary of Mediaeval Judaeo-Arabic Texts* (Jerusalem 2006), 140 cf. KM 796.

raries, Can. Or. 88, fols. 76b–77a): דרציני ... יועיל מכסוי הראות והחשכה ([Arab.] *dārṣīnī*: Cinnamon [*Cinnamomum verum* J. Presl]: ...: It is beneficial for dullness and dimness [of sight]). Hebr. חֲשֵׁכָה is not attested in this sense in the current dictionaries. Anonymous I renders Arab. ظلمة (البصر) as מחשך באפלה. Moses ibn Tibbon translates Arab. ظلمة البصر as חשיכות העינים in his trans. of Ibn al-Jazzār's *Zād al-musāfir* (i.e., *Sefer Ṣedat ha-Derakhim*) I.10.14 (cf. NM 5:85f.; IJZ 1–2:555).

• **חשכת העין · I. dimness of sight**: Arab. غشاوة (Gr. ἀμβλυωπία; cf. UW 99f.) · Ibn Sīnā, *K. al-Qānūn* II · trans. Nathan ha-Me'ati, *Sefer ha-Qanun* (Ms Oxford, Bodleian Libraries, Can. Or. 88, fol. 71b):[147] בקלה אלחמקה ... יועיל מהאפר הנקרא רמד בערבי ומערבים אותו בכוחלים והרבוי ממנו יוליד חשכת העין ([Arab.] [*al-*]*baqla al-ḥamqā'* [lit. 'the stupid vegetable']: Common purslane [*Portulaca oleracea* L.]: ... It is useful in ophthalmia, called *ramad* in Arab., and it is included in collyria. Its excessive use, however, causes dimness of sight). Hebr. חשכת העין is not attested in the current dictionaries. Synonyms used by Nathan are כסוי הראות and הכסוי על העין (see entry כִּסּוּי). Anonymous I renders Arab. غشاوة as סְנֵוֶר (see entry) and Zeraḥyah Ḥen has סנורים (see also entry סַנְוֵר).

· **II. black eye**: Arab. كمودة العين (Gr. ὑπώπιον;[148] cf. UW2:561f.; LSG 1904) · Ibn Sīnā, *K. al-Qānūn* II · trans. Nathan ha-Me'ati, *Sefer ha-Qanun* (Ms Oxford, Bodleian Libraries, Can. Or. 88, fols. 72b–73a): באקלי ... אם עושין ממנו תחבשת בתלתן הנקרא חלבה יועיל מחשכת העין והחולי הנקרא טרפה ועם הלבונה ולובן הביצה והורדים אם עושין ממנו תחבשת לבליטת העין ([Arab.] *bāqillā*: Broad bean [*Vicia faba* L.]: ... Prepared as a plaster with fenugreek, it is useful for a black eye and a blood spot in the eye, called [in Arab.] *ṭarfa*, and as a plaster with frankincense, egg white, and roses, it is [useful] for protrusion of the eye). Zeraḥyah Ḥen translates Arab. كمودة العين as שחרות העין (see entry שַׁחֲרוּת) and Anonymous I has כהות העין (see entry כֵּהוּת).

חִתּוּךְ · tear [of a muscle]: Arab. هتك (Gr. ῥῆξις, ῥῆγμα; cf. UWS 2:248) · Ibn Sīnā, *K. al-Qānūn* II · trans. Nathan ha-Me'ati, *Sefer ha-Qanun* (Ms Oxford, Bodleian Libraries, Can. Or. 88, fol. 109a): סכבינג' ... יועיל ממכאו' הרגלים ובער' נקרס ומחתוך העצלים ([Arab.] *sakbīnaj*: Sagapenum [i.e., i.e., the gum resin of the Persian giant fennel [*Ferula persica* Willd.]]: It is useful for podagra, [called] in Arab. *niqris*, and for muscle tear). In medieval medical literature Hebr. חִתּוּךְ features in BM 1818 in the sense of 'a sharp pain in the organs.' Zeraḥyah Ḥen translates Arab. هتك as חִתּוּךְ, just like Nathan, but also as נִתּוּק (see entry). Anonymous I renders Arab. هتك as רִסּוּק (see entry for his use

147 The same Hebr. term features on fol. 83b, entry זיתון '[Arab.] *zaytūn*: Olive [*Olea europaea* L.].'

148 Cf. the parallel entry on 'broad bean' [*Vicia faba* L.] in the Arab. trans. of Dioscorides' *De materia medica* (Ms Paris, BnF, arabe 2849, fol. 43a): كمودة لون الموضع ويسمى باليونانية اوقوفيا. The term اوقوفيا (read: اوفوفيا) is Gr. ὑπώπιον, *Plur.* ὑπώπια.

of the term רסוק האזן 'tear (puncture) in the ear'). The Arab. synonym فسخ is translated by Nathan as בְּקוּעַ, בְּקִיעָה, and פְּתִיחָה (see entries), and the Arab. synonym وهن also as בְּקוּעַ (see entry).

[חתך] • *Part. Pi'el* מְחַתֵּךְ • הסם המחתך → סַם.

• הרפואה המחתכת → רְפוּאָה.

חָתַם • *Part.* חוֹתֵם • הסם החותם → סַם.

• הרפואה החותמות → רְפוּאָה.

ט

טאעון · **plague boil (plague)**: Arab. طاعون, *Plur.* طواعين (Gr. λοιμός; cf. UW 397) · Ibn Sīnā, *K. al-Qānūn* II · trans. Anonymous I, *Sefer ha-Qanun* (Ms Paris, BnF, héb. 1142, fols. 126b–127a):[149] טין[150] ארמיני ... מועיל מן הטאעון בשתיה ורטיה ומונע התפשט עפוש האיברים ([Arab.] *ṭīn armīnī*: Armenian bole: ... It is useful for plague boils (plague), either when taken orally or when rubbed [on the affected spot]. It prevents putrefaction of the organs from spreading). Hebr. טאעון is a non-attested loan word from Arab. *Sing.* طاعون. The latter term is rendered by Anonymous I as הטאעון והדבר (cf. entry דֶּבֶר). Nathan ha-Me'ati translates Arab. طاعون, *Plur.* طواعين as *Plur.* טאעונים, but also as דֶּבֶר (see entry). Zeraḥyah Ḥen translates Arab. طواعين as אנדראש (i.e., Rom. *antras* / Lat. *anthrax* 'maligant boil') and Anonymous II renders the Arab. term as המורסות אשר יקרו בעת המגפה (see entry מֻרְסָה).

טֶבַע • מטבעו ש- · **being of someone's business, property, nature to ...**: Arab. من شأنه أن (cf. Lane 1491) · Ibn Sīnā, *K. al-Qānūn* II · trans. Zeraḥyah Ḥen, *Sefer ha-Qanun* (Ms Oxford, Bodleian Libaries, Opp. Add. Fol. 12, fol. 160a): והמבשלת היא הרפואה אשר מטבעה שתקנה לליחה בישול כי היא מחממת במיצוע וביושר ויש בו כח מקבץ עוצר הליחה עד שתתבשל ולא תתיך בעוצם ((A ripening (coctive) [drug is a drug] that—by its nature—ripens (concocts) the humor because of its moderate heat; it has an astringent property that retains the humor until it is ripe and does not dissolve it forcefully). Hebr. מטבעו ש- is not attested in the current dictionaries. Nathan ha-Me'ati translates Arab. من شأنه أن as מנהגו ש- (see entry מִנְהָג) and Anonymous I as דרכו ל- (see entry דֶּרֶךְ).

טֳהֳרָה · **detergent; cleansing property**: Arab. جلاء (Gr. σμῆξις; cf. UWS2:305) · Ibn Sīnā, *K. al-Qānūn* II · trans. Zeraḥyah Ḥen, *Sefer ha-Qanun* (Ms Oxford, Bodleian Libaries, Opp. Add. Fol. 12, fol. 265b): קַנְטוּרִיוֹן צֶנְטוֹרֶיַאה ... יש בו טהרה וקיבוץ וחריפות ומעט מתיקות וייבש בלא עקיצה ([Arab.] *qanṭūriyūn*; [i.e., Rom.] ṢeNəṬWəReYa'H [i.e., Lat. *centaurea*]: Knapweed [*Centaurea centaurium* L.] or common centaury [*Centaurium erythraea* Rafn.]: ...: It is detergent, astringent, pungent, and somewhat sweet; it dries without causing irritation). Hebr. טֳהֳרָה is attested in medieval medical literature in the sense of 'evacuation' (for Arab. استفراغ); 'purification' (for Lat. *mundificatio*), and 'purgation' (for Lat. *purgatio*) (cf. NM 5:88). In his trans. of Maimonides' *Medical Aphorisms* (i.e., *Sefer ha-Peraqim*), Zeraḥyah translates Arab. جلاء as טהרה ונקוי, כוח מטהר, לטהר, מטהר, and ריחוץ (cf. BMMG no. 667). Anonymous I renders Arab. جلاء as מֵרוּק (see entry).

---

149 The same term טאעון features, in addition to הטאעון והדבר, on fol. 234a, entry ריבאס '[Arab.] *ribās*: Syrian rhubarb [*Rheum ribes* L.].'

150 טין ארמיני: בול ארמניק Ms¹.

טוּחַ • *Part.* **טָח** • **טח בדבקות** · **agglutinant**: Arab. مغرّ · Ibn Sīnā, *K. al-Qānūn* II · trans. Anonymous I, *Sefer ha-Qanun* (Ms Paris, BnF, héb. 1142, fols. 72ᵇ–73ᵃ: גלנאר ... טח בדבקות עוצר לכל הזולה ([Arab.] *jullanār*: The flower of the wild pomegranate [*Punicum granatum* L.]: ... It is agglutinant [and] stops [the flow of] all kinds of fluids). Hebr. טח בדבקות features in the sense of 'to be agglutinant' in BCD 111 (NM 2:50) in an attestation from Nathan ha-Me'ati's trans. of Maimonides' *Medical Aphorisms* (i.e., *Sefer ha-Peraqim*) XIII.43 (cf. BMMN 150, l. 24; BMMG no. 115). Nathan translates Arab. مغرّ as צוֹפֵד (see entry) and Zeraḥyah Ḥen has *Part. Pi'el* מְדַבֵּק (see entry [דבק]).

• **סַם** → **הסם הטח בדבקות**.

• *Inf. Hif'il* **לְהָטִיחַ** • **to apply as a salve**: Arab. لُطُوخ (cf. WKAS 2.2:692) · Ibn Sīnā, *K. al-Qānūn* II · trans. Zeraḥyah Ḥen, *Sefer ha-Qanun* (Ms Oxford, Bodleian Libaries, Opp. Add. Fol. 12, fol. 212ᵃ): חלתית אַשָׁא פֵ׳דֵידָא ... יועל מחולי השועל להטיח בו עם החומץ והפלפל ([Arab.] *ḥiltīt* / [Hebr.] *ḥiltit*; [i.e., Rom.] 'aŠa' FeDeYDa': Resin of asafetida [*Ferula assa-foetida* L.]: ... It is useful for alopecia when it is applied as a salve with vinegar and pepper). Hebr. *Hif'il* הֵטִיחַ does not feature in a medical sense in the current dictionaries. Zeraḥyah uses the verbal noun הֲטָחָה (see entry) to render Arab. لَطُوخ. Nathan ha-Me'ati translates Arab. لُطُوخ as לִכְלֵךְ (see entry) and Anonymous I has רְטִיָּה (see entry).

טָח (*Part.*) → **טוּחַ**.

טִיחָה • **טיחת דבקות** · **agglutination**: Arab. تغرية · Ibn Sīnā, *K. al-Qānūn* II · trans. Anonymous I, *Sefer ha-Qanun* (Ms Paris, BnF, héb. 1142, fol. 13ᵃ): והמבריא החבורות הוא הסם המנגב ומעבה הלחות הנופלת בין שני שטחי החבורה השכנים אל טיחת דבקות והדבקה הנקר׳ וישקושיטאט ויתדבק אחד מהם באחר כמו דם תנין ואלואן (A [drug] that heals wounds is a drug that dries up and thickens the fluid collected between the two layers of a wound that are close to each other. [It does so] to an extent that it [i.e., the fluid] becomes agglutinant and viscous, called WYŠQWŠYṬ'Ṭ, and both the ends [of the wound] adhere to each other; [examples of such a drug are] dragon's blood [i.e., the resin of *Dracaena cinnabari* Balf. f.] and aloes). Hebr. טיחת דבקות is not attested in the current dictionaries. The term טִיחָה on its own features in the sense of 'agglutination' in BCD 112 (NM 4:75) in an attestation from an anonymous trans. of Ibn Sīnā's *K. al-Adwiya al-qalbiyya* (i.e., *Sammim Libbiyim*). Nathan ha-Me'ati translates Arab. تغرية as צֶמֶד (see entry).

טִיט • **תאות הטיט** → **תַּאֲוָה**.

טְנוּפֶת · **mucus discharged from the eyes (rheum[151])**: Arab. رمص (Gr. λήμη; cf. UWS 1:630) · Ibn Sīnā, *K. al-Qānūn* II · trans. Nathan ha-Me'ati, *Sefer ha-Qanun* (Ms Oxford, Bodleian Libraries, Can. Or. 88, fol. 62ᵇ): אנזרות ... יועיל מהדם והטנופת הנקרא רמץ בערבי

151 'rheum': Cf. Wallis, *Medieval Medicine*, 550: 'a morbid discharge of phlegm in the head (e.g., a runny nose), eyes, joints, etc.'

לבד ומנזילות וקל וחומר הנילוש בחלב חמורה[152] ויוציא לפלוף מהעין (Arab. *anzarūt*: Sarcocolla [a resinous gum derived from *Astragalus sarcocolla* Dymock]: … It is useful for ophthalmia and especially for mucus discharged from the eyes (rheum). It is also beneficial for the catarrhal flow [from the eye], especially its preserve [lit. 'what is kneaded'] with the milk of a she-ass; and it removes motes that might have fallen into the eye). Hebr. טְנוֹפֶת is not attested in this sense in the current dictionaries. Zeraḥyah Ḥen transcribes Arab. رمص as רמץ and Anonymous I renders the Arab. term as לִפְלוּף (cf. BCD 138 (NM 2:55f.; 4:92) for attestations from Nathan's trans. of Maimonides' *Medical Aphorisms* (i.e., *Sefer ha-Peraqim*) VI.13 (cf. BMMN 67, l. 15; BMMG no. 2179) and Moses ibn Tibbon's trans. of Ibn al-Jazzār's *Zād al-musāfir* (i.e., *Sefer Ṣedat ha-Derakhim*) II.1.2 (cf. IJZ 1–2:485)).

• **טנופת האזנים** · **earwax**: Arab. أوساخ الأذن · Ibn Sīnā, *K. al-Qānūn* II · trans. Nathan ha-Me'ati, *Sefer ha-Qanun* (Ms Oxford, Bodleian Libraries, Can. Or. 88, fol. 84[a]): זראונד … ינקה טנופת האזנים ויחזק השמע כשמערבים אותו עם דבש ([Arab.] *zarāwand*: Birthwort [*Aristolochia longa* L., *A. rotunda* L., or *A. clematis* L.]: … It removes earwax and strengthens hearing when it is mixed with honey). Hebr. טנופת אזנים is not attested in the current dictionaries. Zeraḥyah Ḥen translates Arab. أوساخ الأذن as ליכלוכי האוזן (see entry לִכְלוּךְ) and Anonymous I has זוהמת האוזן (see entry זהמה).

• **טנופת השנים** · **dirty teeth (dental sordes)**: Arab. أوساخ الأسنان · Ibn Sīnā, *K. al-Qānūn* II · trans. Nathan ha-Me'ati, *Sefer ha-Qanun* (Ms Oxford, Bodleian Libraries, Can. Or. 88, fol. 84[a]): זראונד … יועיל מהבהק וימרוק השנים ויועיל מן הטנופת אשר בהם ([Arab.] *zarāwand*: Birthwort [*Aristolochia longa* L., *A. rotunda* L., or *A. clematis* L.]: … It is useful for *bahaq*[153] (alphos), it cleans the teeth and is useful for dirty teeth (dental sordes)). Hebr. טנופת השנים is not attested in the current dictionaries. Zeraḥyah Ḥen translates Arab. أوساخ الأسنان as ליכלוך השנים (see entry לִכְלוּךְ) and Anonymous I has זוהמת השנים (see entry זהמה).

[טנף] • *Part. Pi'el* **מְטַנֵּף** • **סם המטנף** → **סַם**.

טרפה · **blood spot in the eye**: Arab. طرفة (cf. MMT 195 (253)) · Ibn Sīnā, *K. al-Qānūn* II · trans. Anonymous I, *Sefer ha-Qanun* (Ms Paris, BnF, héb. 1142, fols. 64[b]–65[b]): באקלא[154] … הוא עם דבש ופניגריג תחבשת לכהות העין ולטרפה ועם לבונה וורד וחלבון ביצה תחבשת לבליטה ([Arab.] *bāqillā*: Broad bean [*Vicia faba* L.]: … As a plaster with honey

152 חמורה (= Ms Paris, BnF, héb. 1136, fol. 64a): חמורתה Ms.

153 '*bahaq* (alphos)': There are three varieties of the disease called *bahaq* acc. to Ibn al-Jazzār (cf. IJZ 7:108, n. 196): white, black, and dust-colored. The white variety is perhaps identical with *Vitiligo alba*, while the black variety is possibly a sort of melanoderma. Arab. *bahaq* stands for Gr. ἀλφός, cf. UW 97: 'weiße Hautflecken.' Durling, *Dictionary of Medical Terms*, 34, translates the Gr. term as: 'dull-white leprosy.' See entry בַּהַק: הבהק הלבן.

154 באקלא: פולין והוא מין קטנית Ms[1].

and fenugreek, it is [useful] for a black eye and a blood spot in the eye, and as a plaster with frankincense, roses, and egg white, it is [useful] for protrusion [of the eye]). In the sense of 'a blood spot in the eye,' Hebr. טרפה is a non-attested loan word from Arab. طرفة. Zeraḥyah Ḥen renders the Arab. term as טרפה as well and Nathan ha-Me'ati translates the Arab. term as החולי הנקרא טרפה.

[יבש] • *Part. Pi'el* מְיַבֵּשׁ • הסם המיבש → סַם.

יָבֵשׁ • הקלפה היבשה → קְלִפָּה.

יָד • *Dual* יָדַיִם • יתדות הידים → יָתֵד.

• נעשה בידים → עָשָׂה.

יְדִיעָה • הקדמת הידיעה → הַקְדָּמָה.

יְהוּדִי • אבן יהודית → אֶבֶן.

• קוץ יהודי → קוֹץ

יַיִן • בלבול היין → בִּלְבּוּל.

[ילד] • *Hif'il* הוֹלִיד • הוליד התלאה · **to cause pain**: Arab. كَرَّب · Ibn Sīnā, *K. al-Qānūn* II · trans. Nathan ha-Me'ati, *Sefer ha-Qanun* (Ms Oxford, Bodleian Libraries, Can. Or. 88, fol. 109ª):[155] סקמוניא ... מוליד התלאה והאצטניסות ויסיר תאות המאכל ([Arab.] *saqmūnīyā* [from Gr. σκαμμωνία]: Scammony [*Convolvulus scammonia* L.]: ... It causes pain and nausea. It also suppresses appetite). Hebr. תְּלָאָה is not attested in the sense of 'pain' in the current dictionaries. In his trans. of Maimonides' *Medical Aphorisms* (i.e., *Sefer ha-Peraqim*) XVII.14, Nathan translates Arab. تكرّب as הצטער (cf. BMMN 172, l. 20; BMMG no. 4356). Zeraḥyah Ḥen translates Arab. كَرَّب as סיער and Anonymous I renders the Arab. term as ציער.

• *Part. Hif'il* מוֹלִיד • הסם המוליד הגסות → סַם.

יַלֶּפֶת • ילפת הצור · **lichen growing on rocks** [*Roccella tinctoria* DC]: Arab. حزاز الصخر (cf. DT 559 (IV. 46), n. 4 · Ibn Sīnā, *K. al-Qānūn* II · trans. Zeraḥyah Ḥen, *Sefer ha-Qanun* (Ms Oxford, Bodleian Libaries, Opp. Add. Fol. 12, fol. 219ª): טַחְלָב ... ואמנם הטחלב הצורי הוא ילפת הצור וכבר זכרנונו ([Arab.] *ṭuḥlub*: Common duckweed [*Lemna minor* L.]: ... We have already discussed 'duckweed growing on rocks', i.e., 'lichen growing on rocks'). Hebr. ילפת הצור is a non-attested calque form Arab. حزاز الصخر. For the identification of Arab. حزاز 'scurf; dandruff' as יַלֶּפֶת, cf. BCD 117 (NM 2:12f.). Nathan ha-Me'ati renders Arab. حزاز الصخر as טחלב על הסלעים and Anonymous I has נתק הסלעים (see entry נֶתֶק).

יָם • ארנבת הים → אַרְנֶבֶת.

[יסף] • *Inf. Hif'il* הוֹסִיף · **spreading**: Arab. انتشار · Ibn Sīnā, *K. al-Qānūn* II · trans. Nathan ha-Me'ati, *Sefer ha-Qanun* (Ms Oxford, Bodleian Libraries, Can. Or. 88, fol. 90ᵇ): כנדר ... הוא מסגר מאד וקל וחומר המכות הטריות וימנע הנגעים הרעים מלהוסיף ([Arab.] *kundur*: Frankincense [*Boswellia sacra* Flueck.]: ... It has a strong healing force, especially for fresh wounds; it prevents malignant ulcers from spreading). Hebr. *Inf. Hif'il* הוֹסִיף is not attested in this sense in the current dictionaries. Zeraḥyah Ḥen translates Arab.

---

155 The same Hebr. term features on fol. 78ᵇ, entry דנד '[Arab.] *dand*: Purging croton [*Croton tiglium* L.].'

انتشار as פָּשׁוּט (see entry) and Anonymous I has התפשט. In addition to הוֹסִיף, Nathan translates the Arab. term as תוספת.

• *Part. Nifʿal* נוֹסָף • השער הנוסף → שֵׂעָר.

יָצָא • המיץ היוצא מן החלב → מִיץ.

[יצב] • *Part. Nifʿal* נִצָּב • הנשימה הנצבת → נְשִׁימָה.

• *Part. Hitpaʿel* מִתְיַצֵּב • הנשימה המתיצבת → נְשִׁימָה.

יְצִיאָה • **יציאת העין** · **prolapse of the eye**: Arab. نتوء العين (cf. MMT 205 (263): 'prolapse of the eye (Exophthalmos);' UW 635: 'Prolaps der Uvea (σταφύλωμα)'[156]) · Ibn Sīnā, *K. al-Qānūn* II · trans. Zeraḥyah Ḥen, *Sefer ha-Qanun* (Ms Oxford, Bodleian Libaries, Opp. Add. Fol. 12, fol. 256ᵇ): עֻלַּיְק סנה ... יועיל מיציאת העין ([Arab.] *ʿullayq*; [i.e., Hebr.] *seneh*: Blackberry [*Rubus fruticosus* L.]: ... It is beneficial for prolapse of the eye). Nathan ha-Meʾati translates Arab. نتوء العين as סימני העין and Anonymous I has הצמחים שבעין.

יָרַד • *Inf.* רֶדֶת · **to be evacuated, excreted**: Arab. نزول · Ibn Sīnā, *K. al-Qānūn* II · trans. Zeraḥyah Ḥen, *Sefer ha-Qanun* (Ms Oxford, Bodleian Libaries, Opp. Add. Fol. 12, fol. 253ᵃ⁻ᵇ): סמַךְ דג ... ואמנם הקלוי הוא טוב לבעלי האצטומכא החזקה ועם הבשמים והצלוי על הגחלים הוא יותר מפרנס ויותר מתעכב לרדת והמבושל הוא הפך ([Arab.] *samak*; [i.e., Hebr.] *dag*: Fish: ... Fried fish is good for people having a strong stomach; the same holds good for spiced fish. Fish roasted over charcoal is more nutritious but is slow to be evacuated (excreted), while the reverse is true for cooked fish). Hebr. יָרַד, *Inf.* רֶדֶת, does not feature in a medical context in the current dictionaries. For *Hifʿil* הוֹרִיד in the sense of 'to evacuate,' see NM 5:95. Nathan ha-Meʾati and Anonymous I both render Arab. نزول as רֶדֶת, just like Zeraḥyah.

• המים שירדו בכיס הביצים → מַיִם.

יְרוֹקָה • **ירוקת המים** · **common duckweed** [***Lemna minor*** **L.**]: Arab. طحلب (cf. MIG no. 698) · *Glossary* (Ms Moscow, Russian State Library, Guenzburg 573, fol. 153ᵃ): טחלאב הוא ירוקת המים ([Arab.] *tuḥlub*; i.e, [Hebr.] *yeroqat ha-mayim*). Hebr. ירוקת המים is not attested in the current dictionaries. A synonymous Hebr. term הירוקה שעל פני המים features in NM 5:95f. in an attestation from Zeraḥyah Ḥen's trans. of Maimonides' *Medical Aphorismsm* (i.e., *Sefer ha-Peraqim*) XXI.79 (cf. BMMZ 204, l. 13; BMMG no. 3113), whereas Nathan ha-Meʾati has עדשי המים in XXV.54 (cf. BMMN 258, ll. 14, 16; BMMG no. 3113), a term also featuring in BCD 197 (NM 1:71f.) in an attestation from Moses ibn Tibbon's trans. of Ibn al-Jazzār's *Zād al-musāfir* (i.e., *Sefer Ṣedat ha-Derakhim*) VII.15.4 (cf. IJZ 7:150, l. 5). For Hebr. *Sing.* עדש המים, cf. also SHS 1:377 (Ayin 2).

יָרֵחַ • אבן הירח → אֶבֶן.

יָרֵךְ • *Dual* ירכים • ראשי הירכים → רֹאשׁ.

---

156 'Prolaps der Uvea' is Arab. نتوء العنبية (cf. MMT ibid.).

[ירש] • *Part. Hifʿil* **מוֹרִישׁ** • **מוריש הקרבונקלי** · **causing nausea**: Arab. مغث · Ibn Sīnā, *K. al-Qānūn* II · trans. Zeraḥyah Ḥen, *Sefer ha-Qanun* (Ms Oxford, Bodleian Libaries, Opp. Add. Fol. 12, fol. 253a): סֻמְסֻם שומשמין ... רע לאצטומכא מוריש הקרבונקלי מפיל תאות המזון משביע מהרה וכשהוא נאכל עם הדבש יסור הזקו ויאחר עכולו[157] וירפה הדקים ([Arab.] *simsim*; [i.e., Hebr.] *shumshemin*: Sesame [*Sesamum indicum* L.]: ... It is bad for the stomach and causes nausea. It reduces appetite and satiates quickly. When taken with honey, its harmful effects are removed. It delays digestion and softens the intestines). Hebr. *Hifʿil* הוריש הקרבונקלי is not attested in the current dictionaries.[158] Nathan ha-Me'ati translates Arab. مغث as מוליד האסטנסות (for אִסְטְנִיסוּת 'nausea; sickness in the stomach; urge to vomit,' cf. BCD 24 (NM 2:10, 30; 4:19)) and Anonymous I renders the Arab. term as מעורר אסטניסות (cf. NM 6:158 for an attestation from Nathan's trans. of Ibn Zuhr's *K. al-Aghdhiya* (i.e., *Sefer ha-Mezonot*)). Another synonym featuring in medieval Hebr. medical literature is גרם אסטניסות (cf. BCD 51 (NM 2:9f.)).

[ישן] • *Hitpaʿel* **הִתְיַשֵּׁן** · **to become rancid**: Arab. زنخ · Ibn Sīnā, *K. al-Qānūn* II · trans. Anonymous I, *Sefer ha-Qanun* (Ms Paris, BnF, héb. 1142, fol. 3b): והשקד אע״פ שהוא שוה ודק כשיתישן יחמם בחוזק (Although almond [oil] is moderate and fine, when it becomes rancid, it becomes very hot). Hebr. הִתְיַשֵּׁן is not attested in this sense in the current dictionaries. Synonyms featuring in Anonymous I's trans. are הֵרִיחַ (see entry [ריח]) and קיבל העפוש הנקרא רנציד (see entry [קבל]).

• *Part. Nifʿal* **נוֹשָׁן** · **chronic**: Arab. مزمن · Ibn Sīnā, *K. al-Qānūn*, Hebr. trans. Anonymous I, Ms Paris, BnF, héb. 1142: פראסיון ... סחיטתו לכאב האוזן נושן ומנקה ופותח מעברי השמע ומסיר הנושן מכאביה ([Arab.] *farāsiyūn*: Common horehound [*Marrubium vulgare* L.]: ... Its juice [is beneficial] for chronic earache; it opens and cleanses the auditory channels and relieves chronic pain [in the ear]). In the sense of 'chronic,' Hebr. נוֹשָׁן features in the Bible (Lev 13:11; cf. KB 448). Nathan ha-Me'ati translates Arab. مزمن as יָשָׁן (see next entry) and Zeraḥyah Ḥen renders the Arab. term as קַדְמוֹן and אָרֹךְ (see entries).

יָשָׁן · **chronic**: Arab. مزمن · Ibn Sīnā, *K. al-Qānūn* II · trans. Nathan ha-Me'ati, *Sefer ha-Qanun* (Ms Oxford, Bodleian Libraries, Can. Or. 88, fol. 90b): פראסיון ... מיצו יועיל לכאב האזן הישן ויפתח וינקה מעברי השמע ויסיר כאב האזן הישן ([Arab.] *farāsiyūn*: Common horehound [*Marrubium vulgare* L.]: ... Its juice is beneficial for chronic earache; it cleanses and opens the auditory channels and relieves chronic pain [in the ear]). Hebr. יָשָׁן is not attested in this sense in the current dictionaries. Zeraḥyah Ḥen translates Arab. مزمن as קַדְמוֹן (see entry) and Anonymous I renders the Arab. term as *Part. Nifʿal* נוֹשָׁן (see previous entry). The latter term features also (for Arab. مزمن)

---

157 עכולו: Emend. ed. עקולו Ms.

158 For *Hifʿil* הוֹרִישׁ on its own in the sense of 'to cause,' see NM 6:94. For קרבונקלי in the sense of 'nausea,' see entry below.

in Nathan's trans. of Maimonides, *Medical Aphorisms* (i.e., *Sefer ha-Peraqim*) XIII.30 (cf. BMMN 149, l. 10; BMMG no. 95).

[ישר] • *Pi'el* **יִשֵּׁר** · **to balance**: Arab. عدّل · Ibn Sīnā, *K. al-Qānūn* II · trans. Nathan ha-Me'ati, *Sefer ha-Qanun* (Ms Oxford, Bodleian Libraries, Can. Or. 88, fol. 57[a]): והמחזיק הוא שמנהגו ליישר תכונת האבר ומנהגו עד שימנענו מלקבל היתרונים הנשפכים אליו והפגעים (A tonic [drug] is a drug that—by its nature—balances the consistency and temperament of an organ to an extent that it prevents the absorption of superfluous matter and disorders that move towards it). Hebr. יִשֵּׁר is not attested for medieval medical literature. Zeraḥyah Ḥen translates Arab. عدّل as *Pi'el* מִצַּע (see entry [מצע]) and Anonymous I has *Hif'il* הִשְׁוָה (see entry [שוה]).

יָשָׁר · **moderate**: Arab. معتدل · al-Rāzī, *K. fī al-Faṣd* · trans. Anonymous, *Ma'amar ba-Haqqazah* (Ms Parma, Biblioteca Palatina, Cod. Parm. 2283,4, fol. 95[a]): צריך שיהיה הבית אשר הקיז בו ישר האויר עליון התקרה פתוח אל הצפון שטוח עם סמי הריח הטובים והורדים ומיני הפירות והמגדים (The house in which venesection is carried out should have moderate air, a high ceiling, [should be] open towards the north, with fragrant ingredients, roses, and choice fruit spread out in it). In the sense of 'moderate,' Hebr. יָשָׁר features in BCD 122 (NM 1:156) in an attestation from Zeraḥyah Ḥen's trans. of Maimonides' *Medical Aphorisms* (i.e., *Sefer ha-Peraqim*) VIII.2 (cf. BMMZ 87, l. 2; BMMG no. 1753: החפיפה הישרה 'the moderate massage').

יָתֵד • *Plur.* יתדות • **יתדות הידים** · **bony prominences in the forearms (wrists)**: Lat. *caville manuum* · Guy de Chauliac, *Inventarium sive Chirurgia Magna* (cf. CMM 1:417, ll. 16–17) · trans. Anonymous (Ms Paris, BnF, héb. 1189, fol. 228[a]): המבעבעים באמת מונחים במקומות שבין העור כמו תחת הזקן ואחור הצואר ובכל הפנים וביתדות הידים והרגלים כי לא ימשכו כי אם הליחה שהוא תחת העור (Vesicant medicines are really those that are put between skin [and flesh] (beneath the skin), such as [those that are put] under the chin, and behind the neck, and on the whole face, and on the bony prominences in the forearms (wrists), and the malleoli of the feet (ankles), for they only attract the moisture that is beneath the skin). Hebr. יתדות הידים is not attested in the current dictionaries.

• **יתדות הרגלים** · **the malleoli of the feet (ankles)**: Lat. *caville pedum* (cf. ND 180) · Guy de Chauliac, *Inventarium sive Chirurgia Magna* (cf. CMM 1:417, ll. 16–17) · trans. Anonymous (Ms Paris, BnF, héb. 1189, fol. 228[a]): המבעבעים באמת מונחים במקומות שבין העור כמו תחת הזקן ואחור הצואר ובכל הפנים וביתדות הידים והרגלים כי לא ימשכו כי אם הליחה שהוא תחת העור (Vesicant medicines are really those that are put between skin [and flesh] (beneath the skin), such as [those that are put] under the chin, and behind the neck, and on the whole face, and on the malleoli of the feet (ankles), and the bony prominences in the forearms (wrists), for they attract the moisture that is beneath the skin). Hebr. יתדות הרגלים is not attested in the current dictionaries.

יֶתֶר • **יתר הזרוע** · **funis brachii (median cephalic vein of the arm); vena cephalica pollicis (cephalic vein of the thumb)**: Arab. حبل الذراع (cf. FA no. 1488; DKT 816) · al-

Rāzī, *K. fī al-Faṣd* · trans. Anonymous, *Ma'amar ba-Haqqazah* (Ms Parma, Biblioteca Palatina, Cod. Parm. 2283,4, fol. 94[a]): וב׳[159] גידים בחיצוני מקומות הנקרא אלמעצמין והם האמות בזרוע ונק׳ יתרי הזרוע והם מגיד אלבסליק (Two veins in the place of the wrists in the arms, they are called 'funis brachii (vena cephalica),' they come from the basilic vein). Hebr. יתר הזרוע is not attested in the current dictionaries.

159 וב׳ גידים בחיצוני מקומות הנקרא אלמעצמין והם האמות בזרוע: عرقان في موضع المعصمين في الذراعين a.

כ

[כאב] • *Hifʿil* **הִכְאִיב** • **הכאיב הבטן** · **to cause gripes (colic)**: Arab. أمغص · Ibn Sīnā, *K. al-Qānūn* II · trans. Anonymous I, *Sefer ha-Qanun* (Ms Paris, BnF, héb. 1142, fol. 105[a]): דנד הוא מין קטאפוסיא ... הציני הוא היותר טוב ויותר חזק מן ההנדי והשחרי רע מאוחר המעשה ומצער ומכאיב הבטן וראוי שתקלף הציני בברזל ([Arab.] *dand*; i.e., a kind of [Rom.] QṬʾPWSYʾ [i.e., *catapucia*]: Purging croton [*Croton tiglium* L.]: ... Chinese [croton] is better and stronger than the Indian [variety]. [The variety] that grows among rocks is inferior, slow in action, and is causing pain and gripes (colic). The Chinese [variety] should be peeled off with an iron [knife]). Hebr. הכאיב הבטן is not attested in the current dictionaries. Nathan ha-Meʾati translates Arab. أمغص as עקץ המעים and Zeraḥyah Ḥen has simply עָקַץ (for both terms, see entry עָקַץ).

כְּאֵב • **כאב האזנים** · **ringing in the ears (tinnitus)**: Arab. الدويّ في الأذن · Ibn Sīnā, *K. al-Qānūn* II · trans. Nathan ha-Meʾati, *Sefer ha-Qanun* (Ms Oxford, Bodleian Libraries, Can. Or. 88, fol. 85[b]):[160] חנטל ... ואם יבושל בשמן זית ויטיפו ממנו באזן יועיל לכאה האזנים ([Arab.] *ḥanẓal*: Colocynth [*Citrullus colocynthis* (L.) Schrad.]: ... If it is boiled in olive oil and dripped into the ear, it is useful for ringing in the ears (tinnitus)). Hebr. כאב האזנים does not feature in this specific sense in the current dictionaries. Zeraḥyah Ḥen translates Arab. الدويّ في الأذن as צלילת האזן (for similar terms, cf. BCD 229 (4:172), s.v. צְלִילָה, and NM 5:168, s.v. צִלְצוּל) and Anonymous I, possibly reading Arab. الدود في الأذن as الدويّ في الأذن, renders the Arab. term as תולעת באוזן.

• **כאב חצי הראש** · **migraine; hemicrania**: Arab. شقيقة · Ibn Sīnā, *K. al-Qānūn* II · trans. Nathan ha-Meʾati, *Sefer ha-Qanun* (Ms Oxford, Bodleian Libraries, Can. Or. 88, fol. 123[a]): רכמה והוא רחם ... יטיפו מררתו עם שמן בנפסג בצד המתחלף מכאב חצי הראש והוא שקיקה בער׳ ([Arab.] *rakham*; i.e., [Hebr.] *raḥam*: Vulture: ... Its gallbladder together with violet oil is instilled into the ear opposite to the affected side in case of migraine (hemicrania); i.e., *shaqīqa* in Arab.). Hebr. כאב חצי הראש features in MD 344, s.v. 'hemicrania.' A synonym featuring in Nathan's trans. of Maimonides, *Medical Aphorisms* (i.e., *Sefer ha-Peraqim*) is פלוח הראש (cf. BMMG no. 2711; cf. also NM 6:175 for an attestation from Nathan's trans. of Ibn Zuhr's *K. al-Aghdhiya* (i.e., *Sefer ha-Mezonot*)). Zeraḥyah Ḥen translates Arab. شقيقة as Rom. מגרניאהץ (from Gr. ἡμικρανία / L. Lat. *hemicrania*) and Anonymous I has כאב חצי הראש, just like Nathan.

• **כאב המעים** · **gripes (colic)**: Arab. مغص (Gr. στρόφος; cf. UW 644; FL 4:196: 'tormina') · al-Rāzī, *K. fī al-Faṣd* · trans. Anonymous, *Maʾamar ba-Haqqazah* (Ms Parma, Biblioteca Palatina, Cod. Parm. 2283,4, fol. 96[a]): אלבסליק יועיל ממורסת הצלעות ... ומכאב המעים הנק׳ אלמגץ הבא פתאם ([Bleeding] the basilic vein is beneficial for pleurisy ... and for sudden gripes (colic), called [in Arab.] *al-maghṣ*). In the sense of 'gripes

---

160 Cf. also Hebr. כאב האזן (for Arab. دويّ) on fol. 95[a], entry חרבק 'Hellebore [*Helleborus* sp.]'.

(colic),' Hebr. כאב המעים features as כאב מעים in BCD 123 (NM 2:52f.) in an attestation from Nathan ha-Me'ati's trans. of Maimonides' *Medical Aphorisms* (i.e., *Sefer ha-Peraqim*) XII.7 (cf. BMMN 139, l. 16; BMMG no. 4888). Synonyms for 'colic,' featuring in medieval Hebr. medical literature, are: הֶמְיָה (cf. BCD 67 (NM 3:64)); חבלים (cf. BCD 88 (NM 3:78)); חבלי הבטן (cf. NM 6:70); חִיל (cf. NM 6:72); חֲרָפָּה (cf. NM 5:84f.); חִתּוּךְ (cf. NM 6:83); מָצוֹק (cf. BCD 156f. (NM 3:136)); משברים (cf. NM 6:129f.); עִוּוּת (cf. BCD 197f. (NM 4:142); NM 5:144f.); עֲקִיצָה (cf. BCD 212f. (NM 3:182)); עקיצת המעיים (cf. NM 6:168); צירים (cf. BCD 228 (NM 3:191f.)); צירים בבטן (cf. BCD 228 (NM 4:170)); and צירים וחבלים (cf. BCD 228 (NM 4:170f.)).

• **כאב הצד** · **pleuralgia**: Arab. وجع الجنب · Ibn Sīnā, *K. al-Qānūn* II · trans. Zeraḥyah Ḥen, *Sefer ha-Qanun* (Ms Oxford, Bodleian Libaries, Opp. Add. Fol. 12, bk. 2, fol. 174[a]): אִעַאלוּג'י ... מועיל מכאב הצד ([Arab.] *aghālūjī*: Agarwood [*Aquilaria malaccensis* Lam.]: ... It is beneficial for pleuralgia). Hebr. כאב הצד is not attested in the current dictionaries. For a variant reading כאב הצדדים, see BCD 123 (NM 3:112, corr.) for an attestation from Do'eg ha-Edomi's trans. of Hippocrates' *Aphorisms* (i.e., *Sefer Agur*) III.23. Nathan translates Arab. وجع الجنب as כאב הצלעות. The latter Hebr. term is used by both Zeraḥyah and Nathan for the Arab. synonym وجع الجنبين.

כֹּבֶד • **כבד התנועה** · **numbness**: Arab. خدر · al-Rāzī, *K. fī al-Faṣd* · trans. Anonymous, *Ma'amar ba-Haqqazah* (Ms Parma, Biblioteca Palatina, Cod. Parm. 2283,4, fol. 94[b]): הקזת הקיפאל יועיל ... מכבד התנועה הנקרא אלכדר עם אדמימות המראה ומהזלות הראש הנק' זוכאם (Bleeding the cephalic vein is beneficial ... for numbness, called [in Arab.] *al-khadar*, combined with redness of the face, and for rheum called [in Arab.] *zukām*). Hebr. כבד התנועה is not attested in the current dictionaries. Synonyms featuring in medieval medical literature are: בִּטּוּל (cf. BCD 32 (NM 1:130)); בטול ההרגש (see entry בִּטּוּל above); בטול החוש (cf. BCD 32 (NM 3:31)); צִנּוּן (cf. NM 6:182); רִפְיוֹן (cf. NM 6:204f.); תַּרְדֵּמָה (cf. NM 6:221f.); and תרדמת האיברים (cf. NM 5:205).

[כבה] • *Pu'al* **כֻּבָּה** • **אבן יכבה בשמן** → אֶבֶן.

כֵּהוּת • **כהות העין** · **black eye**: Arab. كمودة العين (Gr. ὑπώπιον;[161] cf. UW2:561f.; LSG 1904) · Ibn Sīnā, *K. al-Qānūn* II · trans. Anonymous I, *Sefer ha-Qanun* (Ms Paris, BnF, héb. 1142, fols. 64[b]–65[b]): באקלא[162] ... הוא עם דבש ופניגריג תחבשת לכהות העין ולטרפה ועם לבונה וורד וחלבון ביצה תחבשת לבליטה ([Arab.] *bāqillā*: Broad bean [*Vicia faba* L.]: ... As a plaster with honey and fenugreek, it is [useful] for a black eye and a blood spot in the eye, and as a plaster with frankincense, roses, and egg white, it is [useful] for protrusion [of the eye]). Hebr. כהות העין is not attested in the current dictionaries. Nathan ha-Me'ati translates Arab. كمودة العين as חשכת העין (see entry חֲשֵׁכָה) and Zer-

---

161 Cf. the parallel entry on 'broad bean' [*Vicia faba* L.] in the Arab. trans. of Dioscorides' *De materia medica* (Ms Paris, BnF, arabe 2849, fol. 43[a]): كمودة لون الموضع ويسمى باليونانية اوقوفيا. The term اوقوفيا (read: اوفوفيا) is Gr. ὑπώπιον, *Plur.* ὑπώπια.

162 באקלא: פולין והוא מין קטנית Ms[1].

aḥyah Ḥen translates the Arab. term as שחרות העין (see entry שַׁחֲרוּת). For Hebr. כהות עיניים in the sense of 'dimsightedness,' featuring in Rabb. literature and in Joseph Delmedigo's trans. of Hippocrates' *Aphorisms* III.31 (for Gr. ἀμβλυώπια), cf. NM 5:100, s.v. כהות הראות.

כָּוָה • *Part.* כּוֹוֶה · **cautery**: Lat. *cauterium* · Guy de Chauliac, *Inventarium sive Chirurgia Magna* (cf. CMM 1:235, ll. 6–7) · trans. Anonymous (Ms Paris, BnF, héb. 1189, fol. 128[b]): ואני ראיתי פעמים רבות שחמימות הכווה היה מקבל הקנה שהחולה לא היה יכול לסבול הפעלה (I have often seen that the cautery caused the windpipe of the patient to become so hot that he could not endure the [surgical] treatment (cauterization)). Hebr. *Part.* כּוֹוֶה is not attested in the current dictionaries.

• **הסם הכווה** → סַם.

• **הרפואה הכווה** → רְפוּאָה.

כּוֹוֶה (*Part.*) → כָּוָה.

כָּווּץ (*Part. Pass.*) → כָּוַץ.

כּוֹזֵב (*Part.*) → כָּזַב.

כְּוִיָּה · I. **burning**: Arab. حرقة · Ibn Sīnā, *K. al-Qānūn* II · trans. Nathan ha-Me'ati, *Sefer ha-Qanun* (Ms Oxford, Bodleian Libraries, Can. Or. 88, fol. 109[a]): סוס ... יועיל מכוית השתן ויועיל מנגעי הכליות וכיס השתן וחדודם ([Arab.] *sūs*: Licorice [i.e., the root of *Glycyrrhiza glabra* L.]: ... It is useful in cases of burning urine, ulcers in the intestines and urinary bladder, and for [relieving irritation in these organs]). Hebr. כְּוִיָּה is attested in MD 141, s.v. 'cauterization, cautery.' Zeraḥyah Ḥen and Anonymous I both translate Arab. حرقة as שריפה.

· II. **cauterization**: Lat. *cauterizacio* · Guy de Chauliac, *Inventarium sive Chirurgia Magna* (cf. CMM 1:413, l. 33) · trans. Anonymous (Ms Paris, BnF, héb. 1189, fol. 225[a]): הכויה היא פועל היד נעשת עם האש בגוף האדם לתועלת מה מוגבל (Cauterization is a manual operation that is carried with fire on a person's body to achieve a certain benefit). See previous entry.

• **כוית המים החמים** · **scald**: Arab. حرق الماء الحار · Ibn Sīnā, *K. al-Qānūn* II · trans. Zeraḥyah Ḥen, *Sefer ha-Qanun* (Ms Oxford, Bodleian Libaries, Opp. Add. Fol. 12, fols. 248[a]–249[a]): סוּסַן גִ'ליו ... והפרדסי יותר משובח משאר הרפואות לכוית המים החמים ([Arab.] *sawsan*; [i.e., Rom.] ǦiLYWu [i.e., Ital.-Rom. *giglio*]: Lily [*Lilium* L.] or iris [*Iris* L.]: ... The cultivated variety is most beneficial for scalds). Hebr. כוית המים החמים is not attested in the current dictionaries. Nathan ha-Me'ati and Anonymous I both render Arab. حرق الماء الحار as שרפת המים החמים (see entry שְׂרֵפָה).

כּוֹכָב • **כוכב כלב** · **Sirius**: Arab. الشعرى العبور[163] · Ibn Sīnā, *K. al-Qānūn* II · trans. Anonymous I, *Sefer ha-Qanun* (Ms Paris, BnF, héb. 1142, fol. 49[a]): בלסאן ... ויוקח שמנו שישרט

163 Cf. Y. Rapoport and E. Savage-Smith (eds.), *An Eleventh-Century Egyptian Guide to the Universe: The* Book of Curiosities (Leiden 2014), 643.

בברזל אחר עליית כוכב כלב הנקר׳ אלשערי ([Arab.] *balasān*: Balsam of Mecca [*Commiphora opobalsamum* (L.) Engl.]: ... Its oil should be obtained through making an incision [in its trunk] with an iron instrument after the rise of Sirius). Hebr. כוכב כלב is not attested in the current dictionaries. Nathan ha-Me'ati renders Arab. الشعرى العبور as הכוכב הנקרא שערא בערבי and Zeraḥyah Ḥen translates Arab. طلوع الشعرى العبور as עלות השמש בימי הקיץ. In their trans. of Maimonides' *Medical Aphorisms* (i.e., *Sefer ha-Peraqim*) III.68, Nathan renders Arab. طلوع الشعرى العبور 'the rise of Sirius' as עלית הכוכב הנקרא אלשערא אל עבור והוא הכלב (BMMN 49, ll. 21–22; BMMG no. 3164) and Zeraḥyah renders the Arab. term as עלות כוכב הכלב (cf. BMMZ 43, l. 7; BMMG no. 3164).

כָּוַץ • *Part. Pass.* כָּווּץ · **curly**: Arab. جَعد (cf. D 1:197) · Ibn Sīnā, *K. al-Qānūn* II · trans. Anonymous I, *Sefer ha-Qanun* (Ms Paris, BnF, héb. 1142, fol. 147[a]): לוף הוא שרפנטינה ... שרש הכווץ ממרק עדשי הפנים והבהק והנמש ... ובייחוד עם דבש ויוטח ביין על בקיעי הקור ([Arab.] *lūf*; [i.e., Rom.] ŠRPNṬYNH [i.e., O. Occ. [*herba*] *serpentina* (cf. BMZ 48f., 89 (Lamed 6))]: Arum [*Arum* sp., e.g., snakeshead [*Arum maculatum* L.]]: ... The root of the curly variety clears freckles, *bahaq*[164] (alphos), and acne ... especially [when applied] with honey. [Mixed] with wine, it is put on chilblains). The term כָּווּץ is a *Part. Pass.* of the verb כָּוַץ, which features in BM 2306 in the sense of 'to shrink' and in Rabb. literature also in the sense of 'to curl' (cf. JD 625). Nathan ha-Me'ati translates Arab. جَعد as שאינו חלק and Zeraḥyah Ḥen has תַּלְתַּלִּי (see entry).

כּוּשִׁי • *Plur.* **כושים • אבן הכושים** → אֶבֶן.

כָּזַב • *Part.* **כּוֹזֵב** · **false; fake**: Arab. كاذب · Ibn Sīnā, *K. al-Qānūn* II · trans. Zeraḥyah Ḥen, *Sefer ha-Qanun* (Ms Oxford, Bodleian Libaries, Opp. Add. Fol. 12, fol. 196[a]): ... דַּאר צִינִי ויש מן הקינמון שהוא נקרא הקינמון הכוזב ויש לו מעט ריח והוא גס וכחו חלוש ([Arab.] *dārṣīnī*: Cinnamon [*Cinnamomum verum* J. Presl]: ... One variety of cinnamon, called 'false cinnamon,' has mild odor, it is hard and its potency is weak). Hebr. *Part.* כּוֹזֵב is not attested in a medical context in the current dictionaries. Anonymous I renders Arab. كاذب as כּוֹזֵב, just like Zeraḥyah, and Nathan ha-Me'ati translates Arab. كاذب as *Part. Pi'el* מְכַזֵּב (see next entry).

• *Part. Pi'el* **מְכַזֵּב** · **false; fake**: Arab. كاذب · Ibn Sīnā, *K. al-Qānūn* II · trans. Nathan ha-Me'ati, Sefer ha-Qanun (Ms Oxford, Bodleian Libraries, Can. Or. 88, fol. 76[v]: דרציני ... ויש מהדרציני מין נקרא דרציני המכזב ולו ריח טוב וכחו חלש ([Arab.] *dārṣīnī*: Cinnamon [*Cinnamomum verum* J. Presl]: One variety of cinnamon, called 'false cinnamon,' is fragrant and its potency is weak). Hebr. *Part. Pi'el* מְכַזֵּב is not attested in a medical

164 '*bahaq* (alphos)': There are three varieties of the disease called *bahaq* acc. to Ibn al-Jazzār (cf. IJZ 7:108, n. 196): white, black, and dust-colored. The white variety is perhaps identical with *Vitiligo alba*, while the black variety is possibly a sort of melanoderma. Arab. *bahaq* stands for Gr. ἀλφός, cf. UW 97: 'weiße Hautflecken.' Durling, *Dictionary of Medical Terms*, 34, translates the Gr. term as: 'dull-white leprosy.' See entry בַּהַק: הבהק הלבן.

context in the current dictionaries. Zeraḥyah Ḥen and Anonymous I both render Arab. كاذب as *Part.* כּוֹזֵב (see previous entry).

כֹּחַ¹ · roughtail rock agama (stellion) [*Stellagama stellio* **(Linnaeus, 1758)]**: Arab. حرذون (cf. MM 235) · Ibn Sīnā, *K. al-Qānūn* II · trans. Nathan ha-Me'ati, *Sefer ha-Qanun* (Ms Oxford, Bodleian Libraries, Can. Or. 88, fol. 78ᵇ): דם ... דם האנקה הנקרא ורל בערבי ודם הכח הנקרא חרדון בערבי יחזקו הראות (Blood: ... The blood of the monitor lizard, called *waral* in Arab., and that of the roughtail rock agama (stellion), called *ḥirdhawn* in Arab., strengthen vision). Hebr. כֹּחַ is attested in the Bible (Lev 11:30) and in the *Diwan* of Samuel ha-Nagid as 'a species of lizard' (cf. KB 469; BM 2312). According to Feliks (FAB 99), it is identical with the 'monitor lizard' (esp. desert monitor [*Varanus griseus* (Daudin, 1803)] and Nile monitor [*Varanus niloticus* (Linnaeus, 1766)]). The identification of Hebr. כֹּחַ as Arab. حرذون already features in Sa'adya's trans. of Lev 11:30[165] and subsequently in Ibn Janāḥ's *K. al-Uṣūl*:[166] והאנקה והכח الحرذون. Zeraḥyah Ḥen translates Arab. حرذون as שגומיל and Anonymous I renders the Arab. term as כֹּחַ, just like Nathan.

כֹּחַ² • כח בורקי · nitrous (alkaline) property: Arab. بورقية · Ibn Sīnā, *K. al-Qānūn* II · trans. Anonymous I, *Sefer ha-Qanun* (Ms Paris, BnF, héb. 1142, fol. 189ᵇ): סלק ... הסלק יש בו כח בורקי מדקדק ובו חתך ופתוח יותר חזק מחתך הירק הנקר' סרמק ([Arab.] *silq*: Beet [*Beta vulgaris* L.]: ... Beet has a nitrous refining property; its dissolving, deobstruant property is stronger than that of garden orach). In the sense of 'nitrous (alkaline) property,' Hebr. כח בורקי is not attested in the current dictionaries. For the Adj. בורקי in the sense of 'nitrous' (for Lat. *nitrosus*), cf. BCD 31 (NM 4:25) for an attestation from Abraham Avigdor's trans. of Arnau de Villanova's *Medicationis Parabole* (i.e., *Pirqei Arnavṭ de-Villa Nova*) IV.13 (50). In their trans. of Maimonides' *Medical Aphorisms* (i.e., *Sefer ha-Peraqim*) XXI.59, Nathan ha-Me'ati and Zeraḥyah Ḥen both translate Arab. الأشياء البورقية والمالحة 'the alkaline and salty things' with the Adj. בורקי as הדברים הבורקיים והמלוחים (cf. BMMN 203, l. 13; BMMZ 201, l. 7; BMMG no. 2783). Anonymous I translates Arab. بورقية as בּוֹרְקִיּוּת (see entry), while Zeraḥyah Ḥen renders the Arab. term as בורקיית.

כְּחִילָה · application [of an ingredient] as a collyrium: Arab. اكتحال · Ibn Sīnā, *K. al-Qānūn* II · trans. Anonymous I, *Sefer ha-Qanun* (Ms Paris, BnF, héb. 1142, fols. 195ᵃ–196ᵃ): סמך ... עור דג סקיאקון[167] יחוכך בו העפעפים בעלי הגרב ויועיל ועור השרוף גם כן נכנס ברפואות בכחולים ומסיר הכחילה בו עם המלה הצפורן ([Arab.] *samak*: Fish: ... Rubbing with skin of sword fish (?) is useful for someone suffering from itching of the eyelids. Its burnt skin is incorporated in collyria for the eye. Application as a collyrium with

165 Cf. Derenbourg (ed.), *Targum Ḥamishah Ḥumshei Torah be-Lashon 'Aravit le-Rabbeinu Sa'adyah Ga'on ben Yoseph ha-Fayyumi*, 158.

166 Col. 310.

167 סקיאקון: سيفيانوس a.

some salt removes pterygium). Hebr. כְּחִילָה features in BM 2322 in attestations from Nathan ben Yo'el Falaquera's *Sefer Ṣori ha-Guf*[168] and Ibn Sīnā's *Sefer ha-Qanun*. Nathan ha-Me'ati and Zeraḥyah Ḥen both translatesArab. اكتحال as כְּחַל.

כִּיס • כיס הרועה · **shepherd's purse [*Capsella bursa-pastoris* (L.) Medik.]**: Lat. *bursa pastoris* · Guy de Chauliac, *Inventarium sive Chirurgia Magna* (cf. CMM 1:235, ll. 18–19) · trans. Anonymous (Ms Paris, BnF, héb. 1189, fol. 128[b]): פוליגיאוני שהוא וירגא פשטוריש או כיס הרועה נקר' בורסא[169] פשטוריש ([Lat.] PWLYGY'WNY [i.e., *poligonia*]; i.e., [Lat.] WYRG' PŠṬWRYŠ [i.e., *virga pastoris*] or [Hebr.] *kis ha-ro'eh*, [also] called [in Lat.] BWRS' PŠṬWRYS [i.e., *bursa pastoris*]). Hebr. כיס הרועה is a non-attested calque from Lat. *bursa pastoris*.

• **המים שירדו בכיס הביצים** → מַיִם.

כֶּלֶב • *Plur.* **כלבים • זנגביל הכלבים** → זַנְגְּבִיל.

• **כוכב כלב** → כּוֹכָב.

כְּלִי • כלי נקוב · **funnel**: Arab. قمع · Ibn Sīnā, *K. al-Qānūn* II · trans. Zeraḥyah Ḥen, *Sefer ha-Qanun* (Ms Oxford, Bodleian Libaries, Opp. Add. Fol. 12, fols. 228[b]–229[a]): ... לַאדַן יתיר מורסות הרחם לסבול אותו עם פתילה ויוציא העובר המת והשליה בעשן בו עם הכלי הנקוב וכשישתנו עם יין ישן יעצור הבטן וירבה השתן ([Arab.] *lādhan*: Ladanum [i.e., the resin of various species of *Cistus* L.]: ... When used as a suppository, it dissolves uterine swellings. Fumigation with a funnel extracts a dead fetus and placenta. When taken orally with old wine, it causes constipation and diuresis). Hebr. כלי נקוב is not attested in the current dictionaries. Nathan renders Arab. قمع as שפופרת and Anonymous I has משפך.

כַּמִּינָה • כמינת הדם תחת העין: **dark blood collected beneath the tissue under the eye (ecchymosis)**: Arab. كهوبة الدم تحت العين · Ibn Sīnā, *K. al-Qānūn* II · trans. Anonymous I, *Sefer ha-Qanun* (Ms Paris, BnF, héb. 1142, fol. 136[a–b]: כמון ... הנה ילעס ויעורב בשמן זית ויוטף על הצפורן ועל כמינת הדם תחת העין ([Arab.] *kammūn* / [Hebr.] *kammon*: Cumin: ... Chewed and mixed with olive oil it is applied for pterygium and for dark blood collected beneath the tissue under the eye (ecchymosis)). Hebr. כמינת הדם תחת העין is not attested in the current dictionaries. Nathan ha-Me'ati translates Arab. كهوبة الدم تحت العين as הטמנת הדם תחת העין (see entry הַטְמָנָה) and Zeraḥyah Ḥen has הסתרת הדם תחת העין (see entry הַסְתָּרָה).

כִּנָּה • *Plur.* **כנים • כנים עגולים** · **ticks**: Arab. قُرَاد · Ibn Sīnā, *K. al-Qānūn* II · trans. Nathan ha-Me'ati, *Sefer ha-Qanun* (Ms Oxford, Bodleian Libraries, Can. Or. 88, fol. 116[b]): פסאקין: אמרו שהוא שרץ דומה אל הכנים העגולים ובערבי קראד ([Arab.] PS'QYN [read: PS'PYS, i.e., *fasāfis*]: Bed bugs: It is said that they are insects similar to ticks, [called] in Arab.

168 See G. Bos and R. Fontaine, 'Medico-Philosophical Controversies in Nathan b. Yo'el Falaquera's *Sefer Ṣori ha-Guf*,' *Jewish Quarterly Review* 90 (1999): 27–60.

169 בורסא: Emend. ed. בוסא Ms.

qurād). Hebr. כנים עגולים is not attested in the current dictionaries. The term כִּנָּה, *Plur.* כנים, on its own features in KB 483, s.v. כֵּן in the sense of 'gnat; louse,' cf. JD 648, s.v. כִּנָּא; BM 2433f., s.v. כֵּן״. Zeraḥyah Ḥen translates Arab. قُراد as קוף (see entry) and Anonymous I renders the Arab. term as פִּשְׁפֵּשׁ (see entry).

• ביצי הכנים → בֵּיצָה •.

כִּסּוּי • כסוי הראות · **dimness of sight**: Arab. غشاوة (Gr. ἀμβλυωπία; cf. UW 99f.) · Ibn Sīnā, *K. al-Qānūn* II · trans. Nathan ha-Me'ati, *Sefer ha-Qanun* (Ms Oxford, Bodleian Libraries, Can. Or. 88, fols. 76b–77a): דרציני ... יועיל מכסוי הראות והחשכה ([Arab.] *dārṣīnī*: Cinnamon [*Cinnamomum verum* J. Presl]: ... It is beneficial for dimness and dullness of sight). Hebr. כסוי הראות is not attested in the current dictionaries. Anonymous I renders Arab. غشاوة as סנור (הנקר' גשאוה) (see entry סַנְוֵר). Synonymous terms used by Nathan are הכסוי על העין (see next entry) and חשכת העין (see entry חֲשֵׁכָה).

• **הכסוי על העין** · **dimness of sight**: Arab. غشاوة · Ibn Sīnā, *K. al-Qānūn* II · trans. Nathan ha-Me'ati, *Sefer ha-Qanun* (Ms Oxford, Bodleian Libraries, Can. Or. 88, bk. 2, fols. 68a–68b):[170] בלסאן ... ימרוק הכסוי על העין הוא ומשיחתו ([Arab.] *balasān*: Balsam of Mecca [*Commiphora opobalsamum* (L.) Engl.]: [Balsam of Mecca] and its oil cleanse dimness of sight). Hebr. הכסוי על העין is not attested in the current dictionaries. Synonymous terms used by Nathan are כסוי הראות (see previous entry) and חשכת העין (see entry חֲשֵׁכָה). Zeraḥyah Ḥen translates Arab. غشاوة as סנורים (see entry סַנְוֵר) and Anonymous I has הסנור (הנקר' גשאוה) (see also entry סַנְוֵר).

כֶּסֶף • כסף חי נמוח · **'killed' quicksilver (mercury)**:[171] Arab. زئبق مقتول · Ibn Sīnā, *K. al-Qānūn* II · trans. Nathan ha-Me'ati, *Sefer ha-Qanun* (Ms Oxford, Bodleian Librar-

---

170 The same Hebr. term features on fol. 88a, entry חגר אלחבש '[Arab.] *ḥajar al-Ḥabash*: Ethiopian stone.'

171 On the application of quicksilver (mercury) as a remedy for a variety of illnesses in medieval Arab. medical literature, cf. N. Bachour, 'Healing with Mercury: The Uses of Mercury in Arabic Medical Literature,' *Asia* 69, no. 4 (2015): 831–866. Bachour gives a detailed description of the application of 'killed mercury' (Arab. *zi'baq maqtūl*) in Ibn Sīnā's *K. al-Qānūn* (ibid., 843–846) and quotes the preparation method described by Ibn Sīnā: 'Mercury is killed (*yuqtal*) by mixing it with ammoniac (*nushādar*), arsenic (*zirnīkh*), sulphur (*kibrīt*) and copper rust (*zinjār*). One part of the prepared mercury is mixed with the same amount of iron shavings (*burādat al-ḥadīd*), a half part of lime mortar (*nūra*) and a half of alkali (*qily*). The mixture is then sublimated in Aludel (*uthāl*) or put in a bottle to be dried, as the alchemists do it (*ahl al-ishtighāl bi-hādhā l-bāb*). It sublimates into a salt (*yaṣ'ad ka-l-milḥ*).' On the basis of this description, Bachour concludes: 'Thus the killed mercury (*zi'baq maqtūl*) is a white corrosive sublimate that must have contained mainly mercuric chloride (HgCy). This result leads to a further unclarity. Since Avicenna mentions sublimated mercury (*zi'baq muṣa''ad*) alongside killed mercury in the very same chapter—i.e. in the chapter on mercury as well as in the chapter on its toxicity—we would expect the two terms to indicate two different derivatives. Since the Canon contains no further preparation methods for mercury derivatives, this ambiguity cannot be solved.' Cf.

ies, Can. Or. 88, fol. 81^a–b^): זיבק ... אמר בולש כי יש מהאנשים שמשקים הכסף חי הנמוח לחולי איליאוש ([Arab.] *zi'baq*: Quicksilver (mercury): ... Paulus said that some people (physicians) administered 'killed' quicksilver (mercury) in the case of the illness [called] *ileus*). Hebr. כסף חי נמוח is not attested in the current dictionaries. Zeraḥyah Ḥen renders Arab. زئبق مقتول as כסף חי מומת (see next entry) and Anonymous I has המומת ממנו.

• **כסף חי מומת** · **'killed' quicksilver (mercury)**: Arab. زئبق مقتول · Ibn Sīnā, *K. al-Qānūn* II · trans. Zeraḥyah Ḥen, *Sefer ha-Qanun* (Ms Oxford, Bodleian Libaries, Opp. Add. Fol. 12, fol. 205^a^): זיבק כסף חי ... זכר בולש כי יש מבני אדם שישקו המומת ממנו בחולי הקוליקא הנק' איליאוס ([Arab.] *zi'baq*; [i.e., Hebr.] *kesef ḥay*: Quicksilver (mercury): ... Paulus said that some people (physicians) administered 'killed' quicksilver (mercury) in the case of [Hebr.-Lat.] *ḥoli ha-colica*, called *ileus*). Hebr. כסף חי מומת is not attested in the current dictionaries. Nathan ha-Me'ati renders Arab. زئبق مقتول as כסף חי נמוח (see previous entry) and Anonymous I has המומת ממנו.

• **קֶצֶף** → **קצף הכסף** •

כֶּרֶךְ • **כרך מחוטים** · **pledget; compress**: Lat. *plagella* · Guy de Chauliac, *Inventarium sive Chirurgia Magna* (cf. CMM 1:228, ll. 15–16) · trans. Anonymous (Ms Paris, BnF, héb. 1189, fol. 124^b^): ואם לא הנה יוכל להניח כרך מחוטים (If this is impossible, he can apply a pledget). Hebr. כרך מחוטים is not attested in the current dictionaries.

כַּרְכֻּמִי • **המים הכרכומיים** → **מַיִם**.

כֶּרֶם • **ורד הכרם** → **וֶרֶד**.

[כתם] • *Part. Nif'al* **נִכְתָּם** · **infected**: Lat. *infectus* · Guy de Chauliac, *Inventarium sive Chirurgia Magna* (cf. CMM 1:227, ll. 22–24) · trans. Anonymous (Ms Paris, BnF, héb. 1189, fol. 124^a^): ואמנם זה רוגייר ... הנה צוה שכל העור משרשו יובדל והגלגלת הנכתם עם המקדח יקדח (But Roger[172] ... ordered that the skin should be totally removed down to the

---

the quotation from an Indian alchemical work called *Rasahṛdayatantra*, dating from the eleventh/twelfth century in D. Wujastik, 'Mercury Tonics in Sanskrit literature,' in: *Soulless Matter, Seats of Energy: Metals, Gems and Minerals in South Asian Religions and Culture*, ed. by F.M. Ferrari and T. Dähnhardt, 94–115 (Sheffield and Bristol 2015), 96: 'After it [i.e., mercury] has been solidified, it cures disease, having been bound, it gives liberation; having been throughly killed, it gives immortality. What is more compassionate than mercury?,' and the commentary by Wujastik (ibid., 97): 'However, in its natural, liquid state, mercury is unstable, can be burnt, or dried up, though not rotted. And to counter these or other unwelcome properties, alchemists developed a series of eighteen procedures that would make mercury stable. The terms 'solidified', 'bound', and 'killed' we saw in the quotation from the *Rasahṛdayatantra* are technical terms that refer to some of these stages in the processing of mercury.'

172 'Roger': I.e., Rogerius Frugardi, author of the *Chirurgia* composed in the second half of the twelfth century. It was later greatly expanded by Roland of Parma (completed in 1230). Guy de Chauliac's quotations are sometimes derived from this expanded version, which was in effect a new book; cf. CMM 2:13f.

bone and that a hole should then be drilled in the infected skull). Hebr. *Part. Nifʿal* נִכְתָּם does not feature in this sense in the current dictionaries.

כֶּתֶם • *Plur.* **כתמים** · I. **freckles**: Arab. كلف · al-Rāzī, *K. fī al-Faṣd* · trans. Anonymous, *Maʾamar ba-Haqqazah* (Ms Parma, Biblioteca Palatina, Cod. Parm. 2283,4, fol. 93[b]): וגיד א׳ בקצה החוטם ותועיל הקזתו מהכתמי׳ הנק׳ אלכלף[173] ומשנוי המראה והחמימות[174] והנגעים והחבורות אשר בחוטם והשפה (One vein in the tip of the nose, bleeding it is beneficial for freckles called [in Arab.] *al-kalaf*, discoloration, dandruff,[175] pustules and ulcers in the nose and the lips). In the sense of 'freckles,' Hebr. *Sing.* כֶּתֶם features in NM 6:105 in an attestation from Nathan's trans. of Ibn Sīnā's *K. al-Qānūn* (i.e., *Sefer ha-Qanun*) II.

· II. **infections**: Lat. *infecciones* · Guy de Chauliac, *Inventarium sive Chirurgia Magna* (cf. CMM 1:416, ll. 25–26) · trans. Anonymous (Ms Paris, BnF, héb. 1189, fol. 227[b]): יעצו הד׳ חכמים הכויה עם[176] השידונש להריק חמר הגוטא רושא ויתר כתמי הפנים והפה (The four magisters advised to cauterize with (and use) a seton[177] to evacuate the [superfluous] matter [causing] *gutta*[178] *rosea* and other infections of the face and nose). Hebr. כֶּתֶם, *Plur.* כתמים, is not attested in this sense in the current dictionaries.

• **הכתמים שבעור** · **pimples in the face; acne**: Arab. نمش (Gr. ἴονθος; cf. UW 310) · Ibn Sīnā, *K. al-Qānūn* II · trans. Zeraḥyah Ḥen, *Sefer ha-Qanun* (Ms Oxford, Bodleian Libaries, Opp. Add. Fol. 12, fol. 213[a]): חֵמְץ זרעונים ... יטהר הכתמים שבעור הנקראים נֶמַש ([Arab.] *ḥimmiṣ*; [i.e., Hebr.] *zerʿonim*: Chickpeas [*Cicer arietinum* L.]: ... They clean pimples in the face (acne), called [in Arab.] *namash*). Hebr. הכתמים שבעור is not attested in the current dictionaries. Nathan ha-Meʾati translates Arab. نمش as עדשים (cf. NM 6:157 for an attestation from his *Sefer ha-Qanun* II) and Anonymous I transcribes Arab. نمش as נמש (cf. ibid.).

[כתש] • *Part. Piʿel f. Plur.* **מְכַתְּשׁוֹת** · **molars**: Arab. ضرس, *Plur.* أضراس · Ibn Sīnā, *K. al-Qānūn* II · trans. Nathan ha-Meʾati, *Sefer ha-Qanun* (Ms Oxford, Bodleian Librar-

---

173 אלכלף: Emend. ed. אלכלוף Ms.

174 והחמימות (= والحرارة): والحزاز a.

175 'dandruff': Trans. acc. to a.

176 עם השידונש: *ad cetonem* L.

177 'Seton': A seton is a thread or piece of cloth passed through the skin, may be introduced by a needle, and left there; it is of course an irritant and there will be continual drainage around it (that could be interpreted as discharge of unwanted humors). A cautery could also be used to open the way for the introduction of the seton, and the cauterization would make it harder for the drain to close. I thank my colleague and friend Michael R. McVaugh for this explanatory note.

178 *'gutta rosea'*: Cf. ND 485: 'Skin sickness involving red discoloration of face, with little or no unevenness and no ulceration; in some texts said to be first sign of leprosy.'

ies, Can. Or. 88, fol. 81b):[179] זאג ... והאדום הנקרא סורי יחזק השנים והמכתשות המתנועעים ([Arab.] *zāj*: Vitriol: ... Red vitriol, called [in Arab.] *sūrī*, strengthens moving teeth and molars). In the sense of 'molars,' Hebr. *Part. Piʿel f. Plur.* מְכַתְּשׁוֹת is possibly a non-attested abbreviated form standing for שנים מכתשות, with the latter term being derived from the verb כָּתַשׁ 'to pound' (cf. BM 2562f.). In his trans. of entry חלתית ([Arab.] *ḥiltīt* / [Hebr.] *ḥiltit*: Resin of asafetida [*Ferula assa-foetida* L.]) on fol. 85b, Nathan translates Arab. أضراس simply as שן. Zeraḥyah Ḥen and Anonymous I both render the Arab. term as מלתעות.

179 The same Hebr. term features on fol. 63b, entry אקחואן '[Arab.] *uqḥuwān*: Feverfew [*Tanacetum parthenium* (L.) Sch. Bip.].'

לָאזוּרְדִּיּוּת · **azure**: Arab. لازورد · Ibn Sīnā, *K. al-Qānūn* II · trans. Anonymous I, *Sefer ha-Qanun* (Ms Paris, BnF, héb. 1142, fol. 123[a]): חגר ארמיני כלומר אבן ארמיני ובלשו׳ לפיש ארמיניק מהות יש בו מעט מראה לאזורדיות ואינה כמראה הלאזורד ולא במקשיותו ([Arab.] *ḥajar armīnī*; i.e., [Hebr.] *even armini*, and in [Lat.] LPYŠ ʾRMYNYQ [read: LPYŠ ʾRMYNWS, i.e., *lapis Armenus*]: Armenian stone: What is it? It is slightly azure in color but its color is not like that of lapis lazuli, nor does it have its compactness). Hebr. לָאזוּרְדִּיּוּת is a non-attested Hebraization of Arab. لازورد. Zeraḥyah Ḥen renders the Arab. term as אֱזוֹר and Nathan ha-Me'ati transcribes it as לאזורד.

לֵבָב · **pulp**: Arab. لبّ · Ibn Sīnā, *K. al-Qānūn* II · trans. Anonymous I, *Sefer ha-Qanun* (Ms Paris, BnF, héb. 1142, fol. 72[a]): גוז הנדי ... בחירה הטרי החזק הלובן ערבים המים אשר בו ואם לא ימצאו המים יורה שהוא ישן וראוי שיוקח ממנו קלפת לבבו ([Arab.] *jawz hindī*: Coconut [*Cocos nucifera* L.]: ... the choicest [coconut] is that which is fresh, extremely white, and is containing sweet water. Lack of water in it indicates that it is old. In such a case, one should only take the skin of its pulp). Hebr. לֵבָב is not attested in the sense of 'pulp' in the current dictionaries. Nathan ha-Me'ati translates Arab. لبّ as פרי פנימי (cf. entry פְּרִי) and Zeraḥyah Ḥen translates the Arab. term as לֵב (cf. NM 5:105 for an attestation from Moses ibn Tibbon's trans. of Ibn al-Jazzār's *Zād al-musāfir* (i.e., *Sefer Ṣedat ha-Derakhim*) III.6). The Arab. synonym لحم is translated by both Anonymous I and Nathan as בָּשָׂר (see entry).

לָבָן • הבחק הלבן → בֹּהַק.

לֹבֶן · **corneal opacity; leucoma**: Arab. بياض (cf. UWS 3:299) · Ibn Sīnā, *K. al-Qānūn* II · trans. Nathan ha-Me'ati, *Sefer ha-Qanun* (Ms Oxford, Bodleian Libraries, Can. Or. 88, fol. 66[a]): אבנוס ... ימרוק החשכה והלובן ([Arab.] *abanūs*: Ebony: ... It acts as a detergent for dimness of sight and leucoma). Hebr. לֹבֶן does not feature in this sense in the current dictionaries. Anonymous I renders Arab. بياض as לֹבֶן, just like Nathan and Zeraḥyah Ḥen translates the Arab. term as לובן שבעין (see next entry).

• **לובן שבעין** · **corneal opacity; leucoma**: Arab. بياض (cf. UWS 3:299) · Ibn Sīnā, *K. al-Qānūn* II · trans. Zeraḥyah Ḥen, *Sefer ha-Qanun* (Ms Oxford, Bodleian Libaries, Opp. Add. Fol. 12, fol. 177[a]): אָבְנוּס הָבְנִים ... יטהר בסנורים והלובן שבעין ([Arab.] *abanūs*; [i.e., Hebr.] *hovnim*: Ebony: ... It acts as a detergent for dimness of sight and leucoma). Hebr. לובן שבעין is only attested as an anat. term for the 'white of the eye (sclera)' (cf. JD 694; BM 2613). See also NM 5:169 for the Hebr. term צמח בלובן העין ('lit. an inflammation of the white of the eye (sclera)); cataract' in an attestation from Shem Tov ben Isaac's *Sefer ha-Shimmush* XXIX, list 1 (cf. SHS 1:439f. (Ṣade 23)). Nathan ha-Me'ati and Anonymous I both render Arab. بياض as לֹבֶן (see previous entry).

לְבָנָה • אבן הלבנה → אֶבֶן.

לוֹבֶן → לֹבֶן.

לֵחָה • *Plur.* לחות • הגרת לחות הרחם → הֲגָרָה.

לַחוּת • *Plur.* **לחויות** • **הלחויות הנחבאות תחת העור** · **edema**: Arab. الرطوبات المحتقنة تحت الجلد · Ibn Sīnā, *K. al-Qānūn* II · trans. Zeraḥyah Ḥen, *Sefer ha-Qanun* (Ms Oxford, Bodleian Libaries, Opp. Add. Fol. 12, fol. 239[b]): מַרְקַשִׁיתָא ... יועיל כשימשחנו עם החומץ על הבוהק והבהרת והנמש ויתיר הלחויות הנחבאות תחת העור וירקק השער ויתלתלנו ([Arab.] *marqashīthā*: Marcasite: ... Rubbing it with vinegar is useful in *bahaq*[180] (alphos), *baraṣ*,[181] and freckles. It dissolves edema. It makes the hair thin and curly.) In the sense of 'edema,' Hebr. הלחויות הנחבאות תחת העור is a non-attested calque from Arab. الرطوبات المحتقنة تحت الجلد. Nathan ha-Me'ati translates the Arab. term as הרוטבות הנעצרות תחת העור (see entry רְטִבָה) and Anonymous I has הלחויות הנעצרות תחת העור (see next entry).

• **הלחויות הנעצרות תחת העור** · **edema**: Arab. الرطوبات المحتقنة تحت الجلد · Ibn Sīnā, *K. al-Qānūn* II · trans. Anonymous I, *Sefer ha-Qanun* (Ms Paris, BnF, héb. 1142, fol. 167[a]): מארקשיתא ... מועיל אם יורטה בחומץ על הבוהק ונגע[182] צרעת ונמש המתיך גם כן הלחויות הנעצרות תחת העור ומרקיק השער ומתלתלו ([Arab.] *marqashīthā*: Marcasite: ... Rubing it with vinegar is useful in *bahaq*[183] (alphos), *baraṣ*,[184] and freckles. It dissolves edema. It makes the hair thin and curly). In the sense of 'edema,' Hebr. הלחויות הנעצרות תחת העור is a non-attested calque from Arab. الرطوبات المحتقنة تحت الجلد. Nathan ha-Me'ati translates the Arab. term as הרוטבות הנעצרות תחת העור (see entry רְטִבָה) and Zeraḥyah Ḥen has הלחויות הנחבאות תחת העור (see previous entry).

• **הגרת לחויות הרחם** → הֲגָרָה.

לְחִיצָה · **abrasion**: Arab. سحج · Ibn Sīnā, *K. al-Qānūn* II · trans. Zeraḥyah Ḥen, *Sefer ha-Qanun* (Ms Oxford, Bodleian Libaries, Opp. Add. Fol. 12, fol. 194[a]): ג׳לד[185] ... דשן עור הפרדים וזולתם ... הוא רפואה ללחיצת הנעל ולחיצת הירכים והפישטולי ([Arab.] *jild*: Skin: ... The ash of the skin of mules and other similar animals ... it is a remedy for abrasion

---

180 '*bahaq* (alphos)': There are three varieties of the disease called *bahaq* acc. to Ibn al-Jazzār (cf. IJZ 7:108, n. 196): white, black, and dust-colored. The white variety is perhaps identical with *Vitiligo alba*, while the black variety is possibly a sort of melanoderma. Arab. *bahaq* stands for Gr. ἀλφός, cf. UW 97: 'weiße Hautflecken.' Durling, *Dictionary of Medical Terms*, 34, translates the Gr. term as: 'dull-white leprosy.' See entry הבהק הלבן :בַּהַק.

181 '*baraṣ*' (cf. IJZ 7:108, n. 195): This disease has two varieties, namely white and black, which are sometimes summarized under the general term *baraṣ*. The white variety is perhaps identical with *Sklerodermia circumscripta*, while the black variety may be *Psoriasis vulgaris* or *Ichthyosis vulgaris*. The Arab. term *baraṣ* stands for Gr. λέπρα ('leprosy') (cf. UW 97, 387f.). As their is no consensus on the exact meaning of the Arab. term, I have retained the Arab. term in my translation.

182 ונגע צרעת: البرص a.

183 See note 180.

184 See note 181.

185 ג׳לד: Emend. ed. ג׳לוד Ms.

caused by [narrow] shoes and for abrasion of the thighs and for fistula). Hebr. לְחִיצָה is not attested in this sense in the current dictionaries.[186] In addition to לְחִיצָה, Zeraḥyah translates Arab. سحج as דְּחִיקָה (see entry). Nathan ha-Me'ati translates Arab. سحج as בְּקוּעַ (see entry) and Anonymous I has הפשט העור (see entry הֶפְשֵׁט).

• **לחיצת האזן** · **tear (puncture) in the ear**: Arab. شدخ الأذن (Arab. شدخ is Gr. ῥῆγμα 'breakage, fracture; laceration, rupture, rent, tear;' cf. UW 587; LSG 1568) · Ibn Sīnā, *K. al-Qānūn* II · trans. Zeraḥyah Ḥen, *Sefer ha-Qanun* (Ms Oxford, Bodleian Libraries, Opp. Add. Fol. 12, fol. 223[b]): כַּבְּרִית גפרית ... יעצור הָרֵיוּמָא כשיתעשן ויעשנו עם החומץ והדבש על לחיצת האזן ([Arab.] *kibrīt*; [i.e., Hebr.] *gofrit*: Sulphur: ... It stops rheum when it is applied as a fumigation; with vinegar and honey it is used for a tear (puncture) in the ear). Hebr. לחיצת האזן does not feature in this sense in the current dictionaries. Nathan ha-Me'ati translates Arab. شدخ الأذن as רצוץ האזן (see entry רְצוּץ) and Anonymous I has רסוק האזן (see entry רָסוּק). The Hebr. translators probably interpreted the term شَدْخ as derived from شَدَخَ in its general meaning of 'to break, crush, press, squeeze' (cf. Lane 1519) and not in the specific meaning listed above. Arab. شدخ features also as part of the term شدخ العضل 'muscle tear (rupture)' in the *K. al-Qānūn* II and is translated by Zeraḥyah as הפסד המושקלו (cf. NM 6:206, s.v. רצוץ העצלים).

לֶחֶם • **לחם נקודים** · **biscuit; rusk**: Arab. كعك · *Shinnui ha-Shemot ha-Niqra'im Synonimi*, Kaf 52 (Ms Florence, Biblioteca Medicea Laurenziana, Or. 17, fol. 81[a]): כעך[187] ה' לחם נקודים ([Arab.] *ka'k* [i.e., biscuits, rusk, or cake; cf. WKAS 1:234f.; MIG no. 1046); i.e., [Hebr.] *leḥem niqqudim*). Hebr. נָקֹד, *Plur.* נִקֻּדִים, on its own is attested in the Bible (cf. KB 720: 'crumbs, small pastry'); Rabb. literature (cf. LW 3:435: 'Brotkrumen, mica'), and Haskalah literature (Baruch Lindau's *Reshit Limmudim*; cf. BM 3784). The combination לחם נקודים is not attested.

לְטָאָה • **הלטאה המיימי** · **skink**: Arab. اسقنقور (cf. DT 231 (II.52) · Ibn Sīnā, *K. al-Qānūn* II · trans. Nathan ha-Me'ati, *Sefer ha-Qanun* (Ms Oxford, Bodleian Libraries, Can. Or. 88, fol. 66[a]): אסקנקור המהות הוא הלטאה המימי ([Arab.] *isqanqūr*: Skink: What is it? It is [Hebr.] *ha-leṭa'ah ha-meymi* [lit. 'water lizard']). Hebr. הלטאה המיימי is not attested in the current dictionaries. Zeraḥyah Ḥen renders Arab. اسقنقور as אַסְקַנְקוֹר הוא לוג'ירט מיימי ([Arab.] *isqanqūr*, i.e., [Ital.-Rom.-Hebr.] *luserda/lüšerda/lušerda meymi*) and Anonymous I has אשטינקוש and in a marginal gloss: אישטינקוש דג שייט.

186 Hebr. לְחִיצָה also features for Arab. سحج in the sense of 'abrasion' on fol. 238[a], entry מרדאסנג '[Arab.] *murdāsanj*: Litharge,' and fols. 202[b]–203[a], entry ורדים 'Roses [*Rosa* sp.]': יועיל מהנגעים כל שכן הנעשה בעבור לחיצה בירכים ובאצילי הזרועות (They are useful for ulcers and especially those caused by abrasion of the thighs and armpits).

187 כעך: Emend. ed. כטך Ms.

The term אשטינקוש or אישטינקוש is Lat. *stincus*, a deformation of Gr. σκίγκος with the prothetic *e-* typical for Lat. written in Western-Rom. territories such as France or the Iberian Peninsula. The O. Occ.-Hebr. term דג שייט already features (for Arab. اسقنقور) in Moses ibn Tibbon's trans. of Maimonides' *On Hemorrhoids* (i.e., *Ma'amar be-Ṭeḥorim*) VI.9 (cf. BMH 45, l. 13).

לַיְלָה • בנות הלילה → בַּת.

• סנויר לילה → סַנְוֵיר.

• צמח הלילה → צֶמַח.

לִכְלוּךְ • ליכלוך השנים · **dirty teeth (dental sordes)**: Arab. أوساخ الأسنان · Ibn Sīnā, *K. al-Qānūn* II · trans. Zeraḥyah Ḥen, *Sefer ha-Qanun* (Ms Oxford. Opp. Add. Fol. 12, fol. 209[b]): זְרַאוֹנְד אֶשְׁטוּרוּלוּגִ׳יאָה ... יועיל מן הבהק ויטהר השנים ויועיל מן ליכלוכם ([Arab.] *zarāwand*; [i.e., Rom.] 'eŠṬWuRWuLWuǦY'aH: Birthwort [*Aristolochia longa* L., *A. rotunda* L., or *A. clematis* L.]: ... It is useful for *bahaq*[188] (alphos), it cleans the teeth, and it is useful for dirty teeth (dental sordes)). Hebr. ליכלוך השנים is not attested in the current dictionaries. Nathan ha-Me'ati translates Arab. أوساخ الأسنان as טנופת השנים (see entry טִנֹּפֶת) and Anonymous I has זוהמת השנים (see entry זהמה).

Plur. **ליכלוכים • ליכלוכי האוזן** · **earwax**: Arab. أوساخ الأذن · Ibn Sīnā, *K. al-Qānūn* II · trans. Zeraḥyah Ḥen, *Sefer ha-Qanun* (Ms Oxford. Opp. Add. Fol. 12, fol. 201[b]): זְרַאוֹנְד אֶשְׁטוּרוּלוּגִ׳יאָה ... ינקה ליכלוכי האוזן ויחזק השמיעה כשיושם בו עם הדבש ([Arab.] *zarāwand*; [i.e., Rom.] 'eŠṬWuRWuLWuǦY'aH: Birthwort [*Aristolochia longa* L., *A. rotunda* L., or *A. clematis* L.]: ... It removes earwax and strengthens hearing when it is put into [the ear] with honey). Hebr. ליכלוכי האזן features (for Arab. وسخ الأذن) as לכלוך האוזן in Ibn Tibbon's trans. of Ibn al-Jazzār's *Zād al-musāfir* (i.e., *Sefer Ṣedat ha-Derakhim*) VII.27.3 (cf. IJZ 7:169, ll. 15–16; NM 5:40f.; s.v. געול). Nathan ha-Me'ati translates Arab. أوساخ الأذن as טנופת האזנים (see entry טִנֹּפֶת) and Anonymous I has זוהמת האוזן (see entry זהמה).

לִכְלֵךְ (*Pi'el*) · **to apply as a salve**: Arab. لُطُوخ (cf. WKAS 2.2:692) · Ibn Sīnā, *K. al-Qānūn* II · trans. Nathan ha-Me'ati, *Sefer ha-Qanun* (Ms Oxford, Bodleian Libraries, Can. Or. 88, fol. 85[a]): חלתית ... יועיל מחולי השועל אם מלכלכים אותו בחומץ ופלפל ([Arab.] *ḥiltīt* / [Hebr.] *ḥiltit*: Resin of asafetida [*Ferula assa-foetida* L.]: ... It is useful for alopecia when it is applied as a salve with vinegar and pepper). In the sense of 'to apply as a salve,' Hebr. לִכְלֵךְ is a semantic borrowing from Arab. لُطُوخ, which features in BCD 137

---

188 '*bahaq* (alphos)': There are three varieties of the disease called '*bahaq*' acc. to Ibn al-Jazzār: white, black and dustcolored. The white variety is perhaps identical with Vitiligo alba, while the black variety is possibly a sort of melanoderma. Arab. *bahaq* stands for Gr. ἀλφός; cf. UW 97: "weisse Hautflecken." Durling, *Dictionary of Medical Terms*, 34, translates the Gr. term as: "dull-white leprosy."

(NM 1:99) with the trans. 'to spread' in an attestation from Shem Tov ben Isaac's *Sefer ha-Shimmush* XXX.2.13. Zeraḥyah Ḥen translates Arab. لُطُوخ as *Inf. Hif'il* לְהָטִיחַ (see entry טוּחַ) and Anonymous I renders Arab. لُطُوخ as רְטִיָּה (see entry). Nathan also renders Arab. لُطُوخ as מָשַׁח in entry רכמה '[Arab.] *rakham*: Vulture' (fol. 123[a]) (see entry).

• *Part. Pi'el* מְלַכְלֵךְ • הרפואה המלכלכת → רְפוּאָה.

מ

מַאֲדִים (*Part. Hif'il*) → [אדם].
מְאַדֵּם (*Part. Pi'el*) → [אדם].
מְאַוֶּה (*Part. Pi'el*) → [אוה].
מְאוּכָּל → מְאֻכָּל.
מְאוֹרָע → מְאֹרָע.
מְאַכֵּל (*Part. Pi'el*) → אָכַל.
מְאֻכָּל (*Part. Pu'al*) → אָכַל.
מְאֹרָע · **affliction; defect**: Arab. آفة · Ibn Sīnā, *K. al-Qānūn* II · trans. Nathan ha-Me'ati, *Sefer ha-Qanun* (Ms Oxford, Bodleian Libraries, Can. Or. 88, fol. 114[b]): ... פוא אלצבאגין ישקו ממנו במי קראטן ויועיל מגיד הנשה והצינון הנק׳ פלאג שיש ממנו מאורע בהרגש ([Arab.] *fuwwa*[*t*] *al-ṣabbāghīn* [lit. 'dyers' madder']: Common madder [*Rubia tinctorum* L.]: ... When taken with honey water (*melikraton*), it is beneficial for sciatica, hemiplegia, called PL'G [read: P'LG, i.e., Arab. *fālij*], which comes with a sensory defect). Hebr. מְאֹרָע does not feature in this sense in the current dictionaries. In his trans. of Maimonides' *Medical Aphorisms* (i.e., *Sefer ha-Peraqim*), Nathan translates Arab. آفة as פגע (cf. BMMG no. 140), which is also used here by Anonymous I. Zeraḥyah Ḥen renders the Arab. term as חלי (see entry).
מַאֲכָל • מאוה המאכל → [אוה].
מְבוּשָּׁל → מְבֻשָּׁל.
מְבַטֵּל (*Part. Pi'el*) → [בטל].
מְבַעְבֵּעַ (*Part. Pi'el*) → בִּעְבַּע.
מַבְרִיא (*Part. Hif'il*) → [ברא].
מְבַשֵּׁל (*Part. Pi'el*) → [בשל].
מְבֻשָּׁל (*Part. Pu'al*) → [בשל].
מְגַדֵּל (*Part. Pi'el*) → [גדל].
מְגֻדָּל (*Part. Pu'al*) → [גדל].
מְגוּדָּל → מְגֻדָּל.
מָגֵן · **shell**: Arab. صدف, *Plur.* أصداف · Ibn Sīnā, *K. al-Qānūn* II · trans. Anonymous I, *Sefer ha-Qanun* (Ms Paris, BnF, héb. 1142, fol. 98[a]): חלזון מהות הוא מכלל שרץ המים בעלי מגן הנק׳ צדף ([Arab.] *ḥalazūn* / [Hebr.] *ḥilazon*: Snail: What is it? It is a kind of water creature that has a shell, called [in Arab.] *ṣadaf*). Hebr. מָגֵן is not attested in this sense in the current dictionaries. Nathan ha-Mea'ti translates Arab. صدف, *Plur.* أصداف, as קליפות הנק׳ צרף (*צדף) and Zeraḥyah Ḥen has חרסים (see entry חֶרֶס).
מַגֵּפָה • המורסות אשר יקרו בעת המגפה → מֻרְסָה.
מַדְבִּיק (*Part. Hif'il*) → [דבק].
מְדַבֵּק (*Part. Pi'el*) → [דבק].
מִדְבָּרִי • גומא של הרוטא המדברית → גּוֹמָא.

• גִּיד → גיד הרמון המדברי.
• שֹׁרֶשׁ → שרש הרמון המדברי.

מדמע · **the inner canthus (angle) of the eye**: Arab. مأق · Ibn Sīnā, *K. al-Qānūn* II · trans. Zeraḥyah Ḥen, *Sefer ha-Qanun* (Ms Oxford, Bodleian Libaries, Opp. Add. Fol. 12, fol. 264[a–b]): צַבִר אלוֹאֵיי ... יועיל מנגעי העין ומורסותיו וכאביו ומן גרב המדמע וייבש לחותו ([Arab.] *ṣabir*; [Hebr.] *alo'e*: Aloe [*Aloe vera* L.]: ... It is useful for ocular ulcers, swellings, pain, and irritation of the inner canthus (angle) of the eye. It also dries up its moisture). Hebr. מדמע is not attested in the current dictionaries. In addition to this term, Zeraḥyah translates Arab. مأق as דוֹמֵעַ (see entry). The Arab. *Dual* مأقان 'the two canthi (corners) of the eye' is translated by him as הקצוות אשר הדמע יורד מהן and as קצוות העין (cf. BCD 247f. (NM 4:188)) in the *Sefer ha-Qanun* I. Nathan ha-Me'ati translates Arab. مأق as זנב העין (see entry זָנָב) and Anonymous I renders the Arab. term as קצות העין (cf. Zeraḥyah's קצוות העין in BCD 248).

מְדַקְדֵּק (*Part. Pi'el*) → [דקדק].

[מוח] • *Part. Nif'al* נְמוֹחַ • כסף חי נמוח → כֶּסֶף.

מוֹלִיד (*Part. Hif'il*) → [ילד].

מוּמָת (*Part. Hof'al*) → [מות].

מוּקָף → מֻקָּף.

מוּרְיִיס · **a) garum (fermented fish sauce), called *murrī al-ḥūt*; b) a cereal-based preparation, called *murrī al-ḥinṭa***: Arab. مرّي (cf. D 2:576; DT 216f. (II.30); NA 579–582) · Ibn Sīnā, *K. al-Qānūn* II · trans. Anonymous I, *Sefer ha-Qanun* (Ms Paris, BnF, héb. 1142, fol. 195[a–b]): סמך ... והמלוח חם ויבש וכל עוד שיתישן יוסף משניהם ומי הדג המלוח דומה למורייס בענינין ([Arab.] *samak*: Fish: ... Salted [fish] is hot and dry. These two (hot and dry) temperaments develop in intensity with age. Salted fish sauce resembles garum in all respects). Hebr. מוּרְיִיס is a calque from Lat. *muries*, which is attested in the current dictionaries in attestations from Rabb. literature only (cf. JD 750; LW 3:58; SHS 1:435 (Ṣade 12)). Nathan ha-Me'ati and Zeraḥyah Ḥen both translate Arab. مرّي as כּוּתָח (cf. BCD 125 (NM 1:157) for an attestation from Zeraḥyah's trans. of Maimonides' *Medical Aphorisms* (i.e., *Sefer ha-Peraqim*) XVII.33 (cf. BMMN 173, l. 4; BMMG no. 4832); interestingly, Nathan uses the term מורייס in his *Sefer ha-Peraqim* XVII.33, which is used here by Anonymous I for Arab. مرّي (cf. BMMN 175, l. 5; BMMG no. 4832).

מוֹרִישׁ (*Part. Hif'il*) → [ירש].

מוֹרָס → מֹרָס.

מוּרְסָה → מֻרְסָה.

[מות] • *Part.* מֵת • בשר מת → בָּשָׂר.
• *Part. Hof'al* מוּמָת • כסף חי מומת → כֶּסֶף.

מוֹתְרִי · **superfluous**: Arab. فضلي · Ibn Sīnā, *K. al-Qānūn* II · trans. Anonymous I, *Sefer ha-Qanun* (Ms Paris, BnF, héb. 1142, fol. 163[b]): נענאע הוא מינטא הטבע חם ויבש בשניה ויש בו לחות מותריית ([Arab.] *na'na'*; i.e., [Lat.] MYNṬ' [i.e., *mentha*]: Mint, esp. spearmint

[*Mentha spicata* L.]: Its nature: It is hot and dry in the second [degree]. It has superfluous moisture). Hebr. מוֹתְרִי features in BM 2872 in an attestation from Ibn Sīnā's *Sefer ha-Qanun*. Nathan ha-Me'ati translates Arab. فضلي as יִתְרוֹנִי (cf. NM 6:95) and Zeraḥyah Ḥen has עודף (see entry [עדף]).

מְזֻהָם (*Part. Puʿal*) → [זהם].

מְזוּהָם → מְזֻהָם.

מְזוּמָּן → מְזֻמָּן.

מֵזִיב (*Part Hifʿil*) → [זוב].

מַזִּיר (*Part. Hifʿil*) → [נזר].

מִזְמוֹר • **מזמר הרועה** · **European water plantain** [***Alisma plantago-aquatica*** **L.**]: Arab مزمار الراعي · Ibn Sīnā, *K. al-Qānūn* II · trans. Anonymous I, *Sefer ha-Qanun* (Ms Paris, BnF, héb. 1142, fol. 163[b]): מזמאר אלרועי הוא מזמר הרועה ([Arab.] *mizmār al-rāʿī*; i.e., [Hebr.] *mizmor ha-roʿeh*). Hebr. מזמר הרועה is non-attested calque from Arab. مزمار الراعي. Nathan ha-Me'ati transcribes the Arab. term as מזמאר אלראע only and Zeraḥyah Ḥen has זמר הרועה (see entry זֶמֶר).

מְזֻמָּן (*Part Puʿal*) → [זמן].

מֹחַ • **מורסת המוח** → מֻרְסָה.

מְחַבֵּל (*Part. Piʿel*) → [חבל].

מַחֲזִיק (*Part. Hifʿil*) → [חזק].

מְחַזֵּק (*Part. Piʿel*) → [חזק].

מְחַיֶּה (*Part. Piʿel*) → [חיה].

מְחִיצָה • *Plur.* **מחיצות** · **tunics**: Arab. طبقة, *Plur.* طبقات · al-Rāzī, *K. fī al-Faṣd* · trans. Anonymous, *Maʾamar ba-Haqqazah* (Ms Parma, Biblioteca Palatina, Cod. Parm. 2283,4, fol. 94[a]): והם מורכבים מב׳ מחיצות (They [i.e., the pulsatile vessels] consist of two tunics). Hebr. מְחִיצָה, *Plur.* מחיצות, is not attested in this sense in the current dictionaries. For the combined term המחיצה הלבנה and המחיצה המחברת in the sense of 'conjunctiva,' cf. BCD 145 (NM 4:97) and NM 6:117.

מְחַכֵּךְ (*Part Piʿel*) → [חכך].

מַחְלִיק (*Part Hifʿil*) → [חלק].

מַחֲנַק • *Plur.* **מחנקים** · **sore throat; quinsy**: Arab. خوانيق (Gr. συνάγχη; cf. UW 654) · Ibn Sīnā, *K. al-Qānūn* II · trans. Anonymous I, *Sefer ha-Qanun* (Ms Paris, BnF, héb. 1142, fol. 155[r]): וחלב הגמלה יותר מועיל לרקיקת הדם וגם החלב הוא מרפואות שחיני הריאה והשדפון ומועיל המצמוץ וערעור מהמחנקים והזביחה[189] ומורסות הלהאה (Milk of a she-camel is more beneficial in hemoptysis; milk is a [good] drug for pulmonary ulcers and phthisis. Rinsing the mouth and gargling is useful for quinsy, angina, and swollen uvula). Hebr. *Sing.* מַחֲנַק features in BM 2921 in the sense of 'angina,' in an attestation, a.o.,

189 והזביחה: Ms[1] להרוח Ms.

from the *Sefer ha-Qanun*. Nathan ha-Me'ati translates Arab. خوانيق as חניקות (see entry חֲנִיקָה) and Zeraḥyah Ḥen has חֶנֶק (cf. BCD 104f. (NM 1:150f.; corr. 4:229; 3:94f.) for attestations from Zeraḥyah's trans. of Maimonides' *Medical Aphorisms* and *Commentary on Hippocrates'* Aphorisms). Likewise, Shem Tov ben Isaac uses the *Plur.* of the latter term, חנקים, in his *Sefer Almansur* (cf. NM 6:79).

מַחְצָב • אבן המחצב → אֶבֶן.

מַחְשָׁבָה · **anxiety**: Arab. توحّش · Ibn Sīnā, *K. al-Qānūn* II · trans. Zeraḥyah Ḥen, *Sefer ha-Qanun* (Ms Oxford, Bodleian Libraries, Opp. Add. Fol. 12, fol. 201[b]): הַלִילַגְ׳ מִירַבַּלֹנִי ... והחזק יועיל מן הצִינְקוֹפִיץ והמחשבה לשתותו ([Arab.] *halīlaj* [from Pers. *halīlah*]; [Rom.] MiYRaBaLoNiY: (Chebulic) myrobalan: ... When one takes the strong [variety] in a potion, it is useful for treating palpitation and anxiety). In the sense of 'suspicion' (for Arab. تهمة) and 'anxiety' (for Arab. غمّ), Hebr. מַחְשָׁבָה features in BCD 146 (NM 1:162) in attestations from Zeraḥyah's trans. of Maimonides' *Medical Aphorisms* (i.e., *Sefer ha-Peraqim*) VI.95; VII.2 (cf. BMMZ 74, ll. 4, 17; BMMG nos. 5620, 3721). Nathan ha-Me'ati translates Arab. توحّش as השתוממות השכל (see entry הִשְׁתּוֹמְמוּת) and Anonymous I renders the Arab. term as הִשְׁתּוֹמְמוּת (cf. BCD 74 (NM 4:48) for an attestation from an anonymous trans. of Ibn Sīnā's *K. al-Adwiya al-qalbiyya* (i.e., *Sammim Libbiyim*), and NM 5:196 for the variant reading שִׁמָּמוֹן featuring in the anonymous trans. of Isḥāq ibn 'Imrān's *Treatise on Melancholy*). In addition to מַחְשָׁבָה, Zeraḥyah translates Arab. توحّش as אֲנָחָה and תּוּגָה (see entries).

מַחְשָׁךְ • מחשך באפלה · **dimness [of sight]**: Arab. ظلمة (البصر) (Gr. ἀμβλυωπία; cf. UW 99–100) · Ibn Sīnā, *K. al-Qānūn* II · trans. Anonymous I, *Sefer ha-Qanun* (Ms Paris, BnF, héb. 1142, fol. 78rv: דארציני ... מועיל מהסנור הנקר׳ גשאוה ומחשך באפלה ([Arab.] *dārṣīnī*: Cinnamon [*Cinnamomum verum* J. Presl]: ... It is beneficial for dullness, called [in Arab.] *ghashāwa*, and dimness [of sight]). Hebr. מחשך באפלה is not attested in this sense in the current dictionaries. Nathan ha-Me'ati translates Arab. ظلمة (البصر) as חשכה. Abraham ben Isaac translates Arab. ظلمة البصر as חשיכות העינים in his trans. of Ibn al-Jazzār's *Zād al-musāfir* (i.e., *Sefer Ṣedah la-Oreḥim*) I.10.14 (cf. NM 5:85f.; IJZ 1–2:555).

מְחַתֵּךְ (*Part. Pi'el*) → [חתך].

מַטָּה • הנחה למטה → הֲנָחָה.

מְטַנֵּף (*Part. Pi'el*) → [טנף].

מְיַבֵּשׁ (*Part. Pi'el*) → [יבש].

מַיִם • מים ברזליים · **iron water**: Lat. *aqua ferrata* · Guy de Chauliac, *Inventarium sive Chirurgia Magna* (cf. CMM 1:237, ll. 28–29) · trans. Anonymous (Ms Paris, BnF, héb. 1189, fol. 130[a]): וא״כ אם האזנים יצטרכו לרחיצה ירוחץ באוקשימיל או עם יין ודבש ומים ברזליים (Subsequently, if the ears need to be washed, it should be done with oxymel or with wine and honey and iron water). Hebr. מים ברזליים is not attested in the current dictionaries.

• **המים הכרכומיים** · **jaundice**: Arab. الماء الأصفر (Gr. ἴκτερος; cf. UW 308[190]) · Ibn Sīnā, *K. al-Qānūn* II · trans. Anonymous I, *Sefer ha-Qanun* (Ms Paris, BnF, héb. 1142, fols. 169ᵃ–170ᵃ): מר ... מועיל המר המזוקק לרפיון האסטומ׳ ולמים הכרהומיים ולנפח באסטומכא ([Arab.] *murr* / [Hebr.] *mor*: Myrrh: ... Pure myrrh is useful for atony of the stomach, jaundice, and distention of the stomach). In the sense of 'jaundice,' Hebr. המים הכרכומיים is a non-attested calque from Arab. الماء الأصفر. Nathan ha-Me'ati translates Arab. الماء الأصفر as המים הצהובים (see next entry) and Zeraḥyah Ḥen has המים הציטרין (see entry below).

• **המים הצהובים** · **jaundice**: Arab. الماء الأصفر (Gr. ἴκτερος; cf. UW 308[191]) · Ibn Sīnā, *K. al-Qānūn* II · trans. Nathan ha-Me'ati, *Sefer ha-Qanun* (Ms Oxford, Bodleian Libraries, Can. Or. 88, fol. 104ᵃ): מר ... המר[192] יועיל לרפיון האצטומכא ואל המים הצהובים ולנפח האצטו׳ ([Arab.] *murr* / [Hebr.] *mor*: Myrrh: ... Pure[193] myrrh is useful for atony of the stomach, jaundice, and distention of the stomach). In the sense of 'jaundice,' Hebr. המים הצהובים is a non-attested calque from Arab. الماء الأصفر. Zeraḥyah Ḥen translates Arab. الماء الأصفر as המים הציטרין (see next entry) and Anonymous I has המים הכרכומיים (see previous entry).

• **המים הציטרין** · **jaundice**: Arab. الماء الأصفر (Gr. ἴκτερος; cf. UW 308[194]) · Ibn Sīnā, *K. al-Qānūn* II · trans. Zeraḥyah Ḥen, *Sefer ha-Qanun* (Ms Oxford, Bodleian Libraries, Opp. Add. Fol. 12, fol. 240ᵇ): מִירָא ... המירא[195] הטהורה תועיל המירא הטהורה מן רפיון האצטומ׳ והמים הציטרין והנפיחה באצטומכה ([Lat./Rom.] MiYRa' [i.e., Lat. *myrrha* or O. Occ./O. Cat. *mir(r)a*; cf. SHS 1:307 (Mem 8)]: Myrrh: Pure myrrh is useful for atony of the stomach, jaundice, and distention of the stomach). In the sense of 'jaundice,' Hebr.-Lat./Rom. המים הציטרין is a non-attested calque from Arab. الماء الأصفر. Nathan ha-Me'ati translates Arab. الماء الأصفر as המים הצהובים (see previous entry) and Anonymous I has המים הכרכומיים (see entry above).

• **המים שירדו בכיס הביצים** · **hydrocele**: Arab. أدرة الماء (Gr. ὑδροκήλη; cf. UW 697) · Ibn Sīnā, *K. al-Qānūn* II · trans. Zeraḥyah Ḥen, *Sefer ha-Qanun* (Ms Oxford, Bodleian Libraries, Opp. Add. Fol. 12, fol. 171ᵃ⁻ᵇ): אַקְחֻוָאן ... ויועיל ממורסות פי הטבעת החמות ויפתח הטחורים והשמן שלו יועיל[196] מן המים שירדו בכיס הביצים אחר שיבוקעו ([Arab.] *uqḥuwān*: Feverfew [*Tanacetum parthenium* (L.) Sch. Bip.]: ... It is useful for hot swellings of the anus and opens hemorrhoids. Its oil is useful for ruptured hydrocele). Hebr. המים

190 Note that Ullmann also mentions the term in the sense of 'dropsy' in UW 698f.
191 Note that Ullmann also mentions the term in the sense of 'dropsy' in UW 698f.
192 המירא: الخالص add. a.
193 'Pure': Add. acc. to a.
194 Note that Ullmann also mentions the term in the sense of 'dropsy' in UW 698f.
195 המירא הטהורה תועיל מן רפיון האצטומ׳: Emend. ed. תועיל מן רפיון האצטומ׳ המירא הטהורה Ms.
196 יועיל: Emend. ed. ויועיל Ms.

שירדו בכיס הביצים is not attested in the current dictionaries. In addition, Zeraḥyah translates the Arab. synonym قيلة الماء as כיס המים in his trans. of Maimonides *Medical Aphorisms* (i.e., *Sefer ha-Peraqim*) XXIII.57 (cf. BCD 126 (NM 1:159); BMMZ 224, l. 14; BMMG no. 4311). Nathan ha-Me'ati translates Arab. أدرة الماء as אשד המים (see entry אֶשֶׁד) and Anonymous I has הגרת המים באשד (see entry הֲגָרָה).

• **מי הקראטין** · **honey water**: Arab. ماء القراطن (ed. Būlāq 1:367) (read: مالقراطن (Gr. μελίκρατον; cf. D 2:565)) · Ibn Sīnā, *K. al-Qānūn* II · trans. Zeraḥyah Ḥen, *Sefer ha-Qanun* (Ms Oxford, Bodleian Libaries, Opp. Add. Fol. 12, fol. 240[a]): מִיוּבְּזַג׳ אֶשְׁטַפְזִיזַקְרא ... ינתן ממנו לשתות ט״ו גרעינים עם מי הקראטין וינקה כימוסים רעים ויסקוזי ([Arab.] *mayūbazaj* [from Pers. *mawīzak*]; [i.e., Rom.] ʾeŠəṬaPəZiYZaQəRʾ [i.e., O. Occ. *estafizagra*; cf. SHS 1:429f. (Ṣade 2)]: Stavesacre [*Delphinium staphisagria* L]: ... When one ingests fifteen grains with honey water, it cleanses bad viscous chymes). The term מי הקראטין is a combination of Hebr. מים (for Arab. ماء) and קראטין (read: קראטן), a calque from Arab. قراطن. Nathan ha-Me'ati and Anonymous I both render Arab. ماء القراطن as מי הקראטן.

• **אשד המים** → **אֶשֶׁד**.

• **הגרת המים באשד** → **הֲגָרָה**.

• **חולי המים הרעים הבשריי** → **חֳלִי**.

• **ירוקת המים** → **יְרוֹקָה**.

• **כוית המים החמים** → **כְּוִיָּה**.

• **נימות המים** → **נִימָה**.

• **שרפת המים החמים** → **שְׂרֵפָה**.

מֵימִי • **הלטאה המיימי** → **לְטָאָה**.

מִיץ • **המיץ היוצא מן החלב** · **whey**: Lat. *serum* (Arab. ماء الجبن) · Constantinus Africanus, *Viaticum* V.5 · trans. Do'eg ha-Edomi, *Sefer Ya'ir Netiv*: השלישית המטהרת המים האלה היא חלב הגמלים והשתן שלהם והמיץ היוצא מן החלב (The third [therapy] to purge the water [in the case of dropsy] is [to administer the patient] milk or urine of a camel or whey). Hebr. המיץ היוצא מן החלב is not attested in the current dictionaries. Moses ibn Tibbon translates Arab. ماء الجبن as מיץ חלב (cf. BCD 148 (NM 1:71) for an attestation from his trans. of Ibn al-Jazzār's *Zād al-musāfir* (i.e., *Sefer Ṣedat ha-Derakhim*) VII.9.7 (cf. IJZ 7:140, l. 6).

• **מיץ קרוש** · **rob [i.e., fruit or vegetable juice boiled down to syrup]**: Arab. ربّ · Ibn Sīnā, *K. al-Qānūn* II · trans. Anonymous I, *Sefer ha-Qanun* (Ms Paris, BnF, héb. 1142, fols. 143[b]–144[a]): כמתרי ... ולכן ראוי שישתה אחריו מי הדבש עם בשמים ומיצו הקרוש מועיל לשלשול האדומיי ([Arab.] *kummathrā*: Pear [*Pyrus communis* L.]: ... Therefore, after its [consumption] one should drink honey water with aromatics. Its rob is useful for treating bilious diarrhea). Hebr. מיץ קרוש does not feature in the current dictionaries. Nathan ha-Me'ati translates Arab. ربّ as עסיס מבושל (see entry עָסִיס) and Zeraḥyah Ḥen has *Part. Pu'al* מְרוּבָּב (see entry [רבב]). See also the next entry for Zeraḥyah's use of the term מירבב for Arab. ربّ.

מירבב · **rob (fruit or vegetable juice boiled down to syrup)**: Arab. رُبّ · Ibn Sīnā, *K. al-Qānūn* II · translation Zeraḥyah Ḥen, *Sefer ha-Qanun* (Ms Oxford, Bodleian Libraries, Opp. Add. Fol. 12, fol. 254[a]): סַפַּ׳רְגַ׳ל ... כשירחץ דשן ענפיו ועליו יהיה כמו התותיא ומרבבו ינקה לטוב קיבוצו ומירבב התפוחים הוא חמוץ מפני שבו מן הלחות המימיית הקר ([Arab.] *safarjal*: Quince [*Cydonia oblonga* Mill.]: ... If the ashes of its branches and leaves are washed, it becomes like tutty. A rob of quince has a cleansing effect because of its sound astringency, but a rob of apples becomes sour because it contains cold watery moisture). Hebr. מירבב, occurring throughout Zeraḥyah's *Sefer ha-Qanun*,[197] is not attested in the current dictionaries. In addition to מירבב, Zeraḥyah uses *Part. Puʿal* מְרוּבָּב (see entry [רבב]). Nathan ha-Me'ati and Anonymous I both render Arab. رُبّ التفاح as עסיס התפוח(ים). See also entry עָסִיס for the term עסיס מבושל used by Nathan.

מַכְאוֹב • **מכאוב הרגלים** · **podagra; gout**: Arab. نقرس · Ibn Sīnā, *K. al-Qānūn* II · trans. Nathan ha-Me'ati, *Sefer ha-Qanun* (Ms Oxford, Bodleian Libraries, Can. Or. 88, fol. 109[a]): סכבינג׳ ... יועיל ממכאו׳ הרגלים ובער׳ נקרס ומחתוך העצלים ([Arab.] *sakbīnaj*: Sagapenum [i.e., i.e., the gum resin of the Persian giant fennel [*Ferula persica* Willd.]]: It is useful for podagra, [called] in Arab. *niqris*, and for muscle tear). Hebr. מכאוב הרגלים is not attested for medieval medical literature in the current dictionaries. Anonymous I transcribes Arab. نقرس as נקרס. For the synonymous terms נִכְאוּת and נכאות הרגלים, also used by Nathan in his *Sefer ha-Qanun* II, see NM 6:140f.

מַכָּה • *Plur.* **מכות** · **small abscesses; boils**: Arab. دُمّل, *Plur.* دماميل (Gr. δοθίην; cf. UW 203f.) · Ibn Sīnā, *K. al-Qānūn* II · trans. Nathan ha-Me'ati, *Sefer ha-Qanun* (Ms Oxford, Bodleian Libraries, Can. Or. 88, fol. 94[b]): כטמי ... ירכך המורסות וימנע אותם ויתיר המורסות הדמיות ויבשל המכות ויועיל ממורסות הנפח והחזירים ([Arab.] *khiṭmī*: Common marshmallow [*Althaea officinalis* L.]: ... It softens and prevents swellings. It dissolves hematomas, matures small abscesses (boils), and is useful for flatulent swellings and scrofula). Hebr. מַכָּה, *Plur.* מכות, features in the sense of 'wound; plague; stroke; blow' in the Bible and Rabb. literature (cf. KB 579; JD 781). In medieval medical literature it is also attested as 'ulcer' (cf. BCD 149 (NM 1:29)). In his trans. of Maimonides' *Medical Aphorisms* (i.e., *Sefer ha-Peraqim*) XXIII.39a, Nathan transcribes Arab. دمل 'furuncle' as דמאיל (cf. BMMN 223, l. 14; BMMG no. 1790), while Zeraḥyah has שיקולין ובערבי דומלא (cf. BMMZ 221, l. 22; BMMG no. 1790). In the *K. al-Qānūn* II, entry ملح 'salt,' Nathan translates Arab. دماميل as מורסות הנק׳ דמאמיל and Zeraḥyah has שחינים קטנים.

מְכֻזָּב (*Part. Piʿel*) → **כָּזַב**.

מְלוּחַ · **salting; preservation in salt**: Arab. تمليح · Ibn Sīnā, *K. al-Qānūn* II · trans. Zeraḥyah Ḥen, *Sefer ha-Qanun* (Ms Oxford, Bodleian Libaries, Opp. Add. Fol. 12,

---

197 The same term features, e.g., on fol. 186[a], entry בַּנְגְ׳ יוּשְׁקִיאָמוּ '[Arab.] *banj*; [i.e., Rom.] YWuŠəQiY'aMWu [i.e., Ital.-Rom. *iusquiamo*]: Black henbane [*Hyoscyamus niger* L.].' It also features as מי רבב (read: מירבב) in Zeraḥyah's trans. of Maimonides' *Medical Aphorisms* (i.e., *Sefer ha-Peraqim*) XIII.44 (cf. BMMZ 149, l. 12; BMMG no. 2032).

fol. 253[a–b]): סמך דג ... והמשובח שיהיה בו הוא שיבשל המים עד שירתיחו ואחרי כן ישים בו הדג אבל המלוח הוא טוב בעודנו חדש ולא יעמוד הדג במילוחו הרבה ([Arab.] *samak*; [i.e., Hebr.] *dag*: Fish: The best [boiled fish] is that which is put into water once it is boiling; salted fish is [only] good as long as it is fresh and has not been preserved in salt for a long time). Hebr. מְלוּחַ is not attested in the current dictionaries. Nathan ha-Me'ati translates Arab. تمليح as מליחה.

מְלוּי · **rheum:**[198] Arab. زكام · Ibn Sīnā, *K. al-Qānūn* II · trans. Nathan ha-Me'ati, *Sefer ha-Qanun* (Ms Oxford, Bodleian Libraries, Can. Or. 88, fols. 76[a]–77[b]): דרציני ... יועיל מהמלוי הנקרא זכאם בערבי ([Arab.] *dārṣīnī*: Cinnamon [*Cinnamomum verum* J. Presl]: ... It is beneficial for rheum, called *zukām* in Arab.). Hebr. מְלוּי is not attested in this sense in the current dictionaries. In medieval medical literature it features in the sense of 'dyspepsia; indigestion' and 'satiation' in BCD 150f. (NM 1:163; 3:131f.). In addition to מְלוּי, Nathan uses the term מלוי הראש (cf. NM 6:119) in his *Sefer ha-Qanun* II. Zeraḥyah Ḥen transcribes Arab. زكام as זכאם and Anonymous I renders the Arab. term as זכאם הוא קטרא and הזלות הראש (see entry הַזָּלָה).

מֶלַח • **מלח בורצי** · **tanners' salt**: Arab. ملح الصبّاغين (cf. MIG no. 1043) · *Shinnui ha-Shemot ha-Niqra'im Synonimi*, Mem 31 (Ms Florence, Biblioteca Medicea Laurenziana, Or. 17, fol. 83[a]): מלח הוא מינין הרבה מלח זכוכית מלח אינדיאי מלח בורצי מלח מחצבי הנחצב מארץ כנען מלח הנאכל מלח אנטריאני הוא מלח סוכרינו כפי ראזי (Salt: There are many kinds of salt: glass[maker's] salt (potassium or soda), Indian salt, tanners' salt, mineral salt, which is quarried from the land of Canaan, cooking salt, rock salt (MLḤ 'NṬRY'NY [read: MLḤ 'NDR'NY]), that is MLḤ SWKRYNW (?) according to [al-]Rāzī). Hebr. מלח בורצי is a non-attested calque from Arab. ملح الصبّاغين.

• **מלח זכוכית** · **[lit. glass[maker's] salt]; potassium or soda**: Arab. ملح الزجّاجين (cf. MIG no. 908) · *Shinnui ha-Shemot ha-Niqra'im Synonimi*, Mem 31 (Ms Florence, Biblioteca Medicea Laurenziana, Or. 17, fol. 83[a]): מלח הוא מינין הרבה מלח זכוכית מלח אינדיאי מלח בורצי מלח מחצבי הנחצב מארץ כנען מלח הנאכל מלח אנטריאני הוא מלח סוכרינו כפי ראזי (Salt: There are many kinds of salt: glass[maker's] salt (potassium or soda), Indian salt, tanners' salt, mineral salt, which is quarried from the land Canaan, cooking salt, rock salt (MLḤ 'NṬRY'NY [read: MLḤ 'NDR'NY]), that is MLḤ SWKRYNW (?) according to [al-]Rāzī). Hebr. מלח זכוכית is a non-attested calque from Arab. ملح الزجّاجين.

• **פרח המלח** → פֶּרַח.

• **קצף המלח** → קֶצֶף.

מֶלֶךְ • **גרגרי המלך** → גַּרְגַּר.

• **גרעיני המלך** → גַּרְעִין.

מְלַכְלֵךְ (*Part. Pi'el*) → לִכְלֵךְ.

---

198 'rheum': Cf. Wallis, *Medieval Medicine*, 550: 'a morbid discharge of phlegm in the head (e.g., a runny nose), eyes, joints, etc.'

מְמַסְמֵס (*Part. Piʿel*) → **מִסְמֵס**.
מַמְעִיד (*Part Hifʿil*) → [**מעד**].
מְנַגֵּב (*Part. Piʿel*) → [**נגב**].
מְנַגֵּעַ (*Part. Piʿel*) → **נָגַע**.
מְנֻגָּע (*Part. Puʿal*) → **נָגַע**.
מִנְהָג • **מנהגו ש־** · **being of someone's business, property, nature to ...**: Arab. من شأنه أن (cf. Lane 1491) · Ibn Sīnā, *K. al-Qānūn* II · trans. Nathan ha-Me'ati, *Sefer ha-Qanun* (Ms Oxford, Bodleian Libraries, Can. Or. 88, fol. 56[b]): והמבשל הוא אשר מנהגו שיועיל אל התערוב בשול מפני שהוא מחמם ביושר ובו כח קובץ יעצר התערוב עד שיתבשל ולא יתך בכבדות (A ripening (coctive) [drug is a drug] that—by its nature—is good for the ripening (concoction) of the humor because of its moderate heat; it has a astringent property, which retains the humor until it is ripe and does not dissolve it forcefully). Hebr. מנהגו ש־ is not attested in the current dictionaries. Zeraḥyah Ḥen translates Arab. من شأنه أن as מטבעו ש־ (see entry טֶבַע) and Anonymous I has דרכו ל־ (see entry דֶּרֶךְ).
מְנוּגָּע → מְנֻגָּע.
מְנוּחָה · **seat**: Arab. مسكن · al-Rāzī, *K. fī al-Faṣd* · trans. Anonymous, *Ma'amar ba-Haqqazah* (Ms Parma, Biblioteca Palatina, Cod. Parm. 2283,4, fol. 95[a]): וידוע כי סבות העלוף רבות ורפואתו מתחלפת ופעלתו א׳ והוא התכת הכח החיוני ומנוחתו[199] הלב (It is well-known that there are many causes of losing consciousness, its treatment varies, yet its effect is one, i.e., the dissolution of the animal faculty, the seat of which is the heart). Hebr. מְנוּחָה does not feature in this sense in the current dictionaries.
מַנְחִיר (*Part. Hifʿil*) → [**נחר**].
מְנַפֵּחַ (*Part. Piʿel*) → **נָפַח**.
מְסַגֵּר (*Part. Piʿel*) → **סָגַר**.
מְסוּרְטָן → מְסֻרְטָן.
מִסְמֵס • *Part. Piʿel* **מְמַסְמֵס** · **melting**: Arab. مذيب · Ibn Sīnā, *K. al-Qānūn* II · trans. Nathan ha-Me'ati, *Sefer ha-Qanun* (Ms Oxford, Bodleian Libraries, Can. Or. 88, fol. 79[b]): היופאריקון ... מרקיק מפתח ממסמס מתיר ([Arab.] *hayūfārīqūn* [from Gr. ὑπερικόν]: St. John's wort [*Hypericum* sp.]: ... It has a refining, opening, melting, and dissolving [effect]). Hebr. מִסְמֵס features in Rabb. literature, a.o., in the sense of 'to melt, make faint,' but not in a medical context. Zeraḥyah Ḥen translates Arab. مذيب as *Part Hifʿil* מֵזִיב (see entry [זוב]) and Anonymous I has *Part. Hifʿil* מֵמִיס (see entry [מסס]).
מַסְמֵרִיי · **cautery shaped like a round (blunt) nail**: Lat. *clavilis* · Guy de Chauliac, *Inventarium sive Chirurgia Magna* (cf. CMM 1:416, ll. 27–28) · trans. Anonymous (Ms Paris, BnF, héb. 1189, fol. 227[b]): ובמרחב החזה במקורות הזרועות בג׳ אצבעות רחוק מן הפרק עם[200] המסמריי העגול ... ([Cauterization] of the shoulder blade, in the hollows of the

199 ומנוחתו: Emend. ed. ומנוחת Ms ومسكنها a.
200 עם המסמרים העגול: *cum clavili rotundo* L.

arms, three fingers from the joint … with a cautery shaped like a round (blunt) nail). In the sense of 'cautery shaped like a round (blunt) nail,' Hebr. מַסְמֵרִיי is not attested in the current dictionaries.

[מסס] • *Part. Hifʿil* מֵמִיס · **melting**: Arab. مذيب · Ibn Sīnā, *K. al-Qānūn* II · trans. Anonymous I, *Sefer ha-Qanun* (Ms Paris, BnF, héb. 1142, fol. 108[b]): היופאריקון הוא איפריקון … מדקדק פותח ממיס מתיך ([Arab.] *hayūfārīqūn*; i.e., [Gr.] ʾYPRYQWN [i.e., ὑπερικόν]: St. John's wort [*Hypericum* sp.]: … It has a refining, opening, melting, and dissolving [effect]). In the sense of 'to melt,' Hebr. [מסס], *Hifʿil* הֵמִיס, features in BM 3128 in an attestation from the Bible (Deut 1:28) and in EM 986 without attestation. Nathan ha-Meʾati translates Arab. مذيب as *Part. Piʿel* מְמַסְמֵס (see entry מְסָמֵס) and Zeraḥyah Ḥen has *Part Hifʿil* מֵזִיב (see entry [זוב]).

מִסְעָד · **diet**: Lat. *dieta* · Guy de Chauliac, *Inventarium sive Chirurgia Magna* (cf. CMM 1:228, ll. 11–13) · trans. Anonymous (Ms Paris, BnF, héb. 1189, fol. 124[b]): אמנם רפויו מלבד ההנהגה הכוללת מהמסעד והתבלין[201] והנקויים הנאמרים במורסות ובועות אדומות ובנגעים הוירוליוש הוא שירוחץ המקום (Beyond the general regimen consisting of a diet and frequent[202] purging, which we mentioned for swellings, choleric pustules, and virulent ulcers, their cure should consist of washing the spot). Hebr. מִסְעָד features in BM 3131 in attestations from medieval medical literature in the sense of 'food administered to sick people to strengthen them.' It features, as *Plur.* מסעדים, in the sense of 'treatments' in NM 6:121 in an attestation from Samuel Benveniste's trans. of Maimonides' *On Asthma* (i.e., *Maʾamar ʿal ha-Qaṣeret*) XIII.18 (cf. BMA 2:303, l. 7).

מִסְפָּרַיִם · **forceps**: Lat. *forceps* · Guy de Chauliac, *Inventarium sive Chirurgia Magna* (cf. CMM 1:440, ll. 29–31) · trans. Anonymous (Ms Paris, BnF, héb. 1189, fol. 230[a]): וכשנרצה להסיר הבועות יחתכו ויפתחו עם המספרים או עם המחט (If we want to remove blisters, they should be cut and opened with a forceps or with a needle). Hebr. מִסְפָּרַיִם features in BM 3135 in the sense of 'scissors' in attestations from Rabb. literature only (cf. JD 810).

מְסֻרְטָן (*Part. Puʿal*) → [סרטן].

מְסַתֵּם (*Part. Piʿel*) → סָתַם.

מִסְתַּפֵּק (*Part.*) → [ספק].

מְעַבֶּה (*Part. Piʿel*) → [עבה].

[מעד] • *Part Hifʿil* • מַמְעִיד • הסם הממעיד → סַם.

• הרפואה הממעידה → רְפוּאָה.

מְעוּלֶּה → מְעֻלֶּה.

מְעִי • *Plur.* מעים • כאב המעים → כְּאֵב.

---

201 והתבלין והנקויים: *et crebra purgatione* L.

202 'frequent purging': Trans. acc. to L.

- נֶגַע → נגעי המעים.
- עֶקֶץ → עקץ המעים.

מְעִידָה · **slipperiness**: Arab. زلق · Ibn Sīnā, *K. al-Qānūn* II · trans. Nathan ha-Me'ati, *Sefer ha-Qanun* (Ms Oxford, Bodleian Libraries, Can. Or. 88, fol. 111[a]): סליכה ... ויועיל מכאבי הכליות וכיס השתן וכאשר תשב האשה בתבשילו יועיל מרחב הרחם ומעידתו ([Arab.] *salīkha*: Chinese cinnamon [*Cinnamomum cassia* (L.) D. Don]: ... It is good for pain in the intestines and urinary bladder. A sitz bath in the decoction is good for dilation and slipperiness of the uterus). Hebr. מְעִידָה is not attested for medieval Hebr. medical literature. The term features in BCD 155 (cf. NM 1:164) as מעידת המעים (for Arab. زلق الأمعاء) in the sense of 'lientery' in an attestation from Zeraḥyah Ḥen's trans. of Maimonides' *Medical Aphorisms* (i.e., *Sefer ha-Peraqim*) XX.36 (cf. BMMZ 211, l. 13; BMMG no. 2282). Here, Zeraḥyah Ḥen and Anonymous I both render Arab. زلق as הַמְעָדָה (see entry).

מְעַכֵּל (*Part. Pi'el*) → [עכל].

מעלה · **sublimate**: Arab. مصعد · Ibn Sīnā, *K. al-Qānūn* II · trans. Zeraḥyah Ḥen, *Sefer ha-Qanun* (Ms Oxford, Bodleian Libaries, Opp. Add. Fol. 12, fol. 205[a]): זיבק כסף חי ... מעלהו קובץ ([Arab.] *zi'baq*; [i.e., Hebr.] *kesef ḥay*: Quicksilver (mercury): ... Its sublimate is astringent). In the sense of 'sublimate,' Hebr. מעלה is a non-attested calque from Arab. مصعد. A marginal gloss to מעלה reads: שולימאדו. Nathan ha-Me'ati translates Arab. مصعد as עוֹלֶה (see entry עָלָה) and Anonymous I has הנעלה בכלי ההעלאה.

מְעֻלֶּה (*Part. Pu'al*) → עָלָה.

מְעַסֶּה (*Part. Pi'el*) → [עסה].

מְעַפֵּץ (*Part. Pi'el*) → [עפץ].

מְעַפֵּשׁ (*Part. Pi'el*) → [עפש].

מַעֲשֶׂה · **effect**: Arab. أثر · Ibn Sīnā, *K. al-Qānūn* II · trans. Zeraḥyah Ḥen, *Sefer ha-Qanun* (Ms Oxford, Bodleian Libaries, Opp. Add. Fol. 12, fol. 256[a]): עֻנָּאב ... והמאמר הטוב בו הוא מה שאמר בו ג'אלינוס: לא מצאתי לייֻנזובי על שמירת הבריאות בבריאים ולא להשיבה בבריאים מעשה גדול ([Arab.] *'unnāb*: Jujube [*Ziziphus* sp.]: ... The best statement regarding jujube is that by Galen: I did not find that jujube has a significant effect on preserving the health of healthy people and restoring the health of [sick] people). Hebr. מַעֲשֶׂה is not attested in this sense in the current dictionaries. For its different meanings in medieval philosophical literature, cf. PESHAT[203]). Nathan ha-Me'ati translates Arab. أثر as סימן and Anonymous I renders the Arab. term as רֹשֶׁם (see entry).

מְפַגֵּג (*Part. Pi'el*) → [פגג].

מְפוֹצֵץ (*Part. Polel*) → [פצץ].

מְפַזֵּר (*Part. Pi'el*) → [פזר].

---

203 https://peshat.org/display/peshat_lemmas_00002710 (accessed July 27, 2022).

מְפָרֵךְ (*Part. Piʿel*) → [פרך].
מְפַתֵּחַ (*Part. Piʿel*) → פָּתַח.
מְפַתֵּת (*Part. Piʿel*) → [פתת].
[מצא] • *Part. Nifʿal* **נִמְצָא** • **הזמן הנמצא** → זְמַן.
מַצָּב • **מצב הנשימה** · **orthopnea**: Arab. انتصاب النفس (cf. UW 471, s.v. ὀρθόπνοια: نفس (الانتصاب) · Ibn Sīnā, *K. al-Qānūn* II · trans. Nathan ha-Me'ati, *Sefer ha-Qanun* (Ms Oxford, Bodleian Libraries, Can. Or. 88, fol. 73[a]): בול והוא השתן ... יועיל ממצב הנשימה ([Arab.] *bawl*; i.e., [Hebr.] *sheten*: Urine: ... It is good for orthopnea). Hebr. מצב הנשימה is not attested in the current dictionaries. Zeraḥyah Ḥen translates Arab. انتصاب النفس as הצבת הניפוש (see entry הַצָּבָה), while he translates Arab. انتصاب 'orthopnea' as מַצָּב in his trans. of Maimonides' *Medical Aphorisms* (i.e., *Sefer ha-Peraqim*) XXIV.38 (cf. BCD 156 (NM 1:165); BMMZ 238, l. 23; BMMG no. 5143). Anonymous I renders Arab. انتصاب النفس as התיצבות הנשימה (cf. NM 6:60, s.v. הִתְיַצְּבוּת, for an attestation from the anonymous trans. of Maimonides' *On Asthma* (i.e., *Sefer ha-Qaṣeret*) N.2 (cf. BMA 2:388, l. 2)).
מִצְטַעֵר (*Part. Hitpaʿel*) → [צער].
מַצְמִיחַ (*Part. Hifʿil*) → [צמח].
מִצְמֵץ · **to rinse**: Arab. تمضمض · Ibn Sīnā, *K. al-Qānūn* II · trans. Anonymous I, *Sefer ha-Qanun* (Ms Paris, BnF, héb. 1142, fols. 129[b]–130[b]): יתוע ... ואם יבושל שרשו בחומץ וימצמץ בו ישקיט כאב השנים ([Arab.] *yattūʿ*: Spurge [*Euphorbia* sp.]: ... If one boils its root with vinegar and rinses [the mouth] with it, it alleviates toothache). Hebr. מִצְמֵץ features in the sense of 'to rinse' in BM 3252 in attestations from the *Sefer ha-Qanun*. Nathan ha-Me'ati translates Arab. تمضمض as שכשך and Zeraḥyah Ḥen has קִשְׁקֵשׁ (cf. NM 6:195).
[מיצע] • *Piʿel* **מִיצַּע** · **to balance**: Arab. عدّل · Ibn Sīnā, *K. al-Qānūn* II · trans. Zeraḥyah Ḥen, *Sefer ha-Qanun* (Ms Oxford, Bodleian Libaries, Opp. Add. Fol. 12, fol. 160[b]): והמחזקת היא הרפואה אשר מדרכה שתמצע עצמות האבר ומזגו עד שימנע מקבלת המותרות והחליים (A tonic [drug] is a drug that—by its nature—balances the substance and temperament of an organ to an extent that it prevents the absorption of superfluous matters and disorders). Hebr. *Piʿel* מִצַּע is not attested for medieval medical literature. Nathan ha-Me'ati translates Arab. عدّل as *Piʿel* יִשֵּׁר (see entry [ישר]) and Anonymous I has *Hifʿil* הִשְׁוָה (see entry [שוה]).
מִצְרִי • **קוץ מצרי** → קוֹץ.
מִקְוֶה • **אבן המקוה** → אֶבֶן.
מַקִּיף (*Part. Hifʿil*) → [נקף].
מָקוֹר • **אבן המקור** → אֶבֶן.
מְקַלֵּף (*Part. Piʿel*) → קִלֵּף.
מֻקָּף (*Part. Hofʿal*) → [נקף].
מַרְדִּים (*Part. Hifʿil*) → [רדם].
מְרוּבָּב (*Part. Puʿal*) → [רבב].

מֵרוּק · **detergent; cleansing property**: Arab. جلاء (Gr. σμῆξις; cf. UWS 2:305) · Ibn Sīnā, *K. al-Qānūn* II · trans. Anonymous I, *Sefer ha-Qanun* (Ms Paris, BnF, héb. 1142, fols. 219b–220a): קונטריון ... יש בו מרוק וקביצות וחריפות ומעט מתיקות ומנגב בלי עקיצה ([Arab.] *qanṭūriyūn*: Knapweed [*Centaurea centaurium* L.] or common centaury [*Centaurium erythraea* Rafn.]: ... It is detergent, astringent, pungent, and somewhat sweet; it dries without causing irritation). Hebr. מֵרוּק features in BM 3321 in an attestation, a.o., from the *Sefer ha-Qanun* and is explained by Ben Yehudah as נקיון וצחצוח. Zeraḥyah Ḥen translates Arab. جلاء as טָהֳרָה (see entry).

מְרוּקָּח (*Part. Pu'al*) → מְרֻקָּח.

מֶרְחָב • **מרחב החזה** · **shoulder blade**: Lat. *homoplate* · Guy de Chauliac, *Inventarium sive Chirurgia Magna* (cf. CMM 1:416, ll. 27–28) · trans. Anonymous (Ms Paris, BnF, héb. 1189, fol. 227b): ובמרחב החזה במקורות הזרועות בג' אצבעות רחוק מן הפרק ... עם המסמרים העגול ([Cauterization] of the shoulder blade, in the hollows of the arms, three fingers from the joint ... with a cautery shaped like a round (blunt) nail). Hebr. מרחב החזה is not attested in the current dictionaries.

מְרָיִם • עשב מרים → עֵשֶׂב.

[מרס] • *Pu'al* מֹרַס · **to be dissolved**: Lat. *dissolvor* · Guy de Chauliac, *Inventarium sive Chirurgia Magna* (cf. CMM 1:231, ll. 32–33) · trans. Anonymous (Ms Paris, BnF, héb. 1189, fol. 126b): וביחוד אמ' א"ס שאם ימורס במי העפצים ... (Ibn Sīnā said that [this recipe is especially effective] when [the mentioned ingredients] are dissolved in gallnut juice). Hebr. מֹרַס features in Rabb. literature in the sense of 'to be crushed, rubbed, stirred' (cf. JD 845); Ben Yehuda mentions it in the sense of 'to be stirred, mixed' (cf. BM 3339: בחש) and in the sense of 'to be dissolved and stirred' (ibid.: מחה ובחש).

מֹרַס (*Pu'al*) → [מרס].

מֻרְסָא (*Aram.*) • **המורסא הפתוחה** · **lachrymal fistula**: Arab. غرب (Gr. αἰγιλώπιον; cf. UWS 1:71) · Ibn Sīnā, *K. al-Qānūn* II · trans. Nathan ha-Me'ati, *Sefer ha-Qanun* (Ms Oxford, Bodleian Libraries, Can. Or. 88, fol. 68a): באבונג' ... ירפא המרסא הפתוחה הנקרא גרב בערבי כשעושין ממנו תחבשת ([Arab.] *bābūnaj*: Camomile [*Matricaria chamomilla* L.]: ... It cures lachrymal fistula, called *gharab* in Arab., when it is applied as a plaster). Aram.-Hebr. המרסא הפתוחה is not attested in the current dictionaries. Zeraḥyah Ḥen transcribes Arab. غرب as גרב and Anonymous I renders the Arab. term as המורסא הנקר' גרב. On fol. 112b, entry ענב אלתעלב '[Arab.] *'inab al-tha'lab*: Common/black nightshade [*Solanum nigrum* L.],' Nathan translates Arab. غرب as הנאצור הנק' גרב בערבי, while on fol. 91a, entry כמאדריוס '[Arab.] *kamādariyūs* [from Gr. χαμαίδρυς]: Wall germander [*Teucrium chamaedrys* L.],' he transcribes the Arab. term as גרב only. The latter term recurs in his trans. of Maimonides' *Medical Aphorisms* (i.e., *Sefer ha-Peraqim*) XV.29 (cf. BMMN 158, l. 15) and XXIII.72 (cf. BMMN 228, l. 4) (see also BMMG no. 3642).

מֻרְסָה • **מורסת המוח** · **phrenitis**: Arab. شرسام (cf. MIG no. 1002) · al-Rāzī, *K. fī al-Faṣd* · trans. Anonymous, *Ma'amar ba-Haqqazah* (Ms Parma, Biblioteca Palatina, Cod.

Parm. 2283,4, fol. 94b): הקזת הקיפאל יועיל מההכאה והנפילה המתחדשות בראש ומכובד הגוף[204] ומכאב הראש ומגלגולו בעת התנועה ומסבוב הראש הנק׳ אלדואר אשר עם אדמימות הפנים ומלוי הגידים וממורסת המוח החמה הנק׳ אלשירסאם (Bleeding the cephalic vein is beneficial for a blow or a fall that occurs to the head, for heaviness of the body and headache, for dizziness while moving, for dizziness, called [in Arab.] *al-dawār*, combined with redness of the face, for overfilling of the veins, and for hot phrenitis called [in Arab.] *al-shirsām*). Hebr. מורסת המוח features in BCD 161 (NM 3:143) in an attestation from Moses ibn Tibbon's trans. of Maimonides' *Commentary on Hippocrates' Aphorisms* (i.e., *Perush Aphorismi shel Apuqraṭ*) IV.72 (cf. BMCH 1:373, l. 23). A synonym featuring in Shem Tov ben Isaac's *Sefer ha-Shimmush* XXIX, list 1 is צמח המוח (cf. NM 5:169; SHS 1:439 (Ṣade 22)).

• **מורסת הצלעות** · **pleurisy**: Arab. شوصة · i. Ibn Sīnā, *K. al-Qānūn* II · trans. Nathan ha-Me'ati, *Sefer ha-Qanun* (Ms Oxford, Bodleian Libraries, Can. Or. 88, fol. 106a–b): נילופאר ... משקהו טוב אל השעול ומורסת הצלעות והוא שוצה בערבי ([Arab.] *nīlūfar*: Water lily (e.g., blue Egyptian water lily [*Nymphaea nouchali* var. *caerulea* (Savigny) Verdc.]; European white water lily [*Nymphaea alba* L.]; yellow water lily [*Nuphar lutea* (L.) Sm.]): ... Its syrup is good in cough and pleurisy, i.e., *shawṣa* in Arab.). Hebr. מורסת הצלעות is not attested in the current dictionaries. Zeraḥyah Ḥen translates Arab. شوصة as Rom. פיאורילישיו and Anonymous I transcribes the Arab. term as שוסה. In his trans. of Maimonides' *Medical Aphorisms* (i.e., *Sefer ha-Peraqim*), Nathan translates/transcribes Arab. شوصة as חולי האלשוצה or שוצה (cf. BMMG no. 2770). Moses ibn Tibbon translates the Arab. term as מורסת המסך in his trans. of Ibn al-Jazzār's *Zād al-musāfir* (i.e., *Sefer Ṣedat ha-Derakhim*) N.4 (cf. BCD 161 (NM 4:105); IJZ 1–2:441). Another Hebr. synonym, featuring in Shem Tov ben Isaac' *Sefer ha-Shimmush* XXIX, list 1, is צמח בטרפשה (cf. NM 5:168f.; SHS 1:438f. (Ṣade 21)).

· ii. al-Rāzī, *K. fī al-Faṣd* · trans. Anonymous, *Ma'amar ba-Haqqazah* (Ms Parma, Biblioteca Palatina, Cod. Parm. 2283,4, fol. 94b): השער הז׳ במשיכת הליחות בעבור היות הליחות בהתחלת החליים אשר מסבת הדם נגרות בעת תכליתם עומדות ונעצרות יתחייב להחליף ולשנות כפי זה מקומות ההקזה משל לזה כי מי שיקרהו חלי מורסת הצלעות הנק׳ אלשוצא מסבת הדם בצד הימין צריך להשתדל לרפאותו בתחלת החלי (Ch. 7: On drawing [superfluous] humors: Since sanguine [superfluous] humors are flowing in the beginning of diseases and are stagnant in the end of them, one should vary the sites of bloodletting accordingly. For instance, someone affected by sanguine pleurisy, called [in Arab.] *al-shawṣa*, on the right side should be treated in the beginning of the disease [as follows ...]).

204 ומכובד הגוף ומכאב הראש: ومن الصداع الذي معه ثقل البدن والرأس a.

• *Plur.* **מורסות • המורסות הפרים** · **spreading ulcers**: Arab. الأورام الساعية · Ibn Sīnā, *K. al-Qānūn* II · trans. Nathan ha-Me'ati, *Sefer ha-Qanun* (Ms Oxford, Bodleian Libraries, Can. Or. 88, fol. 81[b]): זאג ... הקלקטר יועיל מן האודם והמורסות הפרים ([Arab.] *zāj*: Vitriol: ... Yellow vitriol is useful for erysipelas and spreading ulcers). Hebr. *Sing.* המורסה הפרה is not attested in the current dictionaries. Zeraḥyah Ḥen translates Arab. الأورام الساعية as המורסות המתפשטות (see next entry) and Anonymous I renders the Arab. term as המורסות המתרחבות (see entry below). The synonymous Arab. term القروح الساعية is translated by Nathan as הנגעים הפרים (cf. NM 6:137).

• **המורסות המתפשטות** · **spreading ulcers**: Arab. الأورام الساعية · Ibn Sīnā, *K. al-Qānūn* II · trans. Zeraḥyah Ḥen, *Sefer ha-Qanun* (Ms Oxford. Opp. Add. Fol. 12, fol. 205[a–b]): זַאגְ׳ וִיטְרִיאוֹל ... הקלקטאר יועיל מן האודם והמורסות המתפשטות ([Arab.] *zāj*; [i.e., Lat./Rom.] WeYṬRiY'WoL: Vitriol: ... Yellow vitriol is useful for erysipelas and spreading ulcers). Hebr. המורסה המתפשטת, *Plur.* המורסות המתפשטות, is a non-attested calque from Arab. الأورام الساعية. Nathan ha-Me'ati translates Arab. الأورام الساعية as המורסות הפרים (see previous entry) and Anonymous I has המורסות המתרחבות (see next entry). In his trans. of Maimonides' *Medical Aphorisms* (i.e., *Sefer ha-Peraqim*) II.25, Zeraḥyah translates Arab. الورم الساعي 'shingles' as המורסא השורצת כלומר המתפשטת (cf. BCD 162 (NM 1:191); BMMZ 31, l. 17; BMMG no. 5517), whereas Nathan has המורסא המתרחבת (cf. BCD 162 (NM 2:62); BMMN 39, l. 3; BMMG no. 5517). The synonymous Arab. term القروح الساعية is translated by Zeraḥyah as הנגעים השורצים (cf. NM 6:137).

• **המורסות המתרחבות** · **spreading ulcers**: Arab. الأورام الساعية · Ibn Sīnā, *K. al-Qānūn* II · trans. Anonymous I, *Sefer ha-Qanun* (Ms Paris, BnF, héb. 1142, fols. 115[b]–116[a]): זאג' הוא ויטריאולה ... הקלקטר מועיל מן החמרה והמורסות המתרחבות ([Arab.] *zāj*; i.e., [Lat./Rom.] WYṬRY'WLH: Vitriol: ... Yellow vitriol is useful for erysipelas and spreading ulcers). Hebr. *Sing.* המורסה המתרחבת features as המורסא המתרחבת in BCD 162 (NM 2:62) in an attestation from Nathan ha-Me'ati's trans. of Maimonides' *Medical Aphorisms* (i.e., *Sefer ha-Peraqim*) II.25 (cf. BMMN 39, l. 3; BMMG no. 5517). Nathan ha-Me'ati translates Arab. الأورام الساعية as המורסות הפרים (see entry above) and Zeraḥyah Ḥen has המורסות המתפשטות (see previous entry).

• **מורסות קשות** · **polyps (excrescenses)**: Arab. ناسور, *Plur.* نواسير · al-Rāzī, *K. fī al-Faṣd* · trans. Anonymous, *Ma'amar ba-Haqqazah* (Ms Parma, Biblioteca Palatina, Cod. Parm. 2283,4, fol. 96[a]): אלבסליק יועיל ממורסת הצלעות וממורסות קשות ברחם ([Bleeding] the basilic vein is beneficial for pleurisy and for polyps (excrescenses) in the uterus). Hebr. מורסות קשות is not attested in the current dictionaries.

• **המורסות אשר בעקר האזן** · **swellings at the base of the ears (parotitis)**: Arab. الأورام التي في أصل الأذن · Ibn Sīnā, *K. al-Qānūn* II · trans. Nathan ha-Me'ati, *Sefer ha-Qanun* (Ms Oxford, Bodleian Libraries, Can. Or. 88, fol. 110[b]): סמן ... יבשל המורסות וקל וחומר אשר בעקר האזן ויותר הנערים והנשים ולא יוכל לעשות כזה בגופות הקשות ([Arab.] *samn*: (Fresh) butter: ... It matures swellings, especially at the base of the ears (parotitis). This is especially the case in children and women but it does not have the same effect in hard bodies). Hebr. *Sing.* המורסה אשר בעקר האזן is not attested in the current dictionaries. Zeraḥyah Ḥen translates Arab. الأورام التي في أصل الأذن as המורסות אשר בשורש האזנים (see entry below) and Anonymous I has a similar *Sing.* term המרסה שהיא בשרש האזנים.

• **המורסות אשר יקרו בעת המגפה · plague boils (plague)**: Arab. طاعون, *Plur.* طواعين · Ibn Sīnā, *K. al-Qānūn* II · trans. Anonymous II, *Sefer ha-Qanun* (Ms Parma, Biblioteca Palatina, Cod. Parm. 3045, fol. 48ᵃ): לוטוס ארמיני ... יועיל למורסות אשר יקרו בעת המגפה אם ישתה או ימשח ומונע העיפוש מן האברים ([Lat.-Arab.] LWṬWS (*lutus*) *arminī*: Armenian bole: ... It is useful for plague boils (plague), either when taken orally or when rubbed [on the affected spot]. It prevents putrefaction of the organs). Hebr. המורסות אשר יקרו בעת המגפה is not attested in the current dictionaries. Nathan ha-Me'ati renders Arab. *Plur.* طواعين as טאעונים, but *Sing.* طاعون also as דֶּבֶר (see entry). Zeraḥyah Ḥen translates Arab. طواعين as אנדראש (i.e., Rom. *antras* / Lat. *anthrax* 'maligant boil') and Anonymous I renders the Arab. term as טאעון (see entry).

• **המורסות אשר בשורש האזנים · swellings at the base of the ears (parotitis)**: Arab. الأورام التي في أصل الأذن · Ibn Sīnā, *K. al-Qānūn* II · trans. Zeraḥyah Ḥen, Sefer ha-Qanun (Ms Oxford, Bodleian Libaries, Opp. Add. Fol. 12, fol. 252ʳ: סַמַן חמאה ... יבשל המורסות כל שכן אשר בשורש האזנים כל שכן לנערים ולנשים ולא יוכל על כמותו בגופות הקשים ([Arab.] *samn*; [i.e., Hebr.] *ḥem'ah*: (Fresh) butter: ... It matures swellings, especially at the base of the ears (parotitis). This is especially the case in children and women but it does not have the same effect in hard bodies). Hebr. *Sing.* המורסה אשר בשרש האזנים is not attested in the current dictionaries. Nathan ha-Me'ati translates Arab. الأورام التي في أصل الأذن as המורסות אשר בעקר האזן (see entry above) and Anonymous I has *Sing.* המרסה שהיא בשרש האזנים.

מְרַפֶּה (*Part. Pi'el*) → [**רפה**].

מְרֻקָּח (*Part. Pu'al*) → [**רקח**]

מְשֻׁבָּךְ (*Part. Pu'al*) → [**שבך**].

מְשַׁבֵּר (*Part. Pi'el*) → [**שבר**].

מְשׁוּבָךְ → מְשֻׁבָּךְ.

מְשׁוּתָף → מְשֻׁתָּף.

מָשַׁח · to apply as a salve: Arab. لُطُوخ (cf. WKAS 2.2:692) · Ibn Sīnā, *K. al-Qānūn* II · trans. Nathan ha-Me'ati, *Sefer ha-Qanun* (Ms Oxford, Bodleian Libraries, Can. Or. 88, fol. 123ᵃ): רכמה ... ואמרו קצתם כי נסו אותו לנשיכת העקרב והשרף ודבורים[205] והיה מועיל ואני חושב שזה כשמושחים בו ([Arab.] *rakham*: Vulture: ... Some say that they tried it for scorpion stings, snake bites, and wasp[206] stings, and found it to be useful. I think that this is [only the case] when it is applied as a salve). Hebr. מָשַׁח features in the current dictionaries in the sense of 'to smear, anoint' (cf. KB 643f.; JD 850f.; BM 3365f.).

205 ודבורים: زنبور a.
206 'wasp': Trans. acc. to a.

In addition to מְשַׁח, Nathan translates Arab. لُطُوخ as לִכְלֵךְ (see entry). Zeraḥyah Ḥen and Anonymous I both render Arab. لُطُوخ as טִיחָה (cf. BCD 112 for attestations from Shem Tov ben Isaac's *Sefer ha-Shimmush* XXX.2.20 (cf. NM 1:95) and Moses ibn Tibbon's trans. of Ibn al-Jazzār's *Zād al-musāfir* (i.e., *Sefer Ṣedat ha-Derakhim*) VII.16.3 (cf. NM 1:58; IJZ 7:153, l. 1)).

[משך] • *Part. Nif'al* **נִמְשָׁךְ** • **האברים הנמשכים** → **אֵבֶר**.

מְשַׁכֵּךְ (*Part. Pi'el*) → **[שכך]**.

מַשְׁמִין (*Part. Hif'il*) → **[שמן]**.

מַשְׁמָעוּת · **intention:** Lat. *intentio* (Arab. غرض) · Constantinus Africanus, *Viaticum* V.5, trans. Do'eg ha-Edomi, *Sefer Ya'ir Netiv*: אולם בשני ענינים נעזר האינדרופישים כמו שאמר גיאלינוס ומשמעותינו להיות האחד להתחזק הכח המבשל ואשר הדברים המזיקים אליו ימנעו ממנו והאחר הוא אשר טהרתו יאות עוד להחיש ולגרשו מן הגוף (We should treat dropsy with two things, as Galen said, (1) we should intend to strengthen the digestive faculty and to prevent him from [taking] things that harm it, and (2) we should quickly cleanse and evacuate [the fluid] from the body). Hebr. מַשְׁמָעוּת is not attested in this sense in the current dictionaries; cf. BM 3397: 'meaning, sense (of a word);' PESHAT: 'meaning.'[207] Moses ibn Tibbon translates Arab. غرض as כונה.

מִשְׁרָה · **infusion:** Arab. نقيع · Ibn Sīnā, *K. al-Qānūn* II · trans. Zeraḥyah Ḥen, *Sefer ha-Qanun* (Ms Oxford, Bodleian Libaries, Opp. Add. Fol. 12, fol. 222^{a-b}): ... כֻּנְדֻּר אוּלִיבַּנוּ יועיל לשכל ויחזק אותו ויש בני אדם מי שיצוה בשתיית משרתו על הריקנות ([Arab.] *kundur*; [i.e., Rom.] 'WuLiYBaNWu: Frankincense [*Boswellia sacra* Flueck.]: ... It is beneficial for the mind and strengthens it. Some order to drink an infusion of it on an empty stomach). In the sense of 'infusion; steeping,' Hebr. מִשְׁרָה is attested in Rabb. literature and in Maimonides' *Mishneh Torah* (cf. JD 858; BM 3419). The term features (for Arab. مطبوخ) in Moses ibn Tibbon's trans. of Ibn al-Jazzār's *Zād al-musāfir* (i.e., *Sefer Ṣedat ha-Derakhim*) IV.13 in the sense of 'decoction' (cf. NM 6:133). Nathan ha-Me'ati translates Arab. نقيع as שרוי (cf. BCD 285 (NM 1:193), where it features in the sense of 'macerating' in an attestation from Zeraḥyah Ḥen's trans. of Maimonides' *Medical Aphorisms* (i.e., *Sefer ha-Peraqim*) XX.64 (cf. BMMZ 189, l. 24)) and Anonymous I has מִשְׁרָה, just like Zeraḥyah.

מִשְׁתַּחֵן (*Part. Hitpa'el*) → **[שחן]**.

מְשֻׁתָּף (*Part. Pu'al*) → **[שָׁתַף]**.

מֵת (*Part.*) → **[מות]**.

מִתְאַכֵּל (*Part. Hitpa'el*) → **אָכַל**.

מִתְבָּרֵק (*Part. Hitpa'el*) → **[ברק]**.

מְתוּקָּן → מְתֻקָּן.

מִתְחַבֶּרֶת (*Part. Hitpa'el f.*) → **[חבר]**.

---

207 https://peshat.org/display/peshat_lemmas_00019567 (accessed May 11, 2022).

מְתִיחָה · **stretching**: Arab. امتداد · Ibn Sīnā, *K. al-Qānūn* II · trans. Nathan ha-Me'ati, *Sefer ha-Qanun* (Ms Oxford, Bodleian Libraries, Can. Or. 88, fol. 122[a]): ראונד ... אמר אלכוזי המשק׳ ממנו שני זוזים מזוג ביין מבושל וישקו ממנו אל הרצוץ עם יין ריחני וכן כאשר מושחים במשיחתו לרצוץ העצלים ואל מכאוביהם ואל המתיחה ויועיל מההתר ובער׳ פתק ([Arab.] *rāwand*: Rhubarb [*Rheum* sp.]: ... According to al-Khūzī, a potion of two *zuzim*[208] mixed with inspissated grape juice and fragrant boiled wine [is useful for] bruises; the same effect is achieved when its oil is rubbed on bruised and painful or stretched muscles. It is also good for hernia, [called] in Arab. *fatq*). Hebr. מְתִיחָה features in BCD 167 (NM 3:148) in the sense of 'tetanus.' In his trans. of Maimonides' *Medical Aphorisms* (i.e., *Sefer ha-Peraqim*) IX.91, Nathan translates Arab. امتداد as מְתִיחָה as well (cf. BMMN 116, l. 9; BMMG no. 4732), while the synonymous Arab. term تمدّد is translated by him as הִשְׁתַּטְּחוּת (see entry).

מִתְיַצֵּב (*Part. Hitpa'el*) → [**יצב**].

מֹתֶן • *Dual* **מתנים** · **false ribs (the costal cartilages of the false ribs)**: Arab. شرسوف, *Plur.* شراسيف (cf. D 1:744; FA no. 2994) · al-Rāzī, *K. fī al-Faṣd* · trans. Anonymous, *Ma'amar ba-Haqqazah* (Ms Parma, Biblioteca Palatina, Cod. Parm. 2283,4, fol. 96[a]): אלבסליק יועיל ממורסת הצלעות והשוצא וביניהם הפרש גדול כמו שזכרנו ואם יהיה הכאב נוטה אל צד המתנים הנק׳ אלשראסיף יהיה המשלשל תחלה ואחריו ההקזה ([Bleeding] the basilic vein is beneficial for pleurisy and pleuritis, which are very different from each other as we mentioned [before]. If the pain tends towards the false ribs (the costal cartilages of the false ribs), which are called [in Arab.] *al-sharāsīf*, one should at first apply purgation and then bloodletting). Hebr. מֹתֶן, *Dual* מתנים, does not feature in this sense in the current dictionaries.

מִתְפּוֹצֵץ (*Part. Hitpolel*) → [**פצץ**].

מִתְפַּשֵּׁט (*Part. Hitpa'el*) → [**פשט**].

מְתֻקָּן (*Part. Pu'al*) → [**תקן**].

מִתְרַחֵב (*Part. Hitpa'el*) → [**רחב**].

מִתְרַפֵּא (*Part. Hitpa'el*) → [**רפא**].

---

208 For the term *zuz*, a measure of weight equivalent to one *dirham* (= 3.125 g), cf. NM 6:64.

נ

נִבְדָּל (*Part. Nif'al*) → [**בדל**].

[נגב] • *Part. Pi'el* **מְנַגֵּב** • **הסם המנגב** → **סַם**.

• **הרפואה המנגבת** → **רְפוּאָה**.

נָגוּעַ (*Part. Pass.*) → **נָגַע**.

נִגּוּעַ · **ulceration**: Arab. تقريح · i. Ibn Sīnā, *K. al-Qānūn* II · trans. Zeraḥyah Ḥen, *Sefer ha-Qanun* (Ms Oxford, Bodleian Libaries, Opp. Add. Fol. 12, fol. 220[b]): יברוח ... ימשח עם עלהו הברש שבוע אחד ויתרפא בו בלא ניגוע ([Arab.] *yabrūḥ*: Mandrake [*Mandragora officinarum* L.]: ... If [the spot affected by] acne is rubbed with its leaves for one week, it is cured without ulceration). Hebr. נִגּוּעַ is attested in EM 1116 as a modern term in the sense of 'contamination.' In addition to נִגּוּעַ, Zeraḥyah translates Arab. تقريح as הַשְׁחָנָה (see entry) and חַבָּלָה (see entry). Nathan ha-Me'ati translates the Arab. term as *Nif'al* נִגַּע and Anonymous I has הַשְׁחָנָה (see entry).

· ii. Ibn Sīnā, *K. al-Qānūn* II · trans. Nathan ha-Me'ati, *Sefer ha-Qanun* (Ms Oxford, Bodleian Libraries, Can. Or. 88, fol. 56[a]): והאוכל הוא הסם שמנהגו שיגיע בהתוכו ונגועו שיחסיר עצם הבשר כמו הזנגאר (A corrosive [drug] is—by its nature—a drug that has solvent and ulcerative properties, which are so strong that they reduce the substance of the flesh [of the organ]; [an example of such a drug is] verdigris). Zeraḥyah Ḥen translates Arab. تقريح as חַבָּלָה (see entry) and Anonymous I has הַשְׁחָנָה (see entry).

נָגַע • *Part. Pass.* **נָגוּעַ** • **הגרב הנגוע** → **גָּרָב**.

• *Part. Pi'el* **מְנַגֵּעַ** • **הסם המנגע** → **סַם**.

• *Part. Pu'al* **מְנֻגָּע** · **ulcerous**: Lat. *ulcerosus* · Guy de Chauliac, *Inventarium sive Chirurgia Magna* (cf. CMM 1:224, l. 10) · trans. Anonymous (Ms Paris, BnF, héb. 1189, fol. 122[a]): הסרטן המנוגע הוא נגע נראה עגול ומאוס ומוסרח עם שפתים עבות וקשות (An ulcerous cancer is an ulcer that appears to be round, ugly, and fetid with thick, hard lips (margins)). In the sense of 'ulcerous,' Hebr. *Part. Pu'al* מְנֻגָּע features in BCD 170 (NM 3:132) (for Lat. *vulneratus*) in an attestation from Hillel ben Samuel's trans. of Hippocrates' *Aphorisms* V.23.

נֶגַע • **הנגע הדומה לדבש** · **favus**: Arab. القروح الشهدية · Ibn Sīnā, *K. al-Qānūn* II · trans. Zeraḥyah Ḥen, *Sefer ha-Qanun* (Ms Oxford, Bodleian Libaries, Opp. Add. Fol. 12, fol. 166[a–b]): אִכְלִיל אַלְמַלִךְ מַלִילוֹטָה ... יועיל מן המורסות הקשות והחמות וכל שכן הנגע הדומה לדבש ([Arab.] *iklīl al-malik* [lit. 'crown of the king']; [i.e., Lat.] MaLiYLWoṬaH [i.e., *mellilota*]: Melilot [*Melilotus officinalis* L.]: ... It is beneficial for hard, hot swellings, especially for favus). Hebr. הנגע הדומה לדבש is not attested in the current dictionaries. The Arab. synonym الأورام الشهدية is translated by Zeraḥyah as מור׳ הנקרא דבשיית (cf. NM 6:90, s.v. יַעֲרִי, Plur. יעריים). Nathan ha-Me'ati translates Arab. القروح الشهدية as ⟨המורסה⟩ הדבשית (ובער׳ אלשהדה) (cf. NM 6:128) and Anonymous I renders the Arab. term as ⟨השחינים⟩ היעריים (cf. NM 6:90).

• *Plur.* **נגעים** · **pustules**: Arab. بثور · al-Rāzī, *K. fī al-Faṣd* · trans. Anonymous, *Ma'amar ba-Haqqazah* (Ms Parma, Biblioteca Palatina, Cod. Parm. 2283,4, fol. 93[b]): וגיד א׳ בקצה החוטם ותועיל הקזתו מהכתמי׳ הנק׳ אלכלף[209] ומשנוי המראה והחמימות[210] והנגעים והחבורות אשר בחוטם והשפה (One vein in the tip of the nose, bleeding it is beneficial for freckles called [in Arab.] *al-kalaf*, discoloration, dandruff,[211] pustules and ulcers in the nose and the lips). Hebr. *Sing.* נֶגַע is attested in medieval medical literature in the sense of 'fistula' (cf. BCD 170 (NM 1:31f.)), 'ulcer' (cf. BCD 170 (NM 1:62)), and 'wound' (cf. ibid.).
• **נגעי המעים** · **intestinal abrasions**: Arab. سحج (الأمعاء) · Ibn Sīnā, *K. al-Qānūn* II · trans. Nathan ha-Me'ati, *Sefer ha-Qanun* (Ms Oxford, Bodleian Libraries, Can. Or. 88, fol. 78[b]): דם אלאכוין ... ימנע נגעי המעיים ויועיל מבקוע העגבות ([Arab.] *dam al-akhawayn* [lit. 'blood of the two brothers']: The resin of the Socotra dragontree [*Dracaena cinnabari* Balf. f.] (cf. MIG no. 73): It prevents intestinal abrasions and is beneficial for anal fissures). Hebr. נגעי המעים is not attested in this sense in the current dictionaries. Zeraḥyah Ḥen transcribes Arab. سحج (الأمعاء) as צחאג׳ and Anonymous I renders the Arab. term as הפשט המעיים. Synonyms featuring in medieval Hebr. medical literature are גרידה (cf. BCD 50 (NM 3:48), גרידת המעים (cf. BCD 50 (NM 3:48f.)), הפשט (cf. BCD 71 (NM 2:40f.)), חמרמרות המעים (cf. BCD 104 (NM 3:93)), and שלשול המעים (cf. BCD 277 (NM 3:229)).

[נגר] • *Hif'il* **הִגִּיר** • **הגיר השתן** · **to cause diuresis**: Arab. أدرّ البول (Gr. διουρητικός; cf. UWS 1:202) · Ibn Sīnā, *K. al-Qānūn* II · trans. Nathan ha-Me'ati, *Sefer ha-Qanun* (Ms Oxford, Bodleian Libraries, Can. Or. 88, fol. 105[b]): מוז ... יוסיף בתאות המשגל והוא נאות אל הכליות ויגיר השתן ([Arab.] *mawz*: Banana [*Musa paradisiaca* L.]: ... It increases the sexual lust, is suitable for kidney [ailments], and causes diuresis). Hebr. הגיר השתן is attested as הסם המגיר השתן 'the diuretic remedy' in BCD 187 (NM 4:125) in an anynomyous trans. of Ibn Sīnā's *K. al-Adwiya al-qalbiyya* (i.e., *Sammim Libbiyim*) (see also MD 132, s.v. 'diuretic'). Anonymous I renders Arab. أدرّ البول as הגיר השתן, just like Nathan, and Zeraḥyah Ḥen translates the Arab. term as הרבה השתן (see entry [רבה]).

נְדָנָה · **pod; pericarp; seed capsule**: Arab. قمع · Ibn Sīnā, *K. al-Qānūn* II · trans. Anonymous I, *Sefer ha-Qanun* (Ms Paris, BnF, héb. 1142, fol. 137[a–b]): כרסנה ... אמר דיאסקורידס הוא עשב קטן דק העלים וזרעו בנדנה בלע׳ דולשש ([Arab.] *kirsinna*: Bitter vetch [*Vicia ervilia* (L.) Willd.]: ... According to Dioscorides it is a small herb with thin leaves and seeds in pods, in Rom. DWLŠŠ (?)). Hebr. נְדָנָה, coined after Aram. נְדָנָא, is a variant reading of Hebr. נָדָן, which is attested in the current dictionaries as 'sheath, case' (cf. JD 879), or 'scabbard' (BM 3541f.). A synonym used by Anonymous I is פְּטוֹטֶרֶת (see

209 אלכלף: Emend. ed. אלכלוף Ms.
210 והחמימות (= والحرارة): والحزاز a.
211 'dandruff': Trans. acc. to a.

entry). Nathan ha-Me'ati translates Arab. قمع as קוּפְסָא (see entry) and Zeraḥyah Ḥen has פְּצֶלֶת (see entry).

נוֹסָף (*Part. Nif'al*) → [**יסף**].

[נוע] • *Hif'il* **הֵנִיעַ** • **הניע הבטן** · **to trouble the belly**: Arab. حرّك البطن (Gr. ἐκταράσσω τὴν κοιλίαν; cf. DW 2 (V.3); DWB 335[212]) · Ibn Sīnā, *K. al-Qānūn* II · trans. Zeraḥyah Ḥen, *Sefer ha-Qanun* (Ms Oxford, Bodleian Libaries, Opp. Add. Fol. 12, fol. 258^{a-b}): ... ענבים והענבים הקטופים מיד יניע⟨ו⟩ הבטן ויפתח⟨ו⟩[213] (Grapes: ... Freshly picked grapes trouble the belly and are[214] flatulent). In the sense of 'to trouble the belly,' Hebr. הניע הבטן is a non-attested calque from Arab. حرّك البطن. Nathan ha-Me'ati and Anonymous I both render Arab. حرّك البطن as הניע הבטן as well.

נוֹפֵחַ (*Part.*) → **נָפַח**.

נוֹשָׁן (*Part. Nif'al*) → [**ישן**].

נְזִילִי · **catharral (accompanied by a deluxion of humors)**: Lat. *catarrosus* · Guy de Chauliac, *Inventarium sive Chirurgia Magna* (cf. CMM 1:232, l. 33) · trans. Anonymous (Ms Paris, BnF, héb. 1189, fol. 127^{a}): ועל הרוב הוא בא אחר חולי נזילי ([This type] of polyp mostly comes after a catharral illness). Hebr. נְזִילִי is not attested in the current dictionaries.

[נזר] • *Part. Hif'il* **מַזִּיר** · **repellent**: Arab. رادع · Ibn Sīnā, *K. al-Qānūn* II · trans. Zeraḥyah Ḥen, *Sefer ha-Qanun* (Ms Oxford, Bodleian Libaries, Opp. Add. Fol. 12, fol. 231^{a}): לשון הכבש ... עלהו קובץ ומזיר ([Hebr.] *leshon ha-keves* [lit. 'lamb's tongue']: Broadleaf plantain [*Plantago major* L.]: ... Its leaves are astringent and repellent). Hebr. *Part. Hif'il* מַזִּיר does not feature in this sense in the current dictionaries. Nathan ha-Me'ati translates Arab. رادع as מרתיע. Both translators use the same terms to render Arab. رادع in their trans. of Maimonides' *Medical Aphorisms* (i.e., *Sefer ha-Peraqim*) (cf. BMMG nos. 2074/2075) and Nathan's trans. (מרתיע) features also as part of the term הסם המרתיע 'the repellent remedy' in an anonymous trans. of Ibn Sīnā's *K. al-Adwiya al-qalbiyya* (i.e., *Sammim Libbiyim*) (cf. BCD 189 (NM 4:131)). For Hebr. לשון הכבש in the sense of 'broadleaf plantain [*Plantago major* L.],' see NM 6:111.

• **הרפואה המזירה** → **רְפוּאָה**.

נֶחְבָּא (*Part. Nif'al*) → [**חבא**].

נְחוֹשֶׁת → **נְחֹשֶׁת**.

נְחִיר • *Dual* **נחירים** • **באישות הנחירים** → **בְּאִישׁוּת**.

• **באשת הנחירים** → **בְּאָשָׁה**.

• **סרחון הנחירים** → **סִרְחוֹן**.

• **שפע הדם מן הנחירים** → **שֶׁפַע**.

---

212 Note, that trans. Leclerc (IBF no. 480: 'Dioscorides, livre V. Tous les raisins frais relâchent le ventre') is faulty.

213 ויפתח⟨ו⟩ (= ويفتح): وينفخ a.

214 'are flatulent': Trans. acc. to a.

נֶחְנָק (*Part. Nif'al*) → **חָנַק**.

[נחר] • *Part. Hif'il* **מַנְחִיר** • **הסם המנחיר** → **סַם**.

נָחָשׁ • **אבן הנחש** → **אֶבֶן**.

נְחֹשֶׁת • **פרח הנחושת** → **פֶּרַח**.

[נטף] • *Hif'il* **הִטִּיף** • **הטיף באף** · **to drip (pour) a medicine into the nose**: Arab. سعط · Ibn Sīnā, *K. al-Qānūn* II · trans. Anonymous I, *Sefer ha-Qanun* (Ms Paris, BnF, héb. 1142, fols. 189[b]–109[a]): סלק ... יוטף באף מימיה עם מרירת הכרכי ותסיר הלקוה ותועיל לשחיני האף ומימיה פושרים יוטפו באוזן וישקיטו הכאב וירוחץ במימיה הראש ויסיר הסובין ([Arab.] *silq*: Beet [*Beta vulgaris* L.]: ... When one drips [its juice] into the nose along with the gall-bladder of a crane, it removes facial paralysis and is good for nasal ulcers. Its juice dripped into the nose when it is lukewarm relieves earache. When one washes the head with its juice it removes dandruff). Hebr. הטיף באף is not attested in the current dictionaries. The Arab. synonym سعط في الأنف is rendered by Anonymous I as חבש באף (see entry חָבַשׁ). Nathan ha-Me'ati translates Arab. سعط as עשה סעוט and Zeraḥyah Ḥen translates the Arab. term as עשה אישפונגי באף (for both terms, see entry עָשָׂה).

נִימָה • *Plur.* **נימות** • **נימות המים** · **leeches**: Arab. علق · Ibn Sīnā, *K. al-Qānūn* II · trans. Nathan ha-Me'ati, *Sefer ha-Qanun* (Ms Oxford, Bodleian Libraries, Can. Or. 88, fol. 76[b]):[215] גרב ... מיצו יוציא נימות המים הנקרא עלק בערבי ([Arab.] *gharab*: Weeping willow [*Salix babylonica* L.]: ... Its juice extracts leeches, called *'alaq* in Arab.). Hebr. *Sing.* נימת המים is not attested in the current dictionaries. Zeraḥyah Ḥen (entry אתרוג 'lemon/citron,' fol. 176[a]) translates Arab. علق as עלוקה. Parallel/synonymous terms featuring in medieval Hebr. medical literature are Aram. עַלְקָא, featuring in Shem Tov ben Isaac's *Sefer ha-Shimmush* XXVII (cf. BCD 203 (NM 4:146)) and Rom. ארוגש (i.e., *Plur.* of O. Occ. *eruge* (< Lat. HIRŪDO, 'leech (*sangsue*)' (cf. FEW 4:434a, s.v. *hĭrūdo*)),[216] featuring in Moses ibn Tibbon's trans. of Ibn al-Jazzār's *Zād al-musāfir* (i.e., *Sefer Ṣedat ha-Derakhim*) II.6.2 (cf. IJZ 1–2:492).

נִכְתָּם (*Part. Nif'al*) → **[כתם]**.

נָמוֹחַ (*Part. Nif'al*) → **[מוח]**.

נְמִיכוּת • **נמיכות הקול** · **hoarseness of the voice**: Arab. بحّة الصوت · al-Rāzī, *K. fī al-Faṣd* · trans. Anonymous, *Ma'amar ba-Haqqazah* (Ms Parma, Biblioteca Palatina, Cod. Parm. 2283,4, fol. 93[b]): וב' גידים הנק' אלודג'ין ומקומם בצואר ותועיל הקזתם לנמיכות הקול הנק' אלבחוחה אלצות ולכאב הריאה ולקשי הנשימה הנק' אלרבו ולחלי הצרעת[217] (Two veins called 'jugular veins,' their location is in the neck, bleeding them is beneficial for hoarseness of the voice called [in Arab.] *al-buḥūḥa* (sic) *al-ṣawt*, lung pain, breath-

---

215 The same Hebr. term features on fol. 65[b], entry אתרנג '[Arab.] *utrunj*: Lemon [*Citrus limon* (L.) Osbeck] or citron [*Citrus medica* L.]'.

216 I thank Julia Zwink for the explanation of this term.

217 הצערת: Emend. ed. הצער Ms.

ing difficulty (shortness of breath; asthma), called [in Arab.] *al-rabw*, and leprosy). In the sense of 'hoarseness of the voice,' Hebr. נמיכות קול features in BCD 175 (NM 3:157 (corr.)) for Arab. بحوحة in an attestation from an anonymous trans. of Maimonides' *Commentary on Hippocrates'* Aphorisms (i.e., *Perush Aphorismi shel Apuqraṭ*) III.20 (cf. BMCH 1:546, l. 9). A synonym featuring in medieval medical literature is נחור הגרון (cf. NM 6:138f.), featuring in Nathan ha-Me'ati's *Sefer ha-Qanun* II.

נִמְצָא (*Part. Nif'al*) → [מצא].

נִמְשָׁךְ (*Part. Nif'al*) → [משך].

נְסוֹרֶת → נְסֹרֶת.

נְסֹרֶת · **sawdust**: Arab. نشارة · *Glossary* (Ms Moscow, Russian State Library, Guenzburg 573, fol. 156[a]): נשארה הוא נסורת ([Arab.] *nushāra*; i.e., [Hebr.] *nesoret*). In the sense of 'sawdust,' Hebr. נְסֹרֶת features in BM 3699 in attestations from Rabb. literature only (cf. JD 915).

נעיות · **viscosity**: Arab. مخاطية · Ibn Sīnā, *K. al-Qānūn* II · trans. Anonymous I, *Sefer ha-Qanun* (Ms Paris, BnF, héb. 1142, fol. 195[a]): סמך הוא דג ... הטוב שבדגים מה שלא יהיה גדול הרבה ולא קשה הבשר ולא היבש שבהם ואין דשנות בו כאלו יתפתת ואין נעיות בו ולא זוהמא וטעמו ערב ([Arab.] *samak*; i.e., [Hebr.] *dag*: Fish: ... The best fish is that which is not very big, nor hard of its flesh, or dry or greasy; [neither should it be] brittle, nor viscous, nor fetid; its taste should be pleasant). Hebr. נעיות is not attested in the current dictionaries. Ben Yehuda (cf. BM 3649) mentions the noun נִיעַ in the sense of 'Nasenschleim; mucus nasal' featuring in Rabb. and medieval medical literature (*Sefer ha-Qanun*). For the Adj. נעיי in the sense of 'mucous', cf. BCD 176 (NM 4:113) for an attestation from Shem Tov ben Isaac's *Sefer ha-Shimmush* XXVII. Zeraḥyah Ḥen translates Arab. مخاطية as דבקות כמותר האף.

נֶעֱצָר (*Part. Nif'al*) → עָצַר.

נָפַח • *Part.* נוֹפֵחַ • הסם הנופח → סַם.
• *Part. Pi'el* מְנַפֵּחַ • הרפואה המנפחת → רְפוּאָה.

נַפְטִיּוּת · **having the property of naphtha; containing naphtha**: Arab. نفطية · Ibn Sīnā, *K. al-Qānūn* II · trans. Zeraḥyah Ḥen, *Sefer ha-Qanun* (Ms Oxford, Bodleian Libaries, Opp. Add. Fol. 12, fol. 242[a]): מלח ... ויש ממנו הודיי שחור אין שחרותו בעבור נפטיות שבו אבל בעבור עצמותו (Salt: ... It has an Indian [variety]. It is black not because it contains naphtha but because it is natural). Hebr. נַפְטִיּוּת, coined after Arab. نفطية, is not attested in the current dictionaries. Nathan ha-Me'ati translates Arab. نفطية as נפט and Anonymous I has נַפְטִיּוּת, just like Zeraḥyah.

נְפִיחָה · **flatulence**: Arab. نفخ · Ibn Sīnā, *K. al-Qānūn* II · trans. Zeraḥyah Ḥen, *Sefer ha-Qanun* (Ms Oxford, Bodleian Libaries, Opp. Add. Fol. 12, fol. 226[a]): כַּרְפַּס ... מתיר לנפיחה פותח לסתימה מזיע משכך לכאב והמדברי מנגע מחליא והמרובב ממנו יותר ניאות למחוממים (Celery [*Apium graveolens* L.]: ... It relieves flatulence. It opens blockages, induces perspiration, and allays pain. The wild variety is ulcerating and causes pain; its preserve is more suitable for those who have a hot temperament). In the sense of 'flatulence,' Hebr. נְפִיחָה features in BCD 177 (NM 4:114) in an attestation from an anonymous trans. of Ibn Sīnā's *K. al-Adwiya al-qalbiyya* (i.e., *Sammim Libbiyim*). Synonymous terms used by Zeraḥyah in his trans. of Maimonides' *Medical Aphorisms*, are ניפוח ,נפח, and נפיחות (cf. BMMG no. 5209). Nathan ha-Me'ati and Anonymous I both render Arab. نفخ as נֶפַח (cf. BCD 177 (NM 4:114) for an attestation from Nathan's *Sefer ha Qanun* I).

נְפִילָה • נפילת השער · hair loss: Arab. انتشار الشعر · Ibn Sīnā, *K. al-Qānūn* II · trans. Nathan ha-Me'ati, *Sefer ha-Qanun* (Ms Oxford, Bodleian Libraries, Can. Or. 88, fol. 108[b]): סבאדאוראן[218] ... ימנע בפילת השער ([Arab.] *Sādārawān*: A black resin or tar (cf. DT 121 (I.39), n. 5): ... It prevents loss of hair). Hebr. נפילת השער is not attested in the current dictionaries. Zeraḥyah Ḥen and Anonymous I both render the Arab. term as השרת השער (see entry הֲשָׁרָה).

[נפל] • *Hif'il* הִפִּיל · to reduce: Arab. أسقط · Ibn Sīnā, *K. al-Qānūn* II · trans. Zeraḥyah Ḥen, *Sefer ha-Qanun* (Ms Oxford, Bodleian Libaries, Opp. Add. Fol. 12, fol. 251[a–b]):[219] סַדֵאבְ רוּטָא ... ייבש הזרע ויפסיקנו ויפיל תאות התשמיש וישכך הפונטורא ([Arab.] *sadhāb*; [i.e., Lat.] RWuṬ'a [i.e., *ruta*]: Common rue [*Ruta graveolens* L.]: ... It makes the semen dry and stops [its production]. It reduces sexual lust and relieves gripes). In the sense of 'to reduce,' Hebr. *Hif'il* הִפִּיל is a non-attested semantic borrowing from Arab. أسقط. Nathan ha-Me'ati translates Arab. أسقط as *Hif'il* הֵסִיר and Anonymous I renders the Arab. term as הִפִּיל, just like Zeraḥyah.

נִפְסָל (*Part. Nif'al*) → [פסל].

נִפְרָךְ (*Part. Nif'al*) → [פרך].

נֶפֶשׁ • התהפך הנפש → [הפך].

• חדוש הנפש → חִדּוּשׁ.

נִצָּב (*Part. Nif'al*) → [יצב].

נֶקֶב • נקב העורף · hollow of the neck: Arab. نقرة (cf. FA no. 2256) · al-Rāzī, *K. fī al-Faṣd* · trans. Anonymous, *Ma'amar ba-Haqqazah* (Ms Parma, Biblioteca Palatina, Cod. Parm. 2283,4, fol. 93[b]): וב׳ גידים באחורי הראש סמוכי׳ אל נקרת הראש והוא נקב העורף הנק׳ אלנקרא[220] (There are two veins in the back of the head, close to the hollow of the neck [i.e., Hebr. *niqrat ha-rosh*], [also called] *neqev ha-'oref*, called [in Arab.] *al-nuqra*). Hebr. נקב העורף is not attested in the current dictionaries. For the synonymous נקרת הראש, see entry נִקְרָה. In their trans. of Maimonides' *Medical Aphorisms* XII.43, Nathan ha-Me'ati renders Arab. نقرة as הנקרה בעורף (see also entry נִקְרָה) and Zeraḥyah Ḥen has חולית הצואר (see entry חֻלְיָה). Other synonyms featuring in medieval medical literature are חלל העורף (cf. BCD 100 (NM 1:93f.)), העמק אשר מאחורי

---

218 סבאדאוראן: سادوران a.

219 The same Hebr. term features for Arab. أسقط on fol. 253[a], entry סֶמְסֶם שומשמין '[Arab.] *simsim*; [i.e., Hebr.] *shumshemin*: Sesame [*Sesamum indicum* L.]'.

220 אלנקרא: Emend. ed. אלסקרא Ms.

הצואר (cf. BCD 204 (NM 4:147)), העומק אשר בעליון אחורי הצואר (cf. NM 5:150f.), ערף (cf. NM 5:156), and העורף אחרי הצואר (cf. NM 5:156f.).

נָקֵד • *Plur.* **נקודים** • **לחם נקודים** → **לֶחֶם**.

נָקוּב • **כלי נקוב** → **כְּלִי**.

נִקּוּד → **נָקֵד**.

[נקף] • *Part. Hif'il* מַקִּיף • **האברים המקיפים** → **אֵבֶר**.

• **הקדחות המקיפות** → **קַדַּחַת**.

• *Part. Hof'al* מֻקָּף • **האברים המוקפים** → **אֵבֶר**.

נִקְרָה • **הנקרה בעורף** · **the hollow of the neck**: Arab. نقرة (cf. FA no. 2256) · Maimonides, *Medical Aphorisms* XII.43 · trans. Nathan ha-Me'ati (cf. BMMN 144, l. 22; BMMG no. 5256): לפעמים תתלה קרן המציצה על הנקרה בעורף ותמשוך הליחה הנוזלת אל העינים (Sometimes, apply cupping glasses to the hollow of the neck to attract the matter that streams to the eyes). Hebr. הנקרה בעורף is not attested in the current dictionaries. Zeraḥyah Ḥen translates Arab. نقرة as חולית הצואר (see entry חֻלְיָה).

• **נקרת הראש** · **the hollow of the neck**: Arab. نقرة (cf. FA no. 2256) · al-Rāzī, *K. fī al-Faṣd* · trans. Anonymous, *Ma'amar ba-Haqqazah* (Ms Parma, Biblioteca Palatina, Cod. Parm. 2283,4, fol. 96b): זאת ההרקה נחלקת לב׳ חלקים הא׳ עם שריטה והב׳ בלא שריטה והמקומות הנהוגים לעשות שריטה בהם הם נקרת הראש והצדעים הנק׳ אלאחדעין[221] (This [kind of] evacuation [i.e., bloodletting] is divided into two parts: the first with scarification and the second without scarification. The sites that are regulary used for scarification are the hollow of the neck and the lateral parts of the neck called [in Arab.] *al-akhda'ān*). Hebr. נקרת הראש is not attested in the current dictionaries. For the synonymous Hebr. term נקב העורף, also featuring in the *Ma'amar ba-Haqqazah*, see entry נֶקֶב.

נִרְפֶּה (*Part. Nif'al*) → **[רפה]**.

נִשּׁוּף · **absorption; absorbing effect**: Arab. تنشيف (cf. D 2:672) · Ibn Sīnā, *K. al-Qānūn* II · trans. Zeraḥyah Ḥen, *Sefer ha-Qanun* (Ms Oxford, Bodleian Libaries, Opp. Add. Fol. 12, fol. 201b): הַלִילַגְ׳ מִירַבַּלֹנִי ... מועיל לכאב הטחול ויועיל לכלי המזון כלם וכל שכן השחורים כי הם יחזקו האצטומ׳ וכל שכן המגודלים ויחזקו רפיון האצטומ׳ עם העיבוד והנקיון והנישוף ([Arab.] *halīlaj* [from Pers. *halīlah*]; [Rom.] MiYRaBaLoNiY: (Chebulic) myrobalan: ... They are useful for pain in the spleen and for all nutritive organs—especially the black variety—because they strengthen the stomach, above all the preserved ones. They strengthen the lining of the stomach through their astringent, cleansing, and absorbing effect). Hebr. נִשּׁוּף seems to be coined by Zeraḥyah after Arab. تنشيف. Nathan ha-Me'ati translates the Arab. term as ניגב and Anonymous I has נגוב.

221 אלאחדעין: Emend. ed. אל אלארדעין קרא Ms.

נְשִׁימָה • הנשימה המתיצבת · **orthopnea**: Arab. نفس الانتصاب · Ibn Sīnā, *K. al-Qānūn* II · trans. Anonymous I, *Sefer ha-Qanun* (Ms Paris, BnF, héb. 1142, fols. 37^{b}–38^{a}): ... אנגורה אם ישתה במי השעורים מנקה החזה ואם יבושל עלהו במי השעורים יוציא מה שבחזה מהליחות העבות וזרעה יותר חזק והיא מסירה הגניחה והנשימה המתיצבת והקרה מבעלת הצד ([Arab.] *anjura*: Roman nettle [*Urtica pilulifera* L.]: ... When one takes it with barley water, it cleanses the chest, and when one takes its leaves boiled in barley water, it expels the thick humors in the chest. The seeds are more potent and cure asthma, orthopnea, and cold pleurisy). Hebr. הנשימה המתיצבת does not feature in the current dictionaries. Nathan ha-Me'ati translates Arab. نفس الانتصاب as הנשימה הנצבת (see next entry) and Zeraḥyah Ḥen has הצבת הניפוש (cf. NM 6:56f.).

• **הנשימה הנצבת** · **orthopnea**: Arab. نفس الانتصاب · Ibn Sīnā, *K. al-Qānūn* II · trans. Nathan ha-Me'ati, *Sefer ha-Qanun* (Ms Oxford, Bodleian Libraries, Can. Or. 88, fol. 65^{a-b}):[222] אנגרה ... כשמשקים אותו עם השעורים ינקה החזה וכשמבשלים עליו במי השעור יוציא מה שיש בחזה מתערובים הגסים וזרעו יותר חזק ויסיר עוצר[223] הנשימה ויניח הנשימה הנצבת ומחולי[224] הקר אשר מחולי הצלעות ([Arab.] *anjura*: Roman nettle [*Urtica pilulifera* L.]: ... When one takes it with barley water, it cleanses the chest, and when one takes its leaves boiled with barley water, it expels the thick humors in the chest. The seeds are more potent and cure asthma, orthopnea, and cold pleurisy). Hebr. הנשימה הנצבת does not feature in the current dictionaries. Zeraḥyah Ḥen translates Arab. نفس الانتصاب as הצבת הניפוש (cf. NM 6:56f.) and Anonymous I has הנשימה המתיצבת (see previous entry). Hebr. הנשימה הנצבת also features in Nathan's trans. of Maimonides' *Medical Aphorisms* XXIII.79 (cf. BMMN 229, l. 2: הנשימה המיצבת; variant Ms Moscow, Russian State Library, Guenzburg 115: הנשימה הנצבת). The Arab. synonym انتصاب النفس is translated by Nathan as הצבת הנשימה (see entry הַצָּבָה) and מצב הנשימה (see entry מַצָּב). Other synonyms featuring in medieval Hebr. medical literature are הִתְיַצְּבוּת (cf. BCD 75 (NM 2:42)); מַצָּב (cf. BCD 156 (NM 1:165)); נשימת הזקיפה (cf. NM 5:136); צרות הניפוש (cf. BCD 233 (NM 1:182)); and צרות הנשימה (cf. BCD 233f. (NM 4:176); NM 5:172).

• **הצבת הנשימה** → הַצָּבָה.

• **מצב הנשימה** → מַצָּב.

• **עיצור הנשימה** → עִצּוּר.

• **עוצר הנשימה** → עֹצֶר.

• **קצר הנשימה** → קֹצֶר.

• **קשי הנשימה** → קֹשִׁי.

---

222 The same term features on fol. 85^{b}, entry חנטל '[Arab.] *ḥanẓal*: Colocynth [*Citrullus colocynthis* (L.) Schrad.],' and on fol. 97^{a}, entry כל '[Arab.] *khall*: Vinegar.'

223 עוצר הנשימה ויניח הנשימה הנצבת (= Ms Paris, BnF, héb. 1136, fol. 65^{b}): עוצר הנשימה הנצבת Ms الربو ونفس الانتصاب a.

224 ומחולי הקר אשר מחולי הצלעות: والبارد من ذات الجنب a.

נִתּוּק · **tear [of a muscle]**: Arab. هتك (Gr. ῥῆξις, ῥῆγμα; cf. UWS 2:248) · Ibn Sīnā, *K. al-Qānūn* II · trans. Zeraḥyah Ḥen, *Sefer ha-Qanun* (Ms Oxford, Bodleian Libraries, Opp. Add. Fol. 12, fol. 225[b]): כַּפַּרִי ... ויועיל מן הפלג והביטול ויחזק האיברים מפני שבו מן הקיבוץ וכן יועיל מן הניתוק המתחדש בראשי המושקלי ([Rom.] KaPaRiY [i.e., Ital.-Rom. *cap(p)eri*]: Caper [*Capparis spinosa* L.]: ... It is useful in paralysis and numbness. It strengthens the organs due to its astringent property. It is also useful for tear in the ends of the muscles). Hebr. נִתּוּק features in BM 3865 as a medical term in the sense of 'dislocation [of a limb]' in an attestation from the *Sefer ha-Qanun*. Nathan translates Arab. هتك as חִתּוּךְ (see entry) and Anonymous I has רִסּוּק (see entry for his use of the term רסוק האזן 'tear (puncture) in the ear'). The Arab. synonym فسخ is translated by Zeraḥyah as פִּשּׁוּחַ and הֶפְסֵד (see entries) and the synonymous وهن as חֲלִשָׁה (see entry).

נֶתֶק • **נתק הסלעים** · **lichen growing on rocks [*Roccella tinctoria* DC]**: Arab. حزاز الصخر (cf. DT 559 (IV.46), n. 4) ·Ibn Sīnā, *K. al-Qānūn* II · trans. Anonymous I, *Sefer ha-Qanun* (Ms Paris, BnF, héb. 1142, fol. 125[a]): טחלב ... ואמנם הטחלב הסלעיי הוא חזאז אלצכור כלומ' נתק הסלעים וכבר זכרנונו ([Arab.] *ṭuḥlub*: Common duckweed [*Lemna minor* L.]: ... We have already discussed 'duckweed growing on rocks,' i.e., *ḥazāz al-ṣukhūr* [in Arab.], i.e., 'lichen growing on rocks' [*Roccella tinctoria* DC]). Hebr. נתק הסלעים is not attested in the current dictionaries. For נֶתֶק in the sense of 'freckles' and 'cradle cap,' cf. BCD 182 (NM 2:15f., 69). Nathan ha-Me'ati renders Arab. حزاز الصخر as טחלב על הסלעים and Zeraḥyah Ḥen has ילפת הצור (see entry יַלֶּפֶת).

ס

סב • *Plur.* סובין · **scurf; dandruff**: Arab. إبرية (Gr. πίτυρον; UW 119f.) · Ibn Sīnā, *K. al-Qānūn* II · trans. Zeraḥyah Ḥen, *Sefer ha-Qanun* (Ms Oxford, Bodleian Libraries, Opp. Add. Fol. 12, fol. 206ª): זְגַ׳אג׳ זכוכית ... ינקה הסובין כשירחץ בו ויטהר בשנים ([Arab.] *zujāj*; [i.e., Hebr.] *zekhukhit*: Glass: ... If one washes the head with it, it removes dandruff; it also cleanses the teeth). In the sense of 'pityr⟨i⟩asis capitis,' Hebr. סובין features as סובין שבראש in BM 3900 in an attestation from the *Sefer Almansur* (cf. also NM 6:145, where the latter term features in an attestation from Zeraḥyah's *Sefer ha-Qanun* II (for Arab. سعفة)). Nathan ha-Me'ati translates Arab. إبرية as סובי הראש and Anonymous I has הסובין שבראש. Shem Tov ben Isaac translates Arab. إبرية as חֶרֶס in his *Sefer ha-Shimmush* XXVII (cf. BCD 107 (NM 4:73)) and as יַלֶּפֶת in his *Sefer Almansur*, as part of a similar recipe: זכוכית: יש לו סגולה יפרך בה החצץ המתילד בכיס מקוה המים ויסיר הילפת כשרוחצין בו הראש (Glass: It has a specific property to pulverize stones that develop in the urinary bladder; it removes dandruff when the head is washed with it) (cf. BCD 117 (NM 2:12f.); BMZ 34f. (Zayin 9)). Moses ibn Tibbon renders Arab. إبرية as סנפירות in his trans. of Ibn al-Jazzār's *Zād al-musāfir* (i.e., *Sefer Ṣedat ha-Derakhim*) N.4 (cf. BCD 192 (NM 4:137); IJZ 1–2:440). The Hebr. *Plur.* of סְנַפִּיר features (for the parallel Lat. term *furfures*) also as סנפירים in the term סנפירי הראש in Do'eg ha-Edomi's trans. of Constantinus Africanus' *Viaticum* (i.e., *Sefer Ya'ir Netiv*) I.5.0 (cf. NM 5:140f.; IJZ 1–2:606).

• *Double Plur.* **סובינים** · **eschar**: Arab. خشكريشات · Ibn Sīnā, *K. al-Qānūn* II · trans. Zeraḥyah Ḥen, *Sefer ha-Qanun* (Ms Oxford, Bodleian Library, Opp. Add. Fol. 12, fol. 236ʳ): מֵיזַרְיוּן לַרִיאוּלַא ... כל מיניו נעשים לקובא ולנגעים המלוכלכים עם הדבש ויעתיקו הסובינים מפני שבו מן העצם המתיר האוכל ([Arab.] *māzaryūn*; [i.e., Lat./Rom.] LaRiY'WuLa' [i.e., M. Lat. or O. Occ. *laureola*; cf. SHS1:103 (Alef 16)]: February daphne [*Daphne mezereum* L.]: ... All of its varieties are used with honey in cases of eczema and dirty ulcers. It removes eschar because of its dissolving and corrosive substance). Hebr. סובינים is not attested in the current dictionaries.[225] Nathan ha-Me'ati translates Arab. خشكريشات as קלפות יבשות (see entry קְלִפָּה for Nathan's use of *Sing.* הקלפה היבשה) and Anonymous I has צָרֶבֶת (cf. BCD 233 (NM 2:77f.) for an attestation from Nathan's trans. of Maimonides' *Medical Aphorisms* (i.e., *Sefer ha-Peraqim*) XV.9 (cf. BMMN 155, l. 18) (for Arab. خشكريشة)). Zeraḥyah, on the other hand, translates Arab. خشكريشة in his *Sefer ha-Peraqim* as המקום בעצמו אשר שם כעין סובין (XV.9; cf. BMMZ 154, ll. 1–2; BMMG no. 1356) and as Lat./Rom. קרושטא (i.e., *crusta*/*cruste*; cf. ND 264) (XXIII.38; cf. BMMZ 221, l. 13; BMMG no. 1356).

---

225 The same Hebr. term features for Arab. خشكريشات on fol. 239a, entry מום שעוה '[Arab.-Pers.] *mūm*; [i.e., Hebr.] *sha'awah*: Wax.'

[סבב] • *Part. Polel* **סוֹבֵב** • **הקדחות הסובבות** → קַדַּחַת.

סְבִיאָה · **hangover**: Arab. خمار · Ibn Sīnā, *K. al-Qānūn* II · trans. Anonymous I, *Sefer ha-Qanun* (Ms Paris, BnF, héb. 1142, fols. 23ª–24ª): אפסנתין ... ואם ישתה קדם שתית היין יועיל מהסביאה ([Arab.] *afsantīn*: Absinth wormwood [*Artemisia absinthium* L.]: ... It is good for a hangover if one takes it before drinking wine). Hebr. סְבִיאָה is not attested for medieval medical literature. Nathan ha-Me'ati translates Arab. خمار as בלבול היין (see entry בִּלְבּוּל) and Zeraḥyah Ḥen has שכרות.

סָבַל · **to apply as a suppository**: Arab. حمول · Ibn Sīnā, *K. al-Qānūn* II · trans. Nathan ha-Me'ati, *Sefer ha-Qanun* (Ms Oxford, Bodleian Libraries, Can. Or. 88, fols. 75ᵇ–76ª): גזר ... וגזר המדברי אם נדין שהוא ממין גזר הוא מעורר יותר תאות המשגל מהפרדסי וישלשל דם הוסת והשתן ויותר המדברי כשסובלים ממנו או כששותים אותו ([Arab.] *jazar* / [Hebr.] *gezer*: Carrot [*Daucus carota* L.]: ... Wild carrot, if it may be considered as a carrot, is more stimulant for sexual lust than its cultivated variety. When one consumes carrot, especially the wild variety, or applies it as a suppository, it stimulates menstruation and discharge of urine). Hebr. סָבַל does not feature in this sense in the current dictionaries. For a variant reading סבל פתילה מלמטה (for Arab. احتمل فتيلة) featuring in Nathan's *Sefer ha-Qanun* II, cf. NM 6:147 (cf. ibid. for his use of סָבַל (for Arab. احتمل)). Zeraḥyah Ḥen translates Arab. حمول as סָבַל as well and Anonymous I renders the Arab. term as הנחה למטה (see entry הֲנָּחָה).

סָגַר · I. **to heal; to promote cicatrization**: Arab. أدمل (Gr. ἐπουλόω, ἰάομαι, κολλάω; cf. UW 264, 303f., 354f.) · Ibn Sīnā, *K. al-Qānūn* II · trans. Nathan ha-Me'ati, *Sefer ha-Qanun* (Ms Oxford, Bodleian Libraries, Can. Or. 88, fol. 107ª): נחאס ... יסגר הנגעים הרעים המוסיפים וימנעם מלהוסיף ויאכל הבשר הנוסף והרחוץ יסגר המכות ([Arab.] *nuḥās*: Copper: ... It heals malignant spreading ulcers and prevents their further expansion. It corrodes the excessive flesh. Washed [copper] heals the wounds). Hebr. סָגַר does not feature in this sense in the current dictionaries. Zeraḥyah Ḥen translates Arab. أدمل as *Pi'el* חִיָּה (see entry [חיה]) and Anonymous I has *Hif'il* הבריא. Moses ibn Tibbon translates Arab. أدمل as סתם in his trans. of Ibn al-Jazzār's *Zād al-musāfir* (i.e., *Sefer Ṣedat ha-Derakhim*) III.8 (cf. NM 5:142). See also *Part. Pi'el* מְסַגֵּר below.

· II. **to heal; to promote granulation**: Arab. ألحم (Gr. κολλάω; cf. UW 354f.) · Ibn Sīnā, *K. al-Qānūn* II · trans. Nathan ha-Me'ati, *Sefer ha-Qanun* (Ms Oxford, Bodleian Libraries, Can. Or. 88, fol. 107ᵇ): מרקשיתא ... כשיערב עם ראתינג' יסגור הנגעים ויסיר הבשר הנוסף ([Arab.] *marqashīthā*: Marcasite: ... When it is mixed with pine resin, it heals (promotes granulation of) ulcers (wounds) and removes fleshy excrescenses). Hebr. סָגַר does not feature in this sense in the current dictionaries. Zeraḥyah Ḥen translates Arab. ألحم as *Pi'el* דִּבֵּק (cf. NM 6:42, where דִּבֵּק features for both Arab. ألحم and the synonymous (ألزق) and Anonymous I has *Hif'il* הבריא.

• *Inf. Constr.* **סְגוֹר** · **cicatrization**: Arab. ختم (Gr. ἐπουλόω; cf. UW 264) · Ibn Sīnā, *K. al-Qānūn* II · trans. Nathan ha-Me'ati, *Sefer ha-Qanun* (Ms Oxford, Bodleian Libraries, Can. Or. 88, fol. 107[a]): נחאס ... וכשרוחצים אותו הוא סם משובח בסגור הנגעים ([Arab.] *nuḥās*: Copper: ... When it is washed, it is an excellent drug for the cicatrization of wounds). Zeraḥyah Ḥen translates Arab. ختم as חתימה and Anonymous I has לחתום. Both terms, חתימה and לחתום, feature in Nathan's trans. of Maimonides' *Medical Aphorisms* (i.e., *Sefer ha-Peraqim*) IX.95 and XXIII.40 (cf. BMMN 116, l. 24; 224, l. 9; BMMG no. 1289). Moses ibn Tibbon translates Arab. ألحم as *Hif'il* הֶחְתִּים in his trans. of Ibn al-Jazzār's *Zād al-musāfir* (i.e., *Sefer Ṣedat ha-Derakhim*) VII.25.1 (cf. BCD 109, s.v. חָתַם (NM 1:57); IJZ 7:165, l. 15).

• *Part. Pi'el* מְסַגֵּר · **healing; promoting cicatrization**: Arab. مدمل · Ibn Sīnā, *K. al-Qānūn* II · trans. Nathan ha-Me'ati, *Sefer ha-Qanun* (Ms Oxford, Bodleian Libraries, Can. Or. 88, fol. 90[b]): כנדר ... הוא מסגר מאד וקל וחומר המכות הטריות וימנע הנגעים הרעים מלהוסיף ([Arab.] *kundur*: Frankincense [*Boswellia sacra* Flueck.]: ... It has a strong healing force, especially for fresh wounds; it prevents the spread of malignant ulcers). Hebr. *Part. Pi'el* מְסַגֵּר is not attested in this sense in the current dictionaries. See also סָגַר above. Zeraḥyah Ḥen translates Arab. مدمل as *Part. Pi'el* מחייה (see entry [חיה] for *Pi'el* חִיָּה) and Anonymous I has *Part. Hif'il* מבריא.

• סַם → הסם המסגר.

סִדּוּק • סדוק השפתים · **fissures of the lips**: Lat. *fissure labiorum* · Guy de Chauliac, *Inventarium sive Chirurgia Magna* (cf. CMM 1:237, l. 15) · trans. Anonymous (Ms Paris, BnF, héb. 1189, fol. 130[a]): מסדוק השפתים (On lip fissures). Hebr. סִדּוּק is not attested as a medical term in the current dicitonaries (cf. BM 3964; EM 1217).

סוֹב → סַב.

סוֹבֵב (*Part. Polel*) → [סבב].

סוּמָה • *Plur.* סומות · **marks; spots**: Arab. آثار · Ibn Sīnā, *K. al-Qānūn* II · trans. Anonymous II, *Sefer ha-Qanun* (Ms Parma, Biblioteca Palatina, Cod. Parm. 3045, fol. 29[a]): רוקא ... מי רוקא עם מרת פרה יצליח לסומות המורסות ([Lat.] RWQ' [i.e., (*e*)*ruca*]: Rocket [*Eruca sativa* Mill.]: ... Rocket juice with ox bile is useful for removing ulcer marks). In the sense of 'mark; spot,' Hebr. *Sing.* סוּמָה is a non-attested parallel term to Aram. סוּמָא, which features in Rabb. literature (cf. JD 966). Nathan ha-Me'ati translates Arab. آثار as סימנים (cf. NM 6:151), Zeraḥyah Ḥen renders the Arab. term as רישומים (cf. NM 6:207) and Anonymous I has רושם (cf. NM 6:207 for attestations from the *Sefer ha-Qanun* II by both Nathan and Zeraḥyah).

סוּס • זנב הסוס → זָנָב.

סוֹתֵם (*Part.*) → סָתַם.

סִימָן → סִמָּן.

סִירְחוֹן → סִרְחוֹן.

סֶלַע • *Plur.* סלעים • נתק הסלעים → נֶתֶק.

סַם • הסם המאדם · **the rubefacient drug**: Arab. الدواء المحمر · Ibn Sīnā, *K. al-Qānūn* II · trans. Anonymous I, *Sefer ha-Qanun* (Ms Paris, BnF, héb. 1142, fol. 12[b]): והמאדם הוא הסם שדרכו לחמם האבר אשר נוגע בו חמום חזק עד שימשוך הדם אליו משיכה חזקה עד שיגיע

לחיצונו ומאדמו (A rubefacient [drug] is a drug that—by its nature—warms an organ, which it touches [i.e., comes in contact with], so that the blood is strongly attracted towards it [i.e., the organ], reaches its outside, and turns it red). Hebr. הסם המאדם features in BCD 187 (NM 4:123f.) in an attestation from an anonymous trans. of Ibn Sīnā's *K. al-Adwiya al-qalbiyya* (i.e., *Sammim Libbiyim*). Nathan ha-Me'ati translates Arab. الدواء المحمر as הסם המאדים (see next entry) and Zeraḥyah Ḥen has הרפואה המאדימה (see entry רְפוּאָה).

• **הסם המאדים** · **the rubefacient drug**: Arab. الدواء المحمر · Ibn Sīnā, *K. al-Qānūn* II · trans. Nathan ha-Me'ati, *Sefer ha-Qanun* (Ms Oxford, Bodleian Libraries, Can. Or. 88, fol. 56ª): והמאדים הוא אשר מנהגו לחמם האבר אשר בו יפגע חום חזק עד שימשוך הדם[226] אליו משיכה חזקה ויגיע אל השטח ויאדים אותו (A rubefacient [drug] is [a drug], which—by its nature—intensely warms an organ, which it touches [i.e., comes in contact with], so that the blood is strongly attracted towards it [i.e., the organ], reaches its outside, and turns it red). Hebr. הסם המאדים is not attested in the current dictionaries. Zeraḥyah Ḥen translates Arab. الدواء المحمر as הרפואה המאדימה (see entry רְפוּאָה) and Anonymous I has הסם המאדם (see previous entry).

• **הסם האוטם** · **the obstruent drug**: Arab. الدواء المسدّد · Ibn Sīnā, *K. al-Qānūn* II · trans. Nathan ha-Me'ati, *Sefer ha-Qanun* (Ms Oxford, Bodleian Libraries, Can. Or. 88, fol. 57ᵇ): והאוטם הוא היבש העוצר בעביו ויבשותו או שהוא צופד המעברים ויוליד[227] דם אוטם (An obstruent [drug] is a drying, blocking [drug], which—because of its dense, dry, or agglutinating properties—blogs the passages [of the body] and produces[228] blood clogging). Hebr. הסם האוטם is not attested in the current dictionaries. Zeraḥyah Ḥen renders Arab. الدواء المسدّد as הרפואה המסתמת (see entry רְפוּאָה) and Anonymous I has הסם הסותם (see entry below).

• **הסם האוכל** · **the corrosive drug**: Arab. الدواء الأكّال · Ibn Sīnā, *K. al-Qānūn* II · trans. Nathan ha-Me'ati, *Sefer ha-Qanun* (Ms Oxford, Bodleian Libraries, Can. Or. 88, fol. 56ª): והאוכל הוא הסם שמנהגו שיגיע בהתוכו ונגועו שיחסיר עצם הבשר כמו הזנגאר (A corrosive [drug] is—by its nature—a drug that has solvent and ulcerative properties, which are so strong that they reduce the substance of the flesh [of the organ]; [an example of such a drug is] verdigris). Hebr. הסם האוכל is not attested in the current dictionaries. Zeraḥyah Ḥen translates Arab. الدواء الأكّال as הרפואה האוכלת (see entry רְפוּאָה) and Anonymous I has הסם המאכל (see next entry).

• **הסם המאכל** · **the corrosive drug**: Arab. الدواء الأكّال · Ibn Sīnā, *K. al-Qānūn* II · trans. Anonymous I, *Sefer ha-Qanun* (Ms Paris, BnF, héb. 1142, fol. 13ʳ: והמאכל הוא הסם שדרכו להתיך שמגיע מהתכתו או השחנתו שיחסר מעצם הבשר כמו הזנג׳אר (A corrosive [drug] is—by its nature—a drug that has solvent and ulcerative properties, which are so strong

226 הדם (الدم a): Emend. ed. החום Ms.
227 ויוליד דם אוטם: فيحدث فيها السدد a.
228 'produces blood clogging': 'produces obstructions' a.

that they reduce the substance of the flesh [of the organ]; [an example of such a drug is] verdigris). Hebr. הסם המאכל features in BCD 187 (NM 4:124) in an attestation from an anonymous trans. of Ibn Sīnā's *K. al-Adwiya al-qalbiyya* (i.e., *Sammim Libbiyim*). Nathan ha-Me'ati translates Arab. الدواء الأكّال as הסם האוכל (see previous entry) and Zeraḥyah Ḥen has הרפואה האוכלת (see entry רְפוּאָה).

• **הסם המבטל החרגש · the anesthetic (benumbing; soporific; narcotic) drug**: Arab. الدواء المخدر · Ibn Sīnā, *K. al-Qānūn* II · trans. Nathan ha-Me'ati, *Sefer ha-Qanun* (Ms Oxford, Bodleian Libraries, Can. Or. 88, fol. 57[a]): והמבטל ההרגש הנקרא מכדר בערבי הוא הסם אשר יגיע בקרר האבר שישנה עצם הרוח הנושא אותו אליו כח התנועה וההרגש קר במזגו גס בעצמו ולא יפעל בו הכח הנפשיי (An anesthetic (benumbing; soporific; narcotic) [drug], called *mukhaddir* in Arab., is a drug that has such a strong cooling effect on an organ that it makes the substance of the pneuma, which is carried to the organ by the faculty of movement and sensation, cold in temperament and dense in substance. Consequently, the psychical faculty does not have an effect on it anymore).[229] Hebr. הסם המבטל ההרגש does not feature in the current dictionaries. Zeraḥyah Ḥen translates Arab. الدواء المخدر as הרפואה המבטלת (see entry רְפוּאָה) and Anonymous I has הסם המרדים החוש (see entry below).

• **הסם המבריא · the healing drug (a drug that promotes cicatrization)**: Arab. الدواء المدمل · Ibn Sīnā, *K. al-Qānūn* II · trans. Anonymous I, *Sefer ha-Qanun* (Ms Paris, BnF, héb. 1142, fol. 13[a]): והמבריא החבורות הוא הסם המנגב ומעבה הלחות הנופלת בין שני שטחי החבורה השכנים אל טיחת דבקות והדבקה הנקר׳ וישקושיטאט ויתדבק אחד מהם באחר כמו דם תנין ואלואן ((The [drug] that heals wounds is a drug that dries up and thickens the fluid collected between the two layers of a wound, which are close to each other. [It does so] to an extent that it [i.e., the fluid] becomes agglutinant and viscous, called [in. Rom.] WYŠQWŠYṬ'Ṭ, and both the ends [of the wound] adhere to each other; [examples of such a drug are] dragon's blood [i.e., the resin of *Dracaena cinnabari* Balf.f.] and aloes). Hebr. הסם המבריא is not attested in the current dictionaries. For *Hif'il* הִבְרִיא in the sense of 'to heal; to promote cicatrization,' see entry [חיה]. Nathan ha-Me'ati translates Arab. الدواء المدمل as הסם המסגר (see entry below) and Zeraḥyah Ḥen has הרפואה המחיה (see entry רְפוּאָה).

• **הסם המבשל · the ripening (coctive) drug**: Arab. الدواء المنضج · Ibn Sīnā, *K. al-Qānūn* II · trans. Nathan ha-Me'ati, *Sefer ha-Qanun* (Ms Oxford, Bodleian Libraries, Can. Or. 88, fol. 56[r]: והמבשל הוא אשר מנהגו שיועיל אל התערוב בשול מפני שהוא מחמם ביושר ובו כח קובץ יעצר התערוב עד שיתבשל ולא יתך בכבדות (A ripening (coctive) [drug is a drug] that—by its nature—ripens (concocts) the humor because of its moderate heat-

229 In his trans. of Maimonides' *Medical Aphorisms* (i.e., *Sefer ha-Peraqim*) IX.38, Nathan translates Arab. *Plur.* أدوية مخدرة 'soporific drugs' as רפואות מרדימות (cf. BMMN 108, l. 5; BMMG no. 1884).

ing effect; it has an astringent property that retains the humor until it is ripe and does not dissolve it forcefully). Hebr. הסם המבשל features in BCD 187 (NM 4:124) in an attestation from an anonymous trans. of Ibn Sīnā's *K. al-Adwiya al-qalbiyya* (i.e., *Sammim Libbiyim*). Zeraḥyah Ḥen translates Arab. الدواء المنضج as הרפואה המבשלת (see entry רְפוּאָה) and Anonymous I has הסם המבשל, just like Nathan.

• **הסם המחזק** · **the tonic drug**: Arab. الدواء المقوي · Ibn Sīnā, *K. al-Qānūn* II · trans. Anonymous I, *Sefer ha-Qanun* (Ms Paris, BnF, héb. 1142, fol. 13[a]): והמחזק הוא הסם שדרכו להשוות עצם האבר ומזגו עד שימנע מלקבל המותרים הנהפכים אליו והפגעים (A tonic [drug] is a drug that—by its nature—balances the consistency and temperament of an organ to the extent that it prevents the absorption of superfluous matters and disorders that move towards it). Hebr. הסם המחזק features in BCD 188 (NM 4:126) in an attestation from an anonymous trans. of Ibn Sīnā's *K. al-Adwiya al-qalbiyya* (i.e., *Sammim Libbiyim*). Nathan ha-Me'ati translates Arab. الدواء المقوي as הסם המחזיק and Zeraḥyah Ḥen has הרפואה המחזקת (see entry רְפוּאָה).

• **הסם המחכך** · **the pruritic drug**: Arab. الدواء المحكك · Ibn Sīnā, *K. al-Qānūn* II · trans. Nathan ha-Me'ati, *Sefer ha-Qanun* (Ms Oxford, Bodleian Libraries, Can. Or. 88, fol. 56[a]): והמחכך הוא הסם שמנהגו בחדודו וחומו שימשוך אל הנקבים תערובים נושכים מחככים ואינם מנגעים בכדי שינגעו (A pruritic [drug] is a drug that—by its nature—is so sharp and hot that it attracts the irritant itching humors towards the pores, but not to the extent of producing ulcers). Hebr. הסם המחכך features in BCD 188 (NM 4: 126) in an attestation from an anonymous trans. of Ibn Sīnā's *K. al-Adwiya al-qalbiyya* (i.e., *Sammim Libbiyim*). Anonymous I renders Arab. الدواء المحكك as הסם המחכך, just like Nathan and Zeraḥyah Ḥen translates the Arab. term as הרפואה המחככת (see entry רְפוּאָה).

• **הסם המחליק** · **the smoothing drug**: Arab. الدواء المملس · Ibn Sīnā, *K. al-Qānūn* II · trans. Nathan ha-Me'ati, *Sefer ha-Qanun* (Ms Oxford, Bodleian Libraries, Can. Or. 88, fol. 56[a]): והמחליק הוא הסם הדבק שמנהגו להתפשט על שטח האבר התפשטות חלק השטח וישוב שטח אותו הגשם חלק[230] (A smoothing [drug] is a viscous drug that—by its nature—spreads over the surface of an organ and smoothens it. The surface of that body becomes smoother[231]). Hebr. הסם המחליק features in BCD 188 (NM 4:125) as part of the term הסם המדביק או המחליק 'the agglutinant or mollifacient remedy' (for Lat. *inviscativa seu lenificativa medicina*) in an attestation from an anonymous trans. of Ibn Sīnā's *K. al-Adwiya al-qalbiyya* (i.e., *Sefer ha-Refu'ot ha-Libbiyot*). Zeraḥyah Ḥen translates Arab. الدواء المملس as הרפואה המחליקה (see entry רְפוּאָה) and Anonymous I renders the Arab. term as הסם המחליק, just like Nathan.

230 חלק: أملس a.

231 'smoother': Trans. acc. to a.

• **הסם המחתך** · **the cutting, biting, pungent drug**: Arab. الدواء مقطّع · Ibn Sīnā, *K. al-Qānūn* II · trans. Anonymous I, *Sefer ha-Qanun* (Ms Paris, BnF, héb. 1142, fol. 12[a]): והמחתך הוא הסם אשר דרכו שיעבור בדקותו בין שטח הליחה הדבקה ובין השטח אשר נדבקה בו ויפריד אותה ממנו (A cutting (biting, pungent) [drug] is a drug that—by its nature—penetrates because of its tenuity between the surface of the viscous humor and the surface [of the organ] it adheres to, and separates the latter from the former). Hebr. הסם המחתך features in BCD 188 (NM 4:126) in an attestation from an anonymous trans. of Ibn Sīnā's *K. al-Adwiya al-qalbiyya* (i.e., *Sammim Libbiyim*).

• **הסם החותם** · **the cicatrizing drug**: Arab. الدواء الخاتم · Ibn Sīnā, *K. al-Qānūn* II · trans. Nathan ha-Me'ati, *Sefer ha-Qanun* (Ms Oxford, Bodleian Libraries, Can. Or. 88, fol. 57[b]): והחותם ובלעז אלכתאני הוא הסם המיבש אשר ייבש שטח הנגעים עד שתשוב עלוי קלפה יבשה הנקראת חשכרישת בערבי תשמר אותו מן הפגעים עד שיצמח העור הטבעי (A cicatrizing [drug], in Rom. ʾLKTʾNY, is a desiccant drug that dries up the surface of a wound until it forms a dry scab (crust), called *khashkarīsha* (eschar) in Arab. This scab provides protection against injuries until the natural skin regenerates). Hebr. הסם החותם is not attested in the current dictionaries. For חָתַם in the sense of 'to cicatrize,' cf. BCD 109 (NM 1:152f.). Zeraḥyah Ḥen translates Arab. الدواء الخاتم as הרפואה החותמת (see entry רְפוּאָה).

• **הסם הטח בדבקות** · **the agglutinant (clogging) drug**: Arab. الدواء المغري· Ibn Sīnā, *K. al-Qānūn* II · trans. Anonymous I, *Sefer ha-Qanun* (Ms Paris, BnF, héb. 1142, fol. 14[a–b]): והטח בדבקות הנקרא גלוד טיב הוא הסם היבש שיש בה לחות מעטה מתדבק בה על הפיות ויסתמם ויעצר הנזול (An agglutinant (clogging) [drug] called [in Arab.] ǦLWD ṬYB is a dry drug with a small amount of [viscous] fluid with which it adheres to the openings [in the body] and clogs them, and blocks the flow [of the substance]). Hebr. הסם הטח בדבקות is not attested in the current dictionaries. Nathan ha-Me'ati translates Arab. الدواء المغري as הסם הצופד (see entry below) and Zeraḥyah Ḥen has הרפואה המסתמת (see entry רְפוּאָה).

• **הסם המטנף** · **the drug that infects (contaminates)**: Arab. الدواء الموسّخ · Ibn Sīnā, *K. al-Qānūn* II · trans. Anonymous I, *Sefer ha-Qanun* (Ms Paris, BnF, héb. 1142, fol. 14[a]): והמטנף השחינים הוא הסם המרטיב המתערב בלחויות השחינים וישימם יותר רבות וימנע הנגוב וההבראה (A [drug] that infects (contaminates) a wound is a moistening drug that mixes with the moistures (secretions) of the wound and increases them and [thus] prevents the wound from drying and from forming a scar (cicatrization)). Hebr. הסם המטנף is not attested in the current dictionaries. Nathan ha-Me'ati translates Arab. الدواء الموسّخ as הסם המטנף, just like Anonymous I, and Zeraḥyah Ḥen has הרפואה המלכלכת (see entry רְפוּאָה).

• **הסם המיבש** · **the desiccant drug**: Arab. الدواء المجفف · Ibn Sīnā, *K. al-Qānūn* II · trans. Nathan ha-Me'ati, *Sefer ha-Qanun* (Ms Oxford, Bodleian Libraries, Can. Or. 88, fol. 57[b]): והמיבש הוא הסם אשר יכלה הרוטהא בהתכו ורקיקותו (A desiccant [drug] is a drug that destroys fluids through its dissolving and refining [quality]). Hebr. הסם

המיבש is not attested in the current dictionaries. Zeraḥyah Ḥen translates Arab. الدواء المجفف as הרפואה המנגבת (see entry רְפוּאָה) and Anonymous I has הסם המנגב (see entry below).

• **הסם המוליד הגסות** · **the thickening (inspissating) drug**: Arab. الدواء المغلظ · Ibn Sīnā, *K. al-Qānūn* II · trans. Nathan ha-Me'ati, *Sefer ha-Qanun* (Ms Oxford, Bodleian Libraries, Can. Or. 88, fol. 57[a]): והמוליד הגסות הוא בהפך המרקיק והוא הסם מדרכו שישים תכונת הרוטבה יותר גסה אמנם בקפיאתו ואמנם שישיבנו עכור (A thickening (inspissating) [drug] is the opposite of an attenuant one. It is a drug that—by its nature—makes the consistency of humors more dense either by its coagulating or thickening property). Zeraḥyah Ḥen translates Arab. الدواء المغلظ as הרפואה המעבה (see entry רְפוּאָה) and Anonymous I has הסם המעבה (see entry below).

• **הסם הכווה** · **the cauterizing drug**: Arab. الدواء الكاوي · Ibn Sīnā, *K. al-Qānūn* II · trans. Nathan ha-Me'ati, *Sefer ha-Qanun* (Ms Oxford, Bodleian Libraries, Can. Or. 88, fol. 57[a]): והכווה הוא אשר יאכל הבשר וישרף העור שרפה מיבשת (A cauterizing [drug] is [a drug] that corrodes the flesh and burns and dries the skin).[232] Hebr. הסם הכווה is not attested in the current dictionaries. Zeraḥyah Ḥen translates Arab. الدواء الكاوي as הרפואה הכווה (see entry רְפוּאָה) and Anonymous I has הסם הכווה, just like Nathan.

• **הסם הממעיד** · **the lubricant drug**: Arab. الدواء المزلق · Ibn Sīnā, *K. al-Qānūn* II · trans. Anonymous I, *Sefer ha-Qanun* (Ms Paris, BnF, héb. 1142, fol. 14[a]): והממעיד[233] הוא סם שדרכו שיטפיח שטח גשם שיפגעהו במעבר נעצר בו עד שיפרידהו ממנו וישיב חלקיו יותר נכונים מלקבל ההזלה (A [lubricant [drug] is a drug that—by its nature—moistens the surface of a substance that is blocked in the passage, when it [i.e., the drug] encounters it. It [i.e., the drug] releases it [i.e., the substance] and makes its parts more capable of flowing). Hebr. הסם הממעיד features in BCD 188 (NM 4:127f.) in an attestation from an anonymous trans. of Ibn Sīnā's *K. al-Adwiya al-qalbiyya* (i.e., *Sammim Libbiyim*). Zeraḥyah Ḥen translates Arab. الدواء المزلق as הרפואה הממעידה (see entry רְפוּאָה). For the Arab. parallel term الأشياء المزلقة, translated as דברים מחליקים 'laxatives' by Samuel Benveniste in his trans. of Maimonides' *On Asthma* (i.e., *Ma'amar 'al ha-Qaṣeret*) IX.6, cf. NM 6:43f.; BMA 2:272, ll. 22.

• **הסם המנגב** · **the desiccant drug**: Arab. الدواء المجفف · Ibn Sīnā, *K. al-Qānūn* II · trans. Anonymous I, *Sefer ha-Qanun* (Ms Paris, BnF, héb. 1142, fol. 14[a]): והמנגב הוא הסם שמכלה הלחויות בהתכתו ודקדוקו (A desiccant [drug] is a drug that destroys fluids through its dissolving and refining [quality]). Hebr. הסם המנגב is not attested in

---

232 In his trans. of Maimonides' *Medical Aphorisms* (i.e., *Sefer ha-Peraqim*) VIII.43, Nathan translates Arab. الأدوية التي تحرق وتكوي 'the caustic remedies' as הרפואות השורפות והכוות (cf. BMMN 98, l. 12; BMMG no. 1913).

233 והממעיד הוא סם שדרכו שיטפיח שטח גשם שיפגעהו במעבר נעצר בו עד שיפרידהו ממנו וישיב חלקיו יותר נכונים מלקבל ההזלה: والمزلق هو الدواء الذي يبلّ سطح جسم ملاق لمجرى محتبس فيه حتى يبرئه عنه ويصير أجزاء أقبل للسيلان a.

the current dictionaries. Nathan ha-Me'ati translates Arab. الدواء المجفف as הסם המיבש (see entry above) and Zeraḥyah Ḥen has הרפואה המנגבת (see entry רְפוּאָה).

• **הסם המנגע · the ulcerative drug**: Arab. الدواء مقرح · Ibn Sīnā, *K. al-Qānūn* II · trans. Nathan ha-Me'ati, *Sefer ha-Qanun* (Ms Oxford, Bodleian Libraries, Can. Or. 88, fol. 57[a]): והמנגע הוא הסם שמדרכו שיכלה ויתיך הלחויות המגיעות בין חלקי העור וימשוך החומר הוא אליו עד שישוב נגע כמו הבלאדור (An ulcerative [drug] is a drug that—by its nature—destroys and dissolves the humors that come between the parts of the skin and attracts that [harmful] matter towards it until it forms an ulcer, [an example of such a drug is] the marking nut). Hebr. הסם המנגע features in BCD 188f. (NM 4:128) in an attestation from an anonymous trans. of Ibn Sīnā's *K. al-Adwiya al-qalbiyya* (i.e., *Sammim Libbiyim*). Hebr. *Pi'el* נִגֵּעַ (corr.) is attested in the sense of 'to cause ulceration' in BCD 169 (NM 3:150) in an attestation from Moses ibn Tibbon's trans. of Maimonides' *Commentary on Hippocrates' Aphorisms* (i.e., *Perush Aphorismi shel Apuqraṭ*) V.15 (cf. BMCH 1:379, l. 4). Zeraḥyah Ḥen translates Arab. الدواء مقرح as הרפואה המחבלת (see entry רְפוּאָה) and Anonymous I has הסם המשחין.

• **הסם המנחיר · the roughening drug**: Arab. الدواء المخشّن · Ibn Sīnā, *K. al-Qānūn* II · trans. Anonymous I, *Sefer ha-Qanun* (Ms Paris, BnF, héb. 1142, fol. 11[b]): הסם המנחיר הוא אותו שישים שטח האבר מתחלף החלקים בגובה ושפל (A roughening drug is [a drug] that makes the surface of an organ uneven in height and depth). In the sense of 'the roughening remedy,' Hebr. הסם המנחיר features in BCD 189 (NM 4: 128f.) in an attestation from an anonymous trans. of Ibn Sīnā's *K. al-Adwiya al-qalbiyya* (i.e., *Sammim Libbiyim*). Nathan ha-Me'ati translates Arab. الدواء المخشّن as הסם המעבה (see entry below) and Zeraḥyah Ḥen has הרפואה המעבה (see entry רְפוּאָה).

• **הסם הנופח · the flatulent drug**: Arab. الدواء المنفخ · Ibn Sīnā, *K. al-Qānūn* II · trans. Nathan ha-Me'ati, *Sefer ha-Qanun* (Ms Oxford, Bodleian Libraries, Can. Or. 88, fol. 57[a]): והנופח הוא הסם אשר בעצמו רוטבא גסה כשיפעל בה החום העיקרי לא יתך במהירות אבל ישתנה וישוב רוח כמו הלוביא (A flatulent [drug] is a drug whose substance has dense moisture. When innate heat acts on it, it does not dissolve swiftly but is transformed into wind; [an example of such a drug is the] black-eyed pea). Hebr. הסם הנופח features in BCD 190 (NM 4:133) in an attestation from an anonymous trans. of Ibn Sīnā's *K. al-Adwiya al-qalbiyya* (i.e., *Sammim Libbiyim*). Zeraḥyah Ḥen translates Arab. الدواء المنفخ as הרפואה המנפחת (see entry רְפוּאָה) and Anonymous I has הסם הנופח, just like Nathan.

• **הסם המסגר · the healing drug (a drug that promotes cicatrization)**: Arab. الدواء المدمل · Ibn Sīnā, *K. al-Qānūn* II · trans. Nathan ha-Me'ati, *Sefer ha-Qanun* (Ms Oxford, Bodleian Libraries, Can. Or. 88, fol. 57[b]): והמסגר הוא הסם אשר ייבש ויעבה הרוטבא הנופלת בין שני שטחי הנגע הקרובים זה לזה עד שישוב אל הצפד והדבוק וידבק האחד עם האחר כמו דם אל אכוין והצבר (A healing [drug] is a drug that dries up and thickens the fluid collected between the two layers of a wound, which are close to each other. [It does so] to an extent that it [i.e., the fluid] becomes agglutinant and viscous and both the ends [of the wound] adhere to each other; [examples of such a drug are] dragon's blood [i.e., the resin of *Dracaena cinnabari* Balf. f.] and aloes). Hebr. הסם המסגר is not attested in the current dictionaries. For *Part. Piʿel* מְסַגֵּר in the sense of 'to heal; to promote cicatrization,' cf. entry סָגַר. Zeraḥyah Ḥen translates Arab. الدواء المدمل as הרפואה המחיה (see entry רְפוּאָה) Anonymous I renders the Arab. term as הסם המבריא (see entry above).

• **הסם הסותם** · **the obstruent drug**: Arab. الدواء المسدّد · Ibn Sīnā, *K. al-Qānūn* II · trans. Anonymous I, *Sefer ha-Qanun* (Ms Paris, BnF, héb. 1142, fol. 14[a]): והסוטם הוא הסם היבש העוצר לקביצות חלקיו ויבשו או לטיחת דבקותו המעברים ומחדש בהם הסתימה (An obstruent [drug] is a drying, blocking [drug] that—because of its dense, dry or agglutinating properties—blogs the passages [of the body] and produces obstructions in them). Hebr. הסם הסותם features in BCD 190 (NM 4:133) in an attestation from an anonymous trans. of Ibn Sīnā's *K. al-Adwiya al-qalbiyya* (i.e., *Sammim Libbiyim*). Nathan ha-Me'ati translates Arab. الدواء المسدّد as הסם האוטם (see entry above) and Zeraḥyah Ḥen renders the Arab. term as הרפואה המסתמת (see entry רְפוּאָה).

• **הסם המעבה** · I. **the roughening drug**: Arab. الدواء المخشّن · Ibn Sīnā, *K. al-Qānūn* II · trans. Nathan ha-Me'ati, *Sefer ha-Qanun* (Ms Oxford, Bodleian Libraries, Can. Or. 88, fols. 56[b]): והמעבה הוא אשר ישים שטח האבר מחולף החלקים בגובה והשפלות (A roughening [drug] is [a drug] that makes the surface of an organ uneven in height and depth). In the sense of 'the roughening drug,' Hebr. הסם המעבה is not attested in the current dictionaries. For the noun עֳבִי, used by Nathan in the sense of 'roughness' (for Arab. خشونة) in his *Sefer ha-Qanun* II, cf. NM 6:156. Zeraḥyah Ḥen translates Arab. الدواء المخشن as הרפואה המעבה (see entry רְפוּאָה) and Anonymous I has הסם המנחיר (see entry above).

· II. **the thickening (inspissating) drug**: Arab. الدواء المغلظ · Ibn Sīnā, *K. al-Qānūn* II · trans. Anonymous I, *Sefer ha-Qanun* (Ms Paris, BnF, héb. 1142, fol. 13[b]): והמעבה הוא הפך המדקדק והוא הסם שדרכו להשיב עצם הלחות יותר עב אם בהקפאתו אם בדעיכתו[234] (A thickening (inspissating) [drug] is the opposite of an attenuant one. It is a drug that—by its nature—makes the consistency of humors more dense, either by its coagulating or thickening[235] property). In the sense of 'the thickening (inspissating) drug,' Hebr. הסם המעבה features in BCD 189 (NM 4:129) in an attestation from an anonymous trans. of Ibn Sīnā's *K. al-Adwiya al-qalbiyya* (i.e., *Sammim Libbiyim*). Nathan ha-Me'ati translates Arab. الدواء المغلظ as הסם המוליד הגסות (see entry above) and Zeraḥyah Ḥen has הרפואה המעבה (see entry רְפוּאָה).

• **הסם המעכל** · **the digestive drug**: Arab. الدواء الهاضم · Ibn Sīnā, *K. al-Qānūn* II · trans. Nathan ha-Me'ati, *Sefer ha-Qanun* (Ms Oxford, Bodleian Libraries, Can. Or. 88,

---

234 בדעיכתו: שישיבהו עבה Ms[1] بإخثاره a.

235 'thickening': Trans. acc. to Ms[1] and a.

fols. 56[b]–57[a]): והמעבל הוא הסם אשר מנהגו להועיל אל[236] עכול המזון וכבר הודעתי אותו קודם (A digestive drug is [a drug] that—by its nature—helps the digestion of the food. I have already mentioned it before). Hebr. הסם המעבל features in BCD 189 (NM 4:129) in an attestation from an anonymous trans. of Ibn Sīnā's *K. al-Adwiya al-qalbiyya* (i.e., *Sammim Libbiyim*). Zeraḥyah Ḥen translates Arab. الدواء الهاضم as הרפואה המעכלת (see entry רְפוּאָה) and Anonymous I has הסם המעבל, just like Nathan.

• **הסם המעסה** · **the constricting drug**: Arab. الدواء العاصر · Ibn Sīnā, *K. al-Qānūn* II · trans. Anonymous I, *Sefer ha-Qanun* (Ms Paris, BnF, héb. 1142, fol. 14[a]): והמעסה הוא הסם שמגיע מקביצותו ואסיפתו אל החלקים עד שמכריח הלחויות הרקיקות העומדות בחללם להלחץ ולהתפרק (A constricting [drug] is a drug whose astringency and condensing [quality] on the organs is so strong that the thin fluids, which have collected in their interstices, are necessarily compressed and removed). Hebr. הסם המעסה is not attested in the current dictionaries. Nathan ha-Me'ati translates Arab. الدواء العاصر as הסם העוצר (see entry below) and Zeraḥyah Ḥen has הרפואה השוחטת (see entry רְפוּאָה).

• **הסם המעפש** · **the putrefactive drug**: Arab. الدواء المعفن · Ibn Sīnā, *K. al-Qānūn* II · trans. Nathan ha-Me'ati, *Sefer ha-Qanun* (Ms Oxford, Bodleian Libraries, Can. Or. 88, fol. 57[a]): והמעפש הוא אשר יפסיד מזג הרוח ההולך אל האבר ומזג רוטבתו עד שלא יכשר להיות חלק לאותו האבר ולא יגיע שישרפהו ויאכלהו (A putrefactive [drug] is [a drug] that corrupts the temperament of the pneuma, which flows to an organ, and also the temperament of the humor to such an extent that they are not suitable to be parts of the organ, but not to an extent where they are burnt or corroded).[237] Hebr. הסם המעפש does not feature in the current dictionaries. Zeraḥyah Ḥen translates Arab. الدواء المعفن as הרפואה המעפשת (see entry רְפוּאָה) and Anonymous I has הסם המעפש, just like Nathan.

• **הסם העוצר** · **the constricting drug**: Arab. الدواء العاصر · Ibn Sīnā, *K. al-Qānūn* II · trans. Nathan ha-Me'ati, *Sefer ha-Qanun* (Ms Oxford, Bodleian Libraries, Can. Or. 88, fol. 57[b]): והעוצר הוא הסם אשר יגיע בקבוצו ואסיפתו אל החלקים עד שיצטרכו הרוטבות הרקיקות היושבות בתוכן[238] להלחץ[239] (A constricting [drug] is a drug whose astringency and condensing [quality] on the organs is so strong that the thin fluids, which have collected in their interstices,[240] are compressed and[241] removed). Hebr. הסם העוצר features in the sense of 'constrictive remedy' in BCD 190 (NM 4:134) in an

236 אל עכול המזון: Emend. ed. אל הסם עכול Ms.

237 In his trans. of Maimonides' *Medical Aphorisms* (i.e., *Sefer ha-Peraqim*) XXIII.101, Nathan translates Arab. *Plur.* أدوية معفنة 'putrefying remedies' as סמים מעפשים (cf. BMMN 231, ll. 25–26; BMMG no. 1892).

238 בתוכן: في خللها a.

239 להלחץ: والانفصال add. a.

240 'interstices': Trans. acc. to a.

241 'and removed': Trans. acc. to a.

attestation from an anonymous trans. of Ibn Sīnā's *K. al-Adwiya al-qalbiyya* (i.e., *Sammim Libbiyim*). Zeraḥyah Ḥen renders Arab. الدواء العاصر as הרפואה השוחטת (see entry רְפוּאָה) and Anonymous I has הסם המעסה (see entry above).

• **הסם המפגג · the drug that makes crude (unripe)**: Arab. الدواء المفجج · Ibn Sīnā, *K. al-Qānūn* II · trans. Nathan ha-Me'ati, *Sefer ha-Qanun* (Ms Oxford, Bodleian Libraries, Can. Or. 88, fol. 57[a]): והמפגג הוא בהפך המבשל והמעכל והוא הסם אשר יבטל בקרתו מפעל החום העקרי והזר כמו כן במזון והתערוב עד שישאר בלתי מעוכל ומבושל (A [drug] that makes unripe (crude) is the opposite of a ripening (coctive) and digestive [drug]. It is a drug that—by its cold [nature]—makes the action of innate and extraneous heat on both food and humors ineffective so that it remains undigested and uncooked). Hebr. *Pi'el* פִּגֵּג features in BM 4810 in the sense of 'to clot.' Zeraḥyah Ḥen translates Arab. الدواء المفجج as הרפואה המפגגת (see entry רְפוּאָה) and Anonymous I has הסם המפגג, just like Nathan. In the anonymous trans. of Ibn Sīnā's *K. al-Adwiya al-qalbiyya* (i.e., *Sammim Libbiyim*), Arab. الدواء المفجج features as Hebr. הסם המפיג (cf. BCD 189 (NM 4:130)).

• **הסם המפרך · the [stone-]crushing (lithontriptic) drug**: Arab. الدواء المفتت · Ibn Sīnā, *K. al-Qānūn* II · trans. Nathan ha-Me'ati, *Sefer ha-Qanun* (Ms Oxford, Bodleian Libraries, Can. Or. 88, fol. 57[a]): והמפרך הוא הסם שמדרכו כשיפגע תערוב מאובן יקטין חלקיו וירצץ אותם כמו המשבר החצץ וכמו האבן הנקרא חגר אליהודי ובלעדיו (A [stone-]crushing (lithontriptic) [drug] is a drug that—by its nature—, when it comes across a petrified humor, reduces it into small pieces and crushes it, like [a drug] that breaks up stones; [an example of such a drug is] the stone called [in Arab.] *ḥajar al-Yahūdī* [i.e., Jews' stone], a.o.). Hebr. הסם המפרך is not attested in the current dictionaries. Zeraḥyah Ḥen translates Arab. الدواء المفتت as הרפואה המפוצצת (see entry רְפוּאָה) and Anonymous I has הסם המפתת (see entry below).

• **הסם הפותח · the deobstruent drug**: Arab. الدواء المفتّح · Ibn Sīnā, *K. al-Qānūn* II · trans. Anonymous I, *Sefer ha-Qanun* (Ms Paris, BnF, héb. 1142, fol. 12[a]): והפותח הוא הסם אשר דרכו שיניע הליחה העומדת בתוך חללי המעברים לחוץ כדי שישארו המעברים פתוחים וזה יותר חזק מן הממרק כמו הבטראסליון (A deobstruent [drug] is a drug that—by its nature—moves the humoral matter inside the cavities of the passages to the outside so that they stay open. These drugs are stronger than the detergent ones; [an example of such a drug is] [Arab.] *baṭrāsāliyūn* [i.e., parsley]).[242] Hebr. הסם הפותח features in BCD 191 (NM 4:134f.) in an attestation from an anonymous trans. of Ibn Sīnā's *K. al-Adwiya al-qalbiyya* (i.e., *Sammim Libbiyim*). Nathan ha-Me'ati translates Arab. الدواء المفتّح as הסם המפתח (see next entry) and Zeraḥyah Ḥen has הרפואה הפותחת (see entry רְפוּאָה).

242 In his trans. of Maimonides' *Medical Aphorisms* (i.e., *Sefer ha-Peraqim*) IX.3, Nathan translates Arab. *Plur.* الأدوية المفتّحة 'the opening medications' as הרפואות הפותחות (cf. BMMG no. 1931; BMMN 103, l. 12).

• **הסם המפתח** · **the deobstruent drug**: Arab. الدواء المفتّح · Ibn Sīnā, *K. al-Qānūn* II · trans. Nathan ha-Me'ati, *Sefer ha-Qanun* (Ms Oxford, Bodleian Libraries, Can. Or. 88, fol. 56[v]: והמפתח הוא הסם שמנהגו להניע החומר הנולד מבפנים בחלולי המעברים ⟩ב⟨לחוץ כדי שישארו פתוחים וזה יותר חזק מהממרק כמו הברטסליון (A deobstruent [drug] is a drug that—by its nature—moves the [humoral] matter that originates in the cavities of the passages to the outside so that they stay open. These drugs are stronger than the detergent ones; [an example of such a drug is] [Arab.] *baṭrāsāliyūn* [i.e., parsley]). Hebr. הסם המפתח is not attested in the current dictionaries. Zeraḥyah Ḥen translates Arab. الدواء المفتّح as הרפואה הפותחת (see entry רְפוּאָה) and Anonymous I has הסם הפותח (see previous entry).

• **הסם המפתת** · **the [stone-]crushing (lithontriptic) drug**: Arab. الدواء المفتت · Ibn Sīnā, *K. al-Qānūn* II · trans. Anonymous I, *Sefer ha-Qanun* (Ms Paris, BnF, hébr. 1142, fol. 13[a]): והמפתת הוא הסם שאם יפגש ליחה מתאבנת יקטין חלקיה וירצצם כמו מפתת החצץ וכמו אבן יהודי וזולתו (A [stone-]crushing (lithontriptic) [drug] is a drug that, when it comes across a petrified humor, reduces it into small pieces and crushes it, like [a drug] that breaks up stones; [an example of such a drug is] the Jews' stone, a.o.).[243] Hebr. הסם המפתת is not attested in the current dictionaries. Nathan ha-Me'ati translates Arab. الدواء المفتت as הסם המפרך (see entry above) and Zeraḥyah Ḥen has הרפואה המפוצצת (see entry רְפוּאָה).

• **הסם המצמיח הבשר** · **the drug that makes the flesh grow**: Arab. الدواء المنبت للحم Ibn Sīnā, *K. al-Qānūn* II · trans. Nathan ha-Me'ati, *Sefer ha-Qanun* (Ms Oxford, Bodleian Libraries, Can. Or. 88, fol. 57[b]): והמצמיח הבשר הוא הסם שמנהגו לשנות הדם היורד אל הנגעים בשר לפי שמיישר מזגו ומקשה אותו ביבשות (A [drug] that makes the flesh grow is a drug that—by its nature—changes the blood, which streams to a wound, into flesh by moderating the temperament of the blood and coagulating it through desiccation). Hebr. הסם המצמיח הבשר is not attested in the current dictionaries. Zeraḥyah Ḥen translates Arab. الدواء المنبت للحم as הרפואה המצמיחה הבשר (see entry רְפוּאָה) and Anonymous I has הסם המצמיח הבשר, just like Nathan.

• **הסם המקלף** · **the peeling (exfoliating) drug**: Arab. الدواء القاشر · Ibn Sīnā, *K. al-Qānūn* II · trans. Nathan ha-Me'ati, *Sefer ha-Qanun* (Ms Oxford, Bodleian Libraries, Can. Or. 88, fol. 57[a]): והמקלף הוא הסם שמנהגו ברוב תמרוקו שימרוק חלקי העור הנפסדים כמו הקשט (A peeling (exfoliating) [drug] is a drug that—by its nature [and] its intense cleansing property—cleans the decayed parts of the skin, [an example of such a drug is] costus). Hebr. הסם המקלף is not attested in the current dictionaries. Anonymous I renders Arab. الدواء القاشر as הסם המקלף, just like Nathan, and Zeraḥyah Ḥen trans-

---

243 In his trans. of Maimonides' *Medical Aphorisms* (i.e., *Sefer ha-Peraqim*) XXI.65, Nathan translates Arab. *Plur.* الأدوية المفتتة 'the stone-crushing remedies' as ⟨הסמים⟩ המפתתים החצץ (cf. BMMN 204, l. 7; BMMG no. 1930).

lates the Arab. term as הרפואה הקולפת (see entry רְפוּאָה). Arab. مقشّر in the sense of 'peeling (exfoliating)' is translated by Nathan as מְקַלֵּף (see entry קָלַף).

• **הסם הצופד · the agglutinant (clogging) drug**: Arab. الدواء المغري · Ibn Sīnā, *K. al-Qānūn* II · trans. Nathan ha-Me'ati, *Sefer ha-Qanun* (Ms Oxford, Bodleian Libraries, Can. Or. 88, fol. 57[b]): והצופד הוא הסם היבש אשר בו רוטבא מעוטה דבוקה על הפיות ותסגרם ויעצר המוגר (An agglutinant (clogging) [drug] is a dry drug with a small amount of viscous fluid with which it adheres to the openings [in the body] and clogs them and blocks the flow [of the substance]). Hebr. הסם הצופד is not attested in the current dictionaries. Zeraḥyah Ḥen translates Arab. الدواء المغري as הרפואה המסתמת (see entry רְפוּאָה) and Anonymous I has הסם הטח בדבקות (see entry above). For Nathan's use of *Part.* צוֹפֵד in the sense of 'agglutinant; gluey' in his *Sefer ha-Qanun*, see entry צָפַד.

• **הסם המרדים החוש · the anesthetic (benumbing; soporific; narcotic) drug**: Arab. الدواء المخدّر · Ibn Sīnā, *K. al-Qānūn* II · trans. Anonymous I, *Sefer ha-Qanun* (Ms Paris, BnF, héb. 1142, fol. 13[b]): והמרדים החוש הוא הסם הקר שמגיע מקורו לאבר שישים עצם הרוח הנושא אליו כח התנועה וההרגש קר במזגו עב בעצמותו ולא יעשה[244] בו הכחות הנפשיות (An anesthetic (benumbing; soporific; narcotic) [drug] is a cold drug that has such a strong cooling effect on an organ that it makes the substance of the pneuma, which is carried to the organ by the faculty of movement and sensation, cold in temperament and dense in substance. Consequently, the psychical faculty does not have an effect on it anymore). Hebr. הסם המרדים החוש is not attested in the current dictionaries. Nathan ha-Me'ati translates Arab. الدواء المخدّر as הסם המבטל ההרגש (see entry above) and Zeraḥyah Ḥen has הרפואה המבטלת (see entry רְפוּאָה).

• **הסם הרוחץ · the abluent drug**: Arab. الدواء الغسّال · Ibn Sīnā, *K. al-Qānūn* II · trans. Nathan ha-Me'ati, *Sefer ha-Qanun* (Ms Oxford, Bodleian Libraries, Can. Or. 88, fol. 57[b]): והרוחץ הוא הסם שמנהגו למרק ולא בכח פועל אלא בכח מתפעל (An abluent [drug] is a drug that—by its nature—cleanses, not through its active power but through its passive power). Hebr. הסם הרוחץ is attested in BCD 191 (NM 4:135) in an attestation from an anonymous trans. of Ibn Sīnā's *K. al-Adwiya al-qalbiyya* (i.e., *Sammim Libbiyim*). Zeraḥyah Ḥen translates Arab. الدواء الغسّال as הרפואה הרוחצת (see entry רְפוּאָה) and Anonymous I has הסם הרוחץ, just like Nathan.

• **הסם המשבר הרוח · the carminative drug**: Arab. الدواء الكاسر الرياح · Ibn Sīnā, *K. al-Qānūn* II · trans. Anonymous I, *Sefer ha-Qanun* (Ms Paris, BnF, héb. 1142, fol. 12[a]): והמשבר[245] הרוח הוא הסם שדרכו לשים עצם הרוח דקיק אויריי בחומו ונגובו (A carminative [drug] is a drug that—by its nature—dilutes the substance of the gas and makes it airy through its heat and dryness). Hebr. הסם המשבר הרוח is attested in BCD 189f.

244 יעשה: יעשו Ms[1].
245 והמשבר: אלכאסיר Ms[1].

(NM 4:131) in an attestation from an anonymous trans. of Ibn Sīnā's *K. al-Adwiya al-qalbiyya* (i.e., *Sammim Libbiyim*). Nathan ha-Me'ati translates Arab. الدواء الكاسر الرياح as הסם המשבר הרוחות and Zeraḥyah Ḥen has הרפואה המשברת הרוח (see entry רְפוּאָה).

• **הסם השורף** · **the caustic drug**: Arab. الدواء المحرق · Ibn Sīnā, *K. al-Qānūn* II · trans. Nathan ha-Me'ati, *Sefer ha-Qanun* (Ms Oxford, Bodleian Libraries, Can. Or. 88, fol. 56[b]): והשורף הוא הסם שמנהגו להתיך הרקיק מהתערובים והאיברים וינקה[246] אפרם כמו הפרביון (A caustic [drug] is a drug that—by its nature—dissolves the tenuous humors [of] the organs, leaving[247] behind the ashy matter; [an example of such a drug is] [Arab.] *furbiyūn* [i.e., resin spurge]).[248] Hebr. הסם השורף is not attested in the current dictionaries. Zeraḥyah Ḥen translates Arab. الدواء المحرق as הרפואה השורפת (see entry רְפוּאָה) and Anonymous I has הסם השורף, just like Nathan.

סִמּוּר • **סמור השער** · **horripilation**: Arab. قشعريرة · Ibn Sīnā, *K. al-Qānūn* II · trans. Nathan ha-Me'ati, *Sefer ha-Qanun* (Ms Oxford, Bodleian Libraries, Can. Or. 88, fol. 69[b]): בסר ובלח ... אם יסתפקו ממנו הרבה יוליד הנעירה וסמור השער ([Arab.] *busr* and *balaḥ*: Unripe dates: ... If one uses an excessive quantity of them, they cause shivering and horripilation). Hebr. סמור השער is not attested in the current dictionaries. The term סִמּוּר on its own features in the sense of 'shivering' (for Arab. قشعريرة and اقشعرار) in Nathan's trans. of Maimonides' *Medical Aphorisms* (cf. BMMG nos. 4113/4114). Cf. also BCD 192 (NM 2:167) for סִמּוּר in the sense of 'shivering fit; rigor' (corr.) in an attestation from David Caslari's trans. of Galen's *De inaequali intemperie* (i.e., *Sefer Roʿa Mezeg Mitḥallef*) VI.4. Zeraḥyah Ḥen and Anonymous I both translate Arab. قشعريرة as סִמּוּר.

סְמִימָה • *Plur.* **סמימות** · **poisons**: Arab. سموم · Ibn Sīnā, *K. al-Qānūn* II · trans. Zeraḥyah Ḥen (Ms Oxford, Bodleian Libraries, Opp. Add. Fol. 12, fol. 193[b]):[249] גִ׳בְסִין ... הוא מכלל הסמימות החונקים ([Arab.] *jibsīn*: Gypsum: ... It is one of the suffocating poisons). Hebr. סְמִימָה, *Plur.* סמימות, is not attested in the current dictionaries. Nathan ha-Me'ati and Anonymous I both render Arab. سموم as ארסים.

סְמָמִית · **the spider species phalangium or tarantula**: Arab. رتيلاء (cf. Lane 1028; D 1:509; JAD 1:855f., s.v. *rutaylā'*) · Ibn Sīnā, *K. al-Qānūn* II · trans. Anonymous I, *Sefer ha-Qanun* (Ms Paris, BnF, héb. 1142, fols. 262[a]–263[a]): כבאזי ... עליהו משקיט עקיצת הצרעה תחבשת וכל שכן עם שמן וישתה[250] זרעו ויקיא תמיד ויועיל מעקיצת הסממית ([Arab.]

246 וינקה: وتبقى a.

247 'leaving behind': Trans. acc. to a.

248 In his trans. of Maimonides' *Medical Aphorisms* (i.e., *Sefer ha-Peraqim*) XV.6, Nathan translates Arab. الأدوية المحرقة 'the caustic remedies' as הרפואות השורפות (cf. BMMN 155, l. 5; BMMG no. 1914).

249 The same Hebr. term features (for Arab. سموم) on fol. 195[a], entry גַ׳דְוָאר '[Arab.] *jadwār*: Zedoary [*Curcuma zedoaria* (Christm.) Roscoe)],' and on fol. 191[a], entry גַ׳וְז אגוז '[Arab.] *jawz*; [i.e., Hebr.] *egoz*: Walnut [*Juglans regia* L.].'

250 וישתה: ومن السموم يشرب a.

khubbāzā: Common marshmallow [*Althaea officinalis* L.]: … Its leaves applied as a plaster have a soothing effect on wasp bites, particularly so with olive oil. Against[251] poisons one should ingest its seeds, for then one will vomit frequently. It is also good for the bite of the tarantula). Hebr. סְמָמִית features in BM 4112 in an attestation, a.o., from the *Sefer ha-Qanun*; the term is translated by Ben Yehuda as 'poisonous spider.'[252] Nathan ha-Me'ati translates Arab. رتيلاء as השרץ הנק׳ רותילה בערבי.

סִמָּן • *Plur.* **סימנים רכים** • **סימנים** · **soft pimples [in the face] (possibly acne)**: Arab. البثور اللينة · Ibn Sīnā, *K. al-Qānūn* II · trans. Nathan ha-Me'ati, *Sefer ha-Qanun* (Ms Oxford, Bodleian Libraries, Can. Or. 88, fol. 82[a–b]): זבד אלבחר … והשנים[253] האספוגים מערבים אותם בכבוסים ובתרופות הסימנים הרכים והכתם הנקר׳ כלף בערבי והרושם מבפנים[254] ([Arab.] *zabad al-baḥr* [lit. 'sea froth']: Alcyonium: … The two spongy varieties are incorporated in lotions and other medicines to be used in soft pimples [on the face] (acne), freckles, called *kalaf* in Arab., and facial marks). Hebr. סימנים רכים is not attested in the current dictionaries. Anonymous I renders Arab. البثور اللينة as הצמחים הרכים.

סְנֶה • **סנה הכלב** · **dog rose** [***Rosa canina*** **L.**]: Arab. عليق الكلب (cf. DT 146f. (1.63)) · Ibn Sīnā, *K. al-Qānūn* II · trans. Zeraḥyah Ḥen, *Sefer ha-Qanun* (Ms Oxford, Bodleian Libaries, Opp. Add. Fol. 12, fol. 256[b]): עֻלַּיְק סנה … מין בו נקרא סנה הכלב יש בו פרי כמו הזיתים כמו הצמר מבפנים ([Arab.] *'ullayq*; [i.e., Hebr.] *seneh*: Blackberry [*Rubus fruticosus* L.]: … One of its varieties, called 'dog rose,' bears fruits like olives, which contain a wool-like substance). Hebr. סנה הכלב is not attested in the current dictionaries. Nathan ha-Me'ati transcribes Arab. عليق الكلب as עליק אלכלב and Anonymous I renders the Arab. term as עליק הכלבים. For the identification of عليق as סְנֶה, see BMMG no. 3537.

סַנְוֵר · **dimness of sight**: Arab. غشاوة (Gr. ἀμβλυωπία; cf. UW 99f.) · Ibn Sīnā, *K. al-Qānūn* II · trans. Anonymous I, *Sefer ha-Qanun* (Ms Paris, BnF, héb. 1142, fol. 60[b]): בקלה חמקה … מועיל מן הרמד ונכנס בכחולים והריבוי ממנו מחדש הסנור הנקרא גשאוה ([Arab.] *baqla ḥamqā'* [lit. 'the stupid vegetable']: Common purslane [*Portulaca oleracea* L.]: … It is useful in [Arab.] *ramad* [i.e., ophthalmia] and it is included in collyria. Its excessive use, however, causes dimness of sight, called [in Arab.] *ghashāwa*). Hebr. סַנְוֵר features in BM 4128 in the sense of 'night blindness' in an attestation from Pseudo-Ibn Ezra's *Sefer ha-Nisyonot*: אם יצלה כבד העז ותטיף בו העין יועיל מהסנור ר״ל למי שרואה ביום ולא בלילה (If the liver of a goat is roasted and dripped into the eye, it is beneficial for night blindness; i.e., for someone who can see in the daytime but not at night).[255]

---

251 'Against poisons': Transl. acc. to a.

252 For an extensive discussion of the term סְמָמִית and its different interpretations, see L. Lewysohn, *Zoologie des Talmuds* (Frankfurt am Main 1858), 222f., 299f.

253 והשנים (= Ms Paris, BnF, héb. 1136, fol. 77a): והישנים Ms.

254 מבפנים: في الوجه a.

255 Cf. J.O. Leibowitz and S. Marcus (eds.), *Sefer Hanisyonot: The Book of Medical Experiences Attributed to Abraham ibn Ezra* (Jerusalem 1984), 175f.

Nathan ha-Me'ati translates Arab. غشاوة as חשכת העין (see entry חֲשֵׁכָה) and Zeraḥyah Ḥen has סנורים (see entry below).

• סנויר לילה · **night blindness**: Arab. عشا · Ibn Sīnā, *K. al-Qānūn* II · trans. Anonymous I, *Sefer ha-Qanun* (Ms Paris, BnF, héb. 1142, fols. 102[b]–103[a]): דאר פלפל הוא פלפל ארוך ... עם ⟨מי⟩ כבד עז צלוי מועיל מן סנויר לילה הנקרא עשא ([Arab.] *dārfulful*; i.e., [Hebr.] *pilpel arokh*: Long pepper [*Piper longum* L.]: ... [If one eats it] with roasted liver of a goat it is beneficial for night blindness, called [in Arab.] *ʿashan*). Nathan ha-Me'ati translates Arab. عشا as *Plur.* סנורים (see entry below) and Zeraḥyah Ḥen has מי שאינו (רואה) בלילה.

• *Plur.* **סנורים** · I. **dimness of sight**: Arab. غشاوة (Gr. ἀμβλυωπία; cf. UW 99f.) · Ibn Sīnā, *K. al-Qānūn* II · trans. Zeraḥyah Ḥen, *Sefer ha-Qanun* (Ms Oxford, Bodleian Libaries, Opp. Add. Fol. 12, fol. 187[a]): בַּקְלָה חַמְקָה ... יועיל מן הרמד ויכנס בכחלים והריבוי ממנה יחדש הסנורים ([Arab.] *baqla ḥamqā'* [lit. 'the stupid vegetable']: Common purslane [*Portulaca oleracea* L.]: ... It is useful in [Arab.] *ramad* [i.e., ophthalmia] and it is included in collyria. Its excessive use, however, causes dimness of sight). Hebr. סנורים is attested in the sense of 'blindness; dimness' in Rabb. literature, cf. *Yalqut Esther* 1056: שהיה הסנורים על עיניו 'his eye-sight was veiled' (cf. JD 1006). Nathan ha-Me'ati translates Arab. غشاوة as חשכת העין (see entry חֲשֵׁכָה) and Anonymous I has סנור (see entry above).

· II. **night blindness**: Arab. عشا · Ibn Sīnā, *K. al-Qānūn* II · trans. Nathan ha-Me'ati, *Sefer ha-Qanun* (Ms Oxford, Bodleian Libraries, Can. Or. 88, fol. 78[a]): דאר פלפל ... אם יאכלהו עם כבד עז צלוי יועיל מסנורים ובערבי עשא ([Arab.] *dārfulful*: Long pepper [*Piper longum* L.]: ... If one eats it with roasted liver of a goat it is beneficial for night blindness, in Arab. *ʿashan*). In the sense of 'night blindness,' Hebr. סנורים is only attested in this sense as *Sing.* סַנְוֵר in BM 4128. Zeraḥyah Ḥen translates Arab. عشا as מי שאינו (רואה) בלילה and Anonymous I has סנויר לילה (see entry above). Moses ibn Tibbon translates Arab. عشا as לִילִית in his trans. of Ibn al-Jazzār's *Zād al-musāfir* (i.e., *Sefer Ṣedat ha-Derakhim*) II.5.0–1 (cf. BCD 137 (NM 4:91); IJZ 1–2:491).

סעוט • עשה סעוט → עָשָׂה.

סַפִּירִי • אבן ספירית → אֶבֶן.

[ספק] • *Hitpaʿel* הִסְתַּפֵּק · **to use**: Arab. استعمل · Ibn Sīnā, *K. al-Qānūn* II · trans. Nathan ha-Me'ati, *Sefer ha-Qanun* (Ms Oxford, Bodleian Libraries, Can. Or. 88, fol. 69[b]): בסר ובלח ... אם יסתפקו ממנו הרבה יוליד הנעירה וסמור השער ([Arab.] *busr* and *balaḥ*: Unripe dates: ... If one uses an excessive quantity of them they cause shivering and horripilation). In the sense of 'to use,' Hebr. *Hitpaʿel* הִסְתַּפֵּק is only attested in Rabb. and Halakhic literature (in an attestation from the *Halakhot Pesuqot*; cf. BM 4172f.). Zeraḥyah Ḥen translates Arab. استعمل as אכול and Anonymous I has עשיה (cf. BCD 216 (NM 2:74) for an attestation from Nathan's trans. of Maimonides' *Medical Aphorisms* (i.e., *Sefer ha-Peraqim*) III.91 (cf. BMMN 53, l. 2; BMMG no. 3569)).

• *Part.* **מִסְתַּפֵּק • שמן זית המסתפקים ממנו** → **שֶׁמֶן**.

סֵרְחוֹן • סירחון האף · **ozena (foul odor from the nose)**: Arab. نتن الأنف · Ibn Sīnā, *K. al-Qānūn* II · trans. Zeraḥyah Ḥen, *Sefer ha-Qanun* (Ms Oxford, Bodleian Libaries, Opp. Add. Fol. 12, fol. 196[b]): דָּארשִׁיעְשַׁעֵן ... הדארשיעשעאן טוב לסירחון האף ויעשו ממנו פתילה ([Arab.] *dārshīsha'ān*: Broom [*Genista acanthoclada* DC. or *Cytisus spinosus* Lam.] (cf. MIG no. 223): ... Broom is beneficial for ozena when it is used as a wick). Hebr. סרחון האף is not attested in the current dictionaries. Nathan ha-Me'ati translates Arab. نتن الأنف as באישות הנחירים (see entry בְּאָשָׁה), Anonymous I has באשת הנחירים (see also entry בְּאָשָׁה), and Anonymous II has סרחון הנחירים (see next entry).

• **סרחון הנחירים** · **ozena (foul odor from the nose)**: Arab. نتن الأنف · Ibn Sīnā, *K. al-Qānūn* II · trans. Anonymous II, *Sefer ha-Qanun* (Ms Parma, Biblioteca Palatina, Cod. Parm. 3045, fol. 30[a]): דַּרְסֵיסֵיאַם ... הוא מוביר וטוב להועיל לסרחון הנחירים אם יעשה ממנו פתילה ויושם ([Arab.] *dārshīsha'ān*: Broom [*Genista acanthoclada* DC. or *Cytisus spinosus* Lam.] (cf. MIG no. 223): ... It is beneficial for ozena when a wick is made of it and then applied). Hebr. סרחון הנחירים is not attested in the current dictionaries. Nathan ha-Me'ati translates Arab. نتن الأنف as באישות הנחירים (see entry בְּאָשָׁה), Zeraḥyah Ḥen has סירחון האף (see previous entry), and Anonymous I has באשת הנחירים (see also entry בְּאָשָׁה).

[סרטן] • *Part. Pu'al* **מְסֻרְטָן** · **affected by cancer; cancerous**: Lat. *cancrosus* · Guy de Chauliac, *Inventarium sive Chirurgia Magna* (cf. CMM 1:239, l. 34) · trans. Anonymous (Ms Paris, BnF, héb. 1189, fol. 131[a]): אמנם אותם הנעשים באברים הנמשכים כמו באמה וצואר הרחם הם גרידות חימומים ונגעים המימיים[256] עם מוגליות ומעופשים ומאוכלים ומסורטנים ([Ulcers] that occur in organs that can have a prolapse, such as penis and neck of the uterus (cervix), are: excoriations, heating ulcers, virulent ulcers, putrid ulcers, corrosive ulcers, cancerous ulcers). Hebr. *Part. Pu'al* מְסֻרְטָן is not attested in the current dictionaries.

סִתּוּם · **healing**: Arab. اندمال · al-Rāzī, *K. fī al-Faṣd* · trans. Anonymous, *Ma'amar ba-Haqqazah* (Ms Parma, Biblioteca Palatina, Cod. Parm. 2283,4, fol. 94[a]): ויש בהקזת הגידים הדופקים סכנה בסבת עבי עורם וקשי הפסק דמם וסתומם (Bleeding the pulsatile veins is dangerous because of the coarseness of their skin and the difficulty of stopping the blood and healing them). Hebr. סִתּוּם features in the sense of 'obstruction' (for Arab. سدّة) in BCD 195 (NM 4:140) in an attestation from Moses ibn Tibbon's trans. of Ibn al-Jazzār's *Zād al-musāfir* (i.e., *Sefer Ṣedat ha-Derakhim*) N.4 (cf. IJZ 1–2:441). The verb סָתַם features in the same text (III.8) in the sense of 'to promote cicatrization; to heal' (for Arab. أدمل) (cf. NM 5:142).

סָתַם • *Part.* **סוֹתֵם • הסם הסותם** → **סַם**.

• *Part. Pi'el* **מְסַתֵּם • הרפואה המסתמת** → **רְפוּאָה**.

---

256 המימיים עם מוגליות: *virulenta* L.

ע

[עבה] • *Part. Pi'el* **מְעַבֶּה** • **הסם המעבה** → **סַם.**

• **הרפואה המעבה** → **רְפוּאָה.**

עִבּוּד · **astringent quality, effect**: Arab. دبغ (Gr. στῦψις; cf. UW 646f.) · Ibn Sīnā, *K. al-Qānūn* II · trans. Zeraḥyah Ḥen, *Sefer ha-Qanun* (Ms Oxford, Bodleian Libaries, Opp. Add. Fol. 12, fol. 201ᵇ): הַלִילַג' מִירַבַּלֹנִי ... מועיל לכאב הטחול ויועיל לכלי המזון כלם וכל שכן השחורים כי הם יחזקו האצטומ' וכל שכן המגודלים ויחזקו רפיון האצטומ' עם העיבוד והנקיון והנישוף ([Arab.] *halīlaj* [from Pers. *halīlah*]; [Rom.] MiYRaBaLoNiY: (Chebulic) myrobalan: ... They are useful for pain in the spleen and for all nutritive organs—especially the black variety—because they strengthen the stomach, above all the preserved ones. They strengthen the lining of the stomach through their astringent, cleansing, and absorbing effect). Hebr. עִבּוּד is not attested in this sense in the current dictionaries. The verb עבד features in the *Pi'el* conj. as עיבד האצטומכה 'to strengthen the stomach' (for Arab. دبغ المعدة; cf. D 1:423) in BCD 196 (NM 2:16) in an attestation from Shem Tov ben Isaac's *Sefer Almansur* (cf. BMZ 30f. (He 1)). Anonymous I renders Arab. دبغ as עִבּוּד, just like Zeraḥyah, and Nathan ha-Me'ati translates the Arab. term as שרה.

עָגוֹל • *Plur.* **עגולים** • **כנים עגולים** → **כִּנָּה.**

עִגּוּל · **tent; roll; pledget [inserted into a wound or sore]**: Lat. *tuellum* (cf. ND 1123) · Guy de Chauliac, *Inventarium sive Chirurgia Magna* (cf. CMM 1:235, ll. 9–11) · trans. Anonymous (Ms Paris, BnF, héb. 1189, fol. 128ᵇ): אמנם אם החולה יירא חום הברזל אז צוה רוגייר לעשות עגול או פתילה שרויה במרק[257] (But if the patient is afraid of the heat of the [cautery] iron, Roger[258] orders to apply a tent or pledget steeped in a ruptory[259]). As a medical term, Hebr. עִגּוּל features in the sense of 'eye salve (collyrium)' in BCD 196 (NM 1:63) in attestations from Moses Ibn Tibbon's trans. of Ibn al-Jazzār's *Zād al-musāfir* (i.e., *Sefer Ṣedat ha-Derakhim*) II.1.9 (cf. IJZ 1–2:487) and VII.15.3 (cf. IJZ 7:149, l. 22). Synonyms for עִגּוּל in the sense of 'tent; roll; pledget' used by Anonymous are פִּתּוּל and פְּתִילָה (see entries).

עֵדֶן • **גן עדן** → **גַּן.**

[עדף] • *Part.* **עוֹדֵף** · **superfluous**: Arab. فضلي · Ibn Sīnā, *K. al-Qānūn* II · trans. Zeraḥyah Ḥen, *Sefer ha-Qanun* (Ms Oxford, Bodleian Libaries, Opp. Add. Fol. 12, fol. 244ᵇ): נַעְנַע

---

257 במרק: *in ruptorio* L.

258 'Roger': I.e., Rogerius Frugardi, author of the *Chirurgia* composed in the second half of the twelfth century. It was later greatly expanded by Roland of Parma (completed in 1230). Guy de Chauliac's quotations are sometimes derived from this expanded verison, which was in effect a new book; cf. CMM 2:13f.

259 'ruptory' (i.e., a medicine burning and destroying bodily tissue; cf. ND 941): Trans. acc. to L.

מֵינְטָא הטבע חמה ויבשה בשנייה ויש בה לחות עודפת ([Arab.] *naʿnaʿ*; [i.e., Lat.] MeYNəṬaʾ [i.e., *mentha*]: Mint, esp. spearmint [*Mentha spicata* L.]: Its nature: It is hot and dry in the second [degree]. It has superfluous moisture). Hebr. *Part.* עוֹדֵף is not attested in the sense of 'superflous' in medical literature in the current dictionaries. Nathan ha-Meʾati translates Arab. فضلي as יתרוני (cf. NM 6:95) and Anonymous I renders the Arab. term as מוֹתָרִי (see entry).

עֲדָשָׁה[260] • *Plur.* **עדשים** · **freckles**: Arab. عدشيات (cf. D 2:101f.) · Ibn Sīnā, *K. al-Qānūn* II · trans. Zeraḥyah Ḥen, *Sefer ha-Qanun* (Ms Oxford, Bodleian Libaries, Opp. Add. Fol. 12, fol. 267ᵃ): קִנָה גַלְבָנוּ ... יסיר העדשים מן הפנים ([Arab.] *qinna*; [i.e., Rom.] GaLəBaNWu [i.e., Ital.-Rom. *galbano*, from Lat. *galbanum*]: Galbanum [i.e., gum resin from *Ferula gummosa* Boiss.]: ... It removes freckles from the face). In the sense of 'freckles,' Hebr. עדשים is a semantic borrowing from Arab. عدشيات, which features in BM 4350 in an attestation from Karaite literature; for the synonymous עדשי הפנים, cf. BCD 197 (NM 4:142) for an attestation from Moses Ibn Tibbon's trans. of Ibn al-Jazzār's *Zād al-musāfir* (i.e., *Sefer Ṣedat ha-Derakhim*) N.4 (cf. IJZ 1–2:440, n. 20). Nathan ha-Meʾati and Anonymous I both render Arab. عدشيات as עדשים as well.

עוֹדֵף (*Part.*) → [עדף].

עֲוֵור → עִוֵּר.

עוֹלֶה (*Part.*) → עָלָה.

עוֹצֵר (*Part.*) → עָצַר.

עוֹצֶר → עֹצֶר.

עוֹקֶץ → עֹקֶץ.

[עור] • *Polel* **עוֹרֵר** • **עורר השתן** · **to stimulate micturiction (to be diuretic)**: Arab. أدرّ البول · Ibn Sīnā, *K. al-Qānūn* II · trans. Anonymous II, *Sefer ha-Qanun* (Ms Parma, Biblioteca Palatina, Cod. Parm. 3045, fol. 27ᵃ): יינציאנה ... מעורר השתן ועת הנשים ([Lat./Rom.] YYNṢYʾNH: Gentian [*Gentiana lutea* L.]: ... It stimulates micturiction (it is diuretic) and menstruation). Hebr. עורר השתן is not attested in the current dictionaries. Nathan ha-Meʾati translates Arab. أدرّ البول as שלשל השתן (cf. NM 6:212 for his trans. of Arab. إدرار البول as שלשול השתן 'diuresis'), Zeraḥyah Ḥen translates the Arab. term as הרבה השתן (cf. NM 6:196 for his trans. of Arab. إدرار البول as הרבות השתן), and Anonymous I has הגיר השתן (cf. NM 6:212, s.v. שִׁלְשׁוּל, for his trans. of Arab. إدرار البول as הגרת השתן, which is also attested in Moses ibn Tibbon's trans. of Maimonides' *Commentary on Hippocrates' Aphorisms* (i.e., *Perush Aphorismi shel Apuqraṭ*) I.2 (cf. BCD 62 (NM 3:56); BMCH 1:326, l. 6)).

• **עורר עת הנשים** · **to stimulate menstruation**: Arab. أدرّ الطمث · Ibn Sīnā, *K. al-Qānūn* II · trans. Anonymous II, *Sefer ha-Qanun* (Ms Parma, Biblioteca Palatina, Cod. Parm. 3045, fol. 27ᵃ): יינציאנה ... מעורר השתן ועת הנשים ([Lat./Rom.] YYNṢYʾNH: Gentian

260 עֲדָשָׁה: EM 1298; acc. to Ben Yehuda (BM 4349f.), *Sing.* is עדש.

[*Gentiana lutea* L.]: … It stimulates micturiction and menstruation). Hebr. עורר עת הנשים is not attested in the current dictionaries. Nathan ha-Me'ati translates Arab. أدرّ الطمث as שלשל דם הוסת (cf. NM 6:213), Zeraḥyah Ḥen translates the Arab. term as הביא הוסת (see entry [בוא]), and Anonymous I has הגיר הנדות (cf. NM 6:213, s.v. שלשל דם הוסת, for Nathan's use of הגיר הנדות in his trans. of Maimonides' *Medical Aphorisms* (i.e., *Sefer ha-Peraqim*) XII.10; XVI.2; XXI.66 (cf. BMMN 140, l. 1; 165, l. 17; 204, ll. 12–14; BMMG no. 1681).

עוֹר • **הפשט העור** → **הֶפְשֵׁט.**

• **הכתמים שבעור** → **כֶּתֶם.**

• **הלחויות הנחבאות תחת העור** → **לַחוּת.**

• **הלחויות הנעצרות תחת העור** → **לַחוּת.**

• **הרוטבות הנעצרות תחת העור** → **רֵטְבָּה.**

עִוֵּר • **תרנגול עוור** → **תַּרְנְגוֹל.**

עוֹרֵב • **רגל עורב** → **רֶגֶל.**

עוֹרֶף → **עֹרֶף.**

עֵזֶר · **treatment; approach; technique:** Lat. *auxilium* · Guy de Chauliac, *Inventarium sive Chirurgia Magna* (cf. CMM 1:231, ll. 29–32) · trans. Anonymous (Ms Paris, BnF, héb. 1189, fol. 126[a]): והעזר הב' שיושם דרך הנקב קילור עשוי מטוטיא וסרקקקולא אילואין דם תנין בלושטיאש אנטימוני אלום חלקים שוים ומפרח נחשת רביע חלק (The second treatment is to put through the opening in the fistula a collyrium made from equal parts of tutty, sarcocol, aloes, dragon's blood [i.e., the resin of *Dracaena cinnabari* Balf. f.], rose or blossom of the wild pomegranate, antimony, alum, and one fourth of a part of copper oxide). Hebr. עֵזֶר features (for Lat. *cura*) in the sense of 'healing; treatment; cure' in NM 5:147 in an attestation from Do'eg ha-Edomi's trans. of Constantinus Africanus' *Viaticum* (i.e., *Sefer Ya'ir Netiv*) I.16.3 (cf. IJZ 1–21:617)).

עִטְרָן (*Aram.*) · **tar:** Arab. قطران · Ibn Sīnā, *K. al-Qānūn* II · trans. Zeraḥyah Ḥen, *Sefer ha-Qanun* (Ms Oxford, Bodleian Libaries, Opp. Add. Fol. 12, fol. 221[a–b]): יַתּוּע ... יטיף מחלבו על השן המתאכלת ויפוצצה ויפילה ואיפשר שיושם עם עיטראן למען יהיה יותר משבר כחו והיותר טוב הוא שיכסה המקום הבריא עם השעוה ואחרי כן יטיף בו אחר מכן החלב ([Arab.] *yattūʿ*: Spurge [*Euphorbia* sp.]: … When its milky juice (latex) is dripped on decaying teeth, it breaks them into pieces and makes them fall off. It can be applied with tar to make its breaking power stronger. The best way [to do so] is [first] to cover the healthy [teeth] with wax and then to drip the milky juice (latex) on it [i.e., the decaying teeth]). Aram. עִטְרָן is attested in the sense of 'a sort of resin' in Rabb. and modern literature only (cf. JD 1065; EM 1314). Nathan ha-Me'ati renders Arab. قطران as עטראן as well and Anonymous I transcribes the Arab. term as קטראן.

עִיטֶרָאן → **עִטְרָן.**

עַיִן • **בבת העין** → **בָּבָה.**

• **בליטת העין** → **בְּלִיטָה.**

• **בת העין** → **בַּת.**

• דְּפִיקָה → דפיקת העין.
• הַטְמָנָה → הטמנת הדם תחת העין.
• הַסְתָּרָה → הסתרת העין
• זָנָב → זנב העין.
• זָנָב → זנב העין הגדול.
• חֲבָטָה → חבטת העין.
• חֲשֵׁכָה → חשכת העין.
• יְצִיאָה → יציאת העין.
• כֵּהוּת → כהות העין.
• כְּמִינָה → כמינת הדם תחת העין.
• כִּסּוּי → הכסוי על העין.
• לֹבֶן → לובן שבעין.
• שַׁחֲרוּת → שחרות העין.
• שֵׂעָר → שער בעין.

עִיצּוּר → עִצּוּר.

עַכָּבִישׁ • אֲרִיגָה → אריגת העכביש.
• קוּר → קורי העכביש.

עָכוּר • [שׁוּב] → השיב עכור.

[עכל] • *Part. Pi'el* מְעַכֵּל • סַם → הסם המעכל.
• רְפוּאָה → הרפואה המעכלת.

עָלָה • *Part.* עוֹלֶה · **sublimate**: Arab. مصعد · Ibn Sīnā, *K. al-Qānūn* II · trans. Nathan ha-Me'ati, *Sefer ha-Qanun* (Ms Oxford, Bodleian Libraries, Can. Or. 88, fol. 81^{a-b}: ... זיבק העולה ממנו הוא קובץ ([Arab.] *zi'baq*: Quicksilver (mercury): ... Its sublimate is astringent). In the sense of 'sublimate,' Hebr. *Part.* עוֹלֶה is a non-attested calque from Arab. مصعد. Zeraḥyah Ḥen translates Arab. مصعد as מעלה (see entry).
• *Part. Pu'al* מְעֻלֶּה • אֵבֶר → האברים המעולים.

עִלּוּעַ • עלוע הגרון · **rattling sound in the throat**: Arab. حشرجة · Ibn Sīnā, *K. al-Qānūn* II · trans. Nathan ha-Me'ati, *Sefer ha-Qanun* (Ms Oxford, Bodleian Libraries, Can. Or. 88, fol. 112^{a-b}): ענצל ... החומץ העשוי ממנו יכשין[261] הגרון ויקשה בשרו והוא טוב לצרות הנשימה ולעלוע הגרון ובערבי חשרגה והשעול הישן ([Arab.] *'unṣul*: Sea squill [*Drimia maritima* (L.) Stearn]: ... The vinegar prepared from sea squill makes the flesh of the throat rough and hard. It is good for asthma, for a rattling sound in the throat, [called] in Arab. *ḥashrajah*, and for chronic cough). Hebr. עִלּוּעַ features as a modern term in EM 1328 in the sense of 'swallowing' (בְּלִיעָה). Zeraḥyah Ḥen translates Arab. حشرجة as גַּסּוּת (see entry) and Anonymous I renders the Arab. term as גְּנִיחָה (see entry).

---

261 יכשין (= يخشن a): Emend. ed. יכשיר Ms.

עָמֵל • *Part.* **עָמֵל** • *Plur.* **עמלים** · **wrestlers**: Arab. مصارع, *Plur.* مصارعون · Ibn Sīnā, *K. al-Qānūn* II · trans. Nathan ha-Me'ati, *Sefer ha-Qanun* (Ms Oxford, Bodleian Libraries, Can. Or. 88, fol. 80[b]): וסך ... טינופת העמלים שני מינים ([Arab.] *wasakh*: Dirt: ... Dirt [on the bodies] of wrestlers is of two kinds). In the sense of 'wrestler,' Hebr. עָמֵל is not attested in the current dictionaries (cf. BM 4563f.). In his trans. of Maimonides' *Medical Aphorisms* (i.e., *Sefer ha-Peraqim*) XVIII.9, Nathan translates Arab. مصارعون as עמלים as well (cf. BMMN 177, l. 23; BMMG no. 2878). Zeraḥyah Ḥen and Anonymous I both translate Arab. مصارعون as מתאבקים (see entry [אבק]). Synonymous terms, featuring in the anonymous trans. of Maimonides' *Commentary on Hippocrates' Aphorisms* (i.e., *Perush Aphorismi shel Apuqraṭ*) I.3, 15, are טרחנים and טרחניים (cf. BCD 114 (NM 3:101f.); BMCH 1:521, l. 5; 524, l. 14).

עֵנָב • *Plur.* **ענבים** • **ענבי השדים** · **[lit. 'grapes of the demons']; St John's wort [*Hypericum* sp., esp. *H. perforatum* L. or *H. barbatum Jacq.*]**: Arab. عنب الجنة [lit. 'grapes of the female daemon', it seems to be misspelling of عنب الحية lit. 'grapes of the serpent'] · Ibn Sīnā, *K. al-Qānūn* II · trans. Zeraḥyah Ḥen, *Sefer ha-Qanun* (Ms Oxford, Bodleian Libaries, Opp. Add. Fol. 12, fol. 201[b]): הַיוּפַארִיקוּן והערבים קורין אותו אלגַרב ונקרא במזרח ענבי השֵדים ([Arab.] *hayūfārīqūn* [from Gr. ὑπερικόν]: St. Johns wort [*Hypericum* sp., esp. *H. perforatum* L. or *H. barbatum* Jacq.]: The Arabs call it 'LGaRəB [i.e., *['*ushbat*] *al-qalb*, lit. 'heart herb'][262] and in the East it is called *'invei ha-shedim* [lit. 'grapes of the demons']). Hebr. ענבי השדים is not attested in the current dictionaries. The name is connected to the belief that it chases away demons; cf. LF 1:657. Nathan ha-Me'ati transcribes Arab. عنب الجنة as ענב אלגן (*'inab al-jinn*, 'grape of the jinn').

עָנָף · **branch [of a vein]**: Arab. شعبة (cf. FA no. 2990) · al-Rāzī, *K. fī al-Faṣd* · trans. Anonymous, *Ma'amar ba-Haqqazah* (Ms Parma, Biblioteca Palatina, Cod. Parm. 2283,4, fol. 93[b]): והג' הוא אלאכחל והוא ענף מהבסליק וענף מהקיפאל יתחברו במקום אחד (The third [vein] is the median cubital vein, it is a branch of the basilic vein and a branch of the cephalic vein, which come together in one place). In the sense of 'branch' as an anat. term, Hebr. עָנָף features in BCD 280 (NM 4:209) in an attestation from Zeraḥyah Ḥen's *Sefer ha-Qanun*.

[עשה] • *Part. Pi'el* **מְעַשֶּׂה** • **הסם המעשה** → **סַם**.

עָסִיס · **syrup**: Arab. ميبختج (*maybakhtaj*, cf. MIG no. 227; it is the Arabized form of Pers. *may-pukhtah* 'wine boiled down to a consistency; syrup of dates and grapes' (cf. SCP 1359); acc. to Maimonides' description, it is syrup made of must (cf. MSh no. 84)) · Ibn Sīnā, *K. al-Qānūn* II · trans. Nathan ha-Me'ati, *Sefer ha-Qanun* (Ms Oxford, Bodleian Libraries, Can. Or. 88, fol. 87[a]): חב אלצנובר ... הקטן והגדול מהם יועילו לרוטבות הריאה המעופשות והמוגלא ויציאת הדם והשעול וקל וחומר עם העסיס הנק' מיבכתג בער' החדש וזה במרירות מעט שבהם ([Arab.] *ḥabb al-ṣanawbar*: Pine nut [*Pinus* L.]:

262 *'Ushbat al-qalb* is a well-known synonym of *hayūfārīqūn* (cf. MSh no. 115).

... The small and large varieties are beneficial for putrified humors and pus [in the lungs], for hemorrhage and cough. This is especially the case when used with fresh syrup, called *maybakhtaj* in Arab., having some bitterness). Hebr. עָסִיס features in the current dictionaries in the sense of 'pressed out juice' and 'must; young wine' (cf. BM 4607f.). In Shem Tov ben Isaac's *Sefer ha-Shimmush* XXVII, it has the additional meaning of 'rob (i.e., fruit juice boiled down to syrup)' (for Arab. رُبّ; cf. NM 4:149 (BCD 205)). Zeraḥyah Ḥen renders Arab. ميبختج as מיבכתג and Anonymous I has יין מבושל. The latter term already features in Moses ibn Tibbon's trans. of Ibn al-Jazzār's *Zād al-musāfir* (i.e., *Sefer Sedat ha-Derakhim*) III.1 (cf. NM 5:93) and in a synonym list in Ms Vatican, Biblioteca Apostolica, ebr. 550 (cf. NM 6:88). Another synonymous term is עסיס מבושל (see entry below).

• **עסיס אחו** · **acacia gum (Senegal gum) [*Acacia nilotica* (L.) Delile]**: Arab. أقاقيا (cf. IG 51) · *Glossary* (Ms Moscow, Russian State Library, Guenzburg 573, fol. 148ᵃ): אקקיא הוא עסיס אחו לטי' אקאסיא ([Arab.] *aqāqiyā*; i.e., [Hebr.] *ʿasis aḥu* [i.e., acacia gum (Senegal gum)]; Lat. ʾQʾSYʾ [i.e., *acacia*]). For the identification of Arab. أقاقيا (*aqāqiyā*) as Hebr. עסיס אחו (*asis aḥu*), the latter term featuring in the Bible (Gen 41:2) in the sense of 'sedge; marsh plant' (cf. KB 30f.), cf. SHS 1:106 (Alef 19): ... אחו ומן העשב שלו עושין בארץ מצרים האקקיא וב"ל אקאסיא (ʾ*HW* ... from its plant acacia is prepared in the land of Egypt; o.l. ʾ*Q*ʾ*SY*ʾ).

• **עסיס מבושל** · **I. rob [i.e., fruit or vegetable juice boiled down to syrup]**: Arab. رُبّ · Ibn Sīnā, *K. al-Qānūn* II · trans. Nathan ha-Me'ati, *Sefer ha-Qanun* (Ms Oxford, Bodleian Libraries, Can. Or. 88, fols. 93ᵛ–94ʳ: כמתארי ... ולכן יאות לשתות אחריו מי הדבש עם תבלים ועסיסו מבושל ובער' רב יועיל אל השלשול אשר ממרה אדומה ([Arab.] *kummathrā*: Pear [*Pyrus communis* L.]: ... Therefore, after its [consumption] one should drink honey water with aromatics. Its rob, [called] in Arab. *rubb*, is useful for treating bilious diarrhea). Hebr. עסיס מבושל is not attested in the current dictionaries. Zeraḥyah Ḥen translates Arab. رُبّ as *Part. Puʿal* מְרוּבָּב (see entry [רבב]) and Anonymous I renders it as מיץ קרוש (see entry מִיץ). Other synonyms are בשול יין (cf. NM 5:33); עָסִיס (see entry above); רֹב (cf. NM 5:182); and שפא (from Lat. *sapa*, cf. NM 5:198).

· **II. syrup**: Arab. ميبختج (*maybakhtaj*, cf. MIG no. 227; it is the Arabized form of Pers. *may-pukhtah* 'wine boiled down to a consistency; syrup of dates and grapes' (cf. SCP 1359); acc. to Maimonides' description, it is syrup made of must (cf. MSh no. 84)) · *Glossary* (Ms Moscow, Russian State Library, Guenzburg 573, fol. 155ᵛ: מיבכתג'[263] הוא העסיס המבושל ([Arab.] *maybakhtaj*; i.e., [Hebr.] *he-ʿasis ha-mevusshal*). See also entry עָסִיס.

עִפּוּשׁ · **[lit. 'putrefaction']; change; alteration; reaction**: Arab. تكريج (cf. WKAS 1:120, s.v. كرج II: 'to be or become mouldy') · Ibn Sīnā, *K. al-Qānūn* II · trans. Nathan ha-Me'ati,

263 מיבכתג': Emend. ed. מיבכנג' Ms.

Sefer ha-Qanun (Ms Oxford, Bodleian Libraries, Can. Or. 88, fol. 82ᵇ): זנגאר: מיני עשיית הזנגאר הוא בעפוש הנחשת בשמרי החומץ ([Arab.] *zinjār*: Verdigris: One of the ways to produce verdigris is by the change [effected by the contact] between copper and dregs of vinegar). Hebr. עִפּוּשׁ features in both Nathan's and Zeraḥyah Ḥen's trans. of Maimonides' *Medical Aphorisms* XXIII.109 (i.e., *Sefer ha-Peraqim*) in the sense of 'alteration [of one substance into another]' (cf. BMMN 233, l. 1; BMMZ 232, l. 19; BM 4614). The aphorism is a quotation from Galen's *In Timaeum commentarius* II: 'Ancient [physicians] call the alteration (Arab. تغيّر) of a substance to another type of a different variety 'putrefaction' (Arab. عفونة)' (cf. BMMA 5:71). Anonymous I renders Arab. تكريج as עִפּוּשׁ as well.

• **קיבל העפוש** → [קבל].

• **קיבל העפוש הנקרא *רנציד** → [קבל].

[עפץ] • *Part. Pi'el* **מְעַפֵּץ** · **astringent**: Arab. قابض · Ibn Sīnā, *K. al-Qānūn* II · trans. Anonymous II, *Sefer ha-Qanun* (Ms Parma, Biblioteca Palatina, Cod. Parm. 3045, fol. 38ᵃ): פרח נחושת ... מעפץ ואוכל הבשר ונושך תועלתו למור׳ ולחבורות אוכל בשר מת ([Hebr.] *peraḥ neḥoshet* [lit. 'flower of copper']: Copper oxide: ... It is astringent, corrosive, and irritant. Its usefulness for wounds and ulcers: It erodes out excessive flesh). In the sense of 'astringent,' Hebr. עפץ is attested in the *Hif'il* conj. as *Part. Hif'il* מַעֲפִּיץ in NM 6:162 in an attestation from Abraham ben Isaac's trans. of Ibn al-Jazzār's *Zād al-musāfir* (i.e., *Sefer Ṣedah la-Oreḥim*) VI.10. Nathan ha-Me'ati and Anonymous II both translate Arab. قابض as קובץ.

עָפָר • **זוחלי עפר** → זָחַל.

[עפש] • *Part. Pi'el* **מְעַפֵּשׁ** • **הסם המעפש** → סַם.

• **הרפואה המעפשת** → רְפוּאָה.

עָצָב • *Plur.* **עצבים** • **צירי העצבים** → צִיר.

עִצּוּר · **constipation**: Arab. عقل · Ibn Sīnā, *K. al-Qānūn* II · trans. Zeraḥyah Ḥen, *Sefer ha-Qanun* (Ms Oxford, Bodleian Libaries, Opp. Add. Fol. 12, fols. 179ᵇ–180ᵃ: ... אורז וכשיבושל עם החלב ושמן שקדים יזון מאד ויותר מזון טוב ויחסר ממנו יבשו ועיצורו וכל שכן כשישרנו לילה אחת במי הסובין (Rice: ... When cooked with milk and almond oil, it gives more and better nutrition. Its properties of causing constipation and dryness are lost when it is soaked in bran water and left over night). In the sense of 'constipation,' Hebr. עִצּוּר features (for Lat. *constipatio*) in BCD 207 (NM 2:179) in an attestation from an anonymous translation of *On the Treatment of Small Children* XIII, attr. to al-Rāzī. In addition to עִצּוּר, Zeraḥyah translates Arab. عقل as עֲצִירָה (see entry) and Nathan ha-Me'ati translates Arab. عقل as עצירות (cf. NM 6:164).

• **עיצור הנשימה** · **dyspnea**: Arab. عسر النفس · Ibn Sīnā, *K. al-Qānūn* II · trans. Zeraḥyah Ḥen, *Sefer ha-Qanun* (Ms Oxford, Bodleian Libaries, Opp. Add. Fol. 12, fol. 247ᵃ⁻ᵇ): סַרוּ שִׁיפְּרֵיש ... ישתו אגוזו עם היין לרקיקת הדם ולעיצור הנשימה והצבתה ולשעול הישן וכן בישולו ([Arab.] *sarw*; [Rom.] ŠiYPəReYŠ: Mediterranean cypress [*Cupressus sempervirens* L.]: ... Its nuts are taken orally with wine in cases of hemoptysis, dyspnea, orthopnea, and chronic cough. The decoction of cypress possesses similar properties). Hebr. עיצור הנשימה does not feature in the current dictionaries. Nathan ha-Me'ati translates Arab. عسر النفس as עוצר הנשימה (see entry עֹצֶר) and Anonymous I has כובד הנשימה (see NM 6:97).

עֲצִירָה · **constipation**: Arab. عقل · Ibn Sīnā, *K. al-Qānūn* II · trans. Zeraḥyah Ḥen, *Sefer ha-Qanun* (Ms Oxford. Opp. Add. Fol. 12, fol. 176[b]): אִגָ'אץ פְּרוּנְגֵי ... הגומא שלהן חותכות ומדבקות והפרונגי מדמשק יש בו עצירה וקיבוץ לפי דיאסקורידוש וזולתי ג'לינוס ([Arab.] *ijjāṣ*; [i.e., Rom.] PəRWNəGeY: Plum tree [*Prunus domestica* L.]: Its gum is diluting and agglutinant. According to Dioscorides, the Damascus variety is constipating and astringent, but according to Galen it is not so). In the sense of 'constipation,' Hebr. עֲצִירָה features (for Lat. *constipatio*) in BCD 207 (NM 2:72) in a later attestation from Bonfos' trans. of *On the Treatment of Small Children* XII, attr. to al-Rāzī. Nathan ha-Me'ati translates Arab. عقل as עוצר and Anonymous I renders the Arab. term as עֲצִירָה, just like Zeraḥyah.

• **עצירת דם הוסת** · **amenorrhea**: Arab. احتباس الحيض · al-Rāzī, *K. fī al-Faṣd* · trans. Anonymous, *Ma'amar ba-Haqqazah* (Ms Parma, Biblioteca Palatina, Cod. Parm. 2283,4, fol. 96[b]): הקזת אלמבאץ' ואלצפאן מועילים מעצירת דם הוסת קודם עתו בשני ימים (Bleeding from the popliteal fossa and the saphenous vein is beneficial for amenorrhea two days before its time). Hebr. עצירת דם הוסת is not attested in the current dictionaries. For a variant reading עצירת הוסת, see next entry. In his trans. of Maimonides' *Medical Aphorisms* XVI.3–4, Nathan ha-Me'ati renders the Arab. parallel term احتباس دم الطمث as העצר (דם) הנדות (cf. BMMN 165, l. 21; 166, l. 3; BMMG no. 784) and Zeraḥyah Ḥen has כשהוסת נעצר (cf. BMMZ 164, ll. 4, 8; BMMG no. 784).

• **עצירת הוסת** · **amenorrhea**: Arab. احتباس الحيض · al-Rāzī, *K. fī al-Faṣd* · trans. Anonymous, *Ma'amar ba-Haqqazah* (Ms Parma, Biblioteca Palatina, Cod. Parm. 2283,4, fol. 96[a]): אלבסליק יועיל ממורסת הצלעות ... וממורסת הרחם המתחדשת מסבת עצירת הוסת ([Bleeding] the basilic vein is beneficial for pleurisy ... and for the swelling of the uterus that occurs due to amenorrhea). Hebr. עצירת הוסת is not attested in the current dictionaries. For a variant reading עצירת דם הוסת, see previous entry. In his trans. of Maimonides' *Medical Aphorisms* XVI.3–4, Nathan ha-Me'ati renders the Arab. parallel term احتباس دم الطمث as העצר (דם) הנדות (cf. BMMN 165, l. 21; 166, l. 3; BMMG no. 784) and Zeraḥyah Ḥen has כשהוסת נעצר (cf. BMMZ 164, ll. 4, 8; BMMG no. 784).

• **עצירת השתן** · **dysuria**: Arab. حبس البول · Ibn Sīnā, *K. al-Qānūn* II · trans. Anonymous I, *Sefer ha-Qanun* (Ms Paris, BnF, héb. 1142, fols. 248[a]–250[a]): תאנה ... מועיל לכליות ולמקוה הלחים והיבשים ויושמו[264] על עצירת השתן ואינם נאותים לשפיכת הליחות אל המעים וסחיטת העלים פותחת פיות העורקים מהטבעת (Figs: ... Both the fresh and dry figs are useful for kidneys and urinary bladder. They are applied for dysuria, but they are not

264 ויושמו: Ms[1] ומזיקים Ms.

suitable when there is [excessive] flow of matter towards the intestines. The extract of its leaves opens the anal vessels). Hebr. עצירת השתן features in BM 4642 in later attestations, a.o., from Me'ir Aldabi's *Shevilei Emunah*. Nathan ha-Me'ati translates Arab. حبس البول as עוצר השתן (see entry עָצַר).

עֲצִירוּת • עצירות הדם · **cessation of bleeding (hemostasis)**: Arab. حبس الدم · Ibn Sīnā, *K. al-Qānūn* II · trans. Nathan ha-Me'ati, *Sefer ha-Qanun* (Ms Oxford, Bodleian Libraries, Can. Or. 88, fol. 107[b]): סנדרוס יש בו קבוץ וסגלתו עצירות הדם ([Arab.] *sandarūs*: Sandarac [i.e., resin from the sandarac gum tree [*Tetraclinis articulate* (Vahl) Mast.]]: It is astringent and has the specific property to stop bleeding). Hebr. עֲצִירוּת on its own features in BM 4643 in the sense of 'obstruction; constipation' only. Zeraḥyah Ḥen translates Arab. حبس الدم as לעצור הדם and Anonymous I has עצירת הדם.

עֶצֶם • עצם הפיל · **ivory**: Arab. عاج · Ibn Sīnā, *K. al-Qānūn* II · trans. Nathan ha-Me'ati, *Sefer ha-Qanun* (Ms Oxford, Bodleian Libraries, Can. Or. 88, fols. 89[b]–90[a]): ... יברוח ואמרו כי שרשו כשמבשלים ממנו עצם הפיל ובערבי אלעאג שש שעות ירכך אותו ויתיר[265] אסרו ([Arab.] *yabrūḥ*: Mandrake [*Mandragora officinarum* L.]: ... It is said that ivory, in Arab. *al-ʿāj*, if it is decocted with the root of mandrake for six hours, will become soft and manageable). Hebr. עצם הפיל is not attested in the current dictionaries. Zeraḥyah Ḥen translates Arab. عاج as השן הנקרא אוֹרִיפַּנְט and Anonymous I has שן הפיל (see entry שֵׁן).

• *Plur.* **עצמות • פרקי העצמות** → **פֶּרֶק**.

עָצַר • *Part.* **עוֹצֵר • עוצר הטבע** · **constipating**: Arab. عاقل · Ibn Sīnā, *K. al-Qānūn* II · trans. Nathan ha-Me'ati, *Sefer ha-Qanun* (Ms Oxford, Bodleian Libraries, Can. Or. 88, fol. 83[r]: זערור ... הוא עוצר הטבע ועוצר[266] השתן ([Arab.] *zuʿrūr*: Medlar [*Mespilus germanica* L.] or azarole [*Crataegus azarolus* L.] (cf. MIG no. 58): ... It is constipating and retains[267] the urine). Hebr. עצר הטבע, *Part.* עוצר הטבע, is not attested in the current dictionaries. The synonymous terms עצר את הבטן and עצר את המעיים feature in BM 4660f. The term טֶבַע features in the sense of 'defecation' in BM 1843f. in attestations from the *Sefer ha-Qanun*. Zeraḥyah Ḥen and Anonymous I both render Arab. عاقل as עוצר.

• **הסם העוצר** → **סַם**.

• *Part. Nifʿal* **נֶעֱצָר • הלחויות הנעצרות תחת העור** → **לַחוּת**.

• **הרוטבות הנעצרות תחת העור** → **רֵטְבָּה**.

עֹצֶר • עוצר ההריון · **infertility**: Arab. عسر الحبل · Ibn Sīnā, *K. al-Qānūn* II · trans. Zeraḥyah Ḥen, *Sefer ha-Qanun* (Ms Oxford, Bodleian Libaries, Opp. Add. Fol. 12, fols. 195[a–b]): גַ'זָר קרוֹטֵי ... ויועילו זרעו ושרשו לעוצר ההריון ([Arab.] *jazar*; i.e., [Lat./Rom.] QaRWoṬeY [i.e., Lat. Plur. *carotae* / Ital. Plur. *carote*]: Carrot [*Daucus carota* L.]: ... Its seed and

265 ויתיר אסרו: وسلس قياده a.
266 ועוצר: ولا يحبس a.
267 'retains': 'does not retain' a.

roots are beneficial for [women suffering from] infertility). Hebr. עוצר ההריון is not attested in the current dictionaries. Nathan ha-Me'ati and Anonymous I both translate Arab. عسر الحبل as קושי ההריון and Anonymous II renders the Arab. term as חולשת קבול ההריון (see entry חֲלִשָׁה).

• **עוצר הנשימה** · **asthma (dyspnea; panting)**: a) Arab. ربو (UWS 1:180, s.v. ἄσθμα: 'Atemnot, Keuchen') · Ibn Sīnā, *K. al-Qānūn* II · trans. Nathan ha-Me'ati, *Sefer ha-Qanun* (Ms Oxford, Bodleian Libraries, Can. Or. 88, fol. 65^{a-b}: אנגרה ... כשמשקים אותו עם השעורים ינקה החזה וכשמבשלים עליו במי השעור יוציא מה שיש בחזה מתערובים הגסים וזרעו יותר חזק ויסיר עוצר[268] הנשימה ויניח הנשימה הנצבת ומחולי[269] הקר אשר מחולי הצלעות ([Arab.] *anjura*: Roman nettle [*Urtica pilulifera* L.]: ... When one takes it with barley water, it cleanses the chest, and when one takes its leaves boiled with barley water, it expels the thick humors in the chest. The seeds are more potent and cure asthma (dyspnea; panting), orthopnea, and cold[270] pleurisy). Hebr. עוצר הנשימה does not feature in the current dictionaries. In addition, Nathan translates Arab. ربو as קצר הנשימה (see entry קֹצֶר). Zeraḥyah Ḥen translates Arab. ربو as Rom. אזְמו[271] and Anonymous I has גניחה. The latter term also features (for Arab. ربو) in Nathan's trans. of Maimonides' *Medical Aphorisms* VIII.19 (cf. BCD 47 (NM 2:34f.); BMMN 94, l. 18; BMMG no. 2043). Other synonyms featuring in medieval Hebr. medical literature are גוויש (i.e., O. Occ. **gois*; cf. NM 5:36f.); גְּנוּחַ (cf. BCD 47 (NM 1:83)); נזילה על הריאה (cf. BCD 172 (NM 3:151)); עצר הנפוש (cf. BCD 212 (NM 1:178)); צרות הנשימה (cf. NM 6:172); and רנפלי (cf. BCD 262 (NM 2:19)).

· b) Arab. عسر النفس · Ibn Sīnā, *K. al-Qānūn* II · trans. Nathan ha-Me'ati, *Sefer ha-Qanun* (Ms Oxford, Bodleian Libraries, Can. Or. 88, fol. 108^{a}): סרו ... ישקו אגוזיו עם יין לרקיקת הדם ולעוצר הנשימה ואל הנשימה הנצבת והשעול וכן תבשילו ([Arab.] *sarw*: Mediterranean cypress [*Cupressus sempervirens* L.]: ... Its nuts are taken orally with wine in cases of hemoptysis, dyspnea, orthopnea, and [chronic] cough. The decoction of cypress possesses similar properties). Zeraḥyah Ḥen translates Arab. عسر النفس as עיצור הנשימה (see entry עִצּוּר) and Anonymous I has כובד הנשימה (cf. NM 6:97).

• **עוצר השתן** · **dysuria**: Arab. حبس البول · Ibn Sīnā, *K. al-Qānūn* II · trans. Nathan ha-Me'ati, *Sefer ha-Qanun* (Ms Oxford, Bodleian Libraries, Can. Or. 88, fols. 126^{b}–127^{b}): תין והוא תאנים ... יועיל אל הכליות וכיס השתן הרטובים מהם והיבשים ויושמו לעוצר השתן ואינם נאותים להגרת החמרים אל המעים ומיץ עליהם יפתח גידי העגבות ([Arab.] *tīn*; i.e., [Hebr.]

268 עוצר הנשימה ויניח הנשימה הנצבת (= Ms Paris, BnF, héb. 1136, fol. 65^{b}): עוצר הנשימה הנצבת Ms الربو ونفس الانتصاب a.

269 ומחולי הקר אשר מחולי הצלעות: والبارد من ذات الجنب a.

270 'cold pleurisy': Trans. acc. to a.

271 Zeraḥyah also translates Arab. ربو as שִׁעוּל in his *Sefer ha-Qanun* (see entry).

te'enim: Figs [*Ficus carica* L.]: ... Both the fresh and dry figs are useful for kidneys and urinary bladder. They are applied for dysuria, but they are not suitable when there is (excessive) flow of matter towards the intestines. The extract of its leaves opens the anal vessels). Hebr. עוצר השתן also features (for Arab. عسر البول) in BCD 212 (NM 3:181) in an attestation from Moses ibn Tibbon's trans. of Maimonides' *Commentary on Hippocrates'* Aphorisms (i.e., *Perush Aphorismi shel Apuqraṭ*) VI.36 (cf. BMCH 1:400, l. 6). Anonymous I renders Arab. حبس البول as עצירת השתן (see entry עֲצִירָה).

עָקֵב · **malleolus**: Arab. كعب (cf. FA no. 1753) · al-Rāzī, *K. fī al-Faṣd* · trans. Anonymous, *Ma'amar ba-Haqqazah* (Ms Parma, Biblioteca Palatina, Cod. Parm. 2283,4, fol. 94ª): וב׳ גידים הנק׳ וידועים בגיד הנשה ונמצאים בחיצוני העקבים אשר בצד החיצוני (Two veins that are called and known as 'sciatica,' they are found on the outer one of the malleoli, on the outside). Hebr. עָקֵב is not attested in this sense in the current dictionaries.

עִקּוּד · **stiffness**: Arab. تعقّد (Gr. ἀγκύλη; cf. UW 67) · Ibn Sīnā, *K. al-Qānūn* II · trans. Zeraḥyah Ḥen, *Sefer ha-Qanun* (Ms Oxford, Bodleian Libaries, Opp. Add. Fol. 12, fol. 237ª): מֻקְל[272] דֵילִיאוּ יהודי ודֵילִיאוּ מכיי ... יועיל להפסד המושקלו ומן הקווץ וקושי העצבים ועקודם ([Arab.] *muql*;[273] [Rom.-Hebr.] DeYLeY'W *yehudi* and [Rom.-Arab.] DeYLY'W *Makkī*: Judean and Meccan bdellium: ... It is useful in muscle rupture, spasms, hardness and stiffness of the nerves). Hebr. עִקּוּד features in BM 4669, n. 1, with reference to the following quotation from the *Sefer Sod ha-Sodot*: הקשרים הנקראים עקוד ('and the slings (?) which are called *akud*').[274] In his note, Ben Yehuda remarks that the reading עִקּוּד is possibly preferable to עָקוּד. Nathan ha-Me'ati translates Arab. تعقّد as קִשּׁוּר (see entry) and Anonymous I has הִתְקַשְּׁרוּת (see entry). The synonymous Arab. تحجّر, featuring as part of the term تحجّر المفاصل in the *K. al-Qānūn*, is translated by Zeraḥyah as קושי (הפרקים).

• *Plur.* **עקודים** · **1. coagulation**: Arab. تعقّد · Ibn Sīnā, *K. al-Qānūn* II · trans. Zeraḥyah Ḥen, *Sefer ha-Qanun* (Ms Oxford, Bodleian Libaries, Opp. Add. Fol. 12, fol. 239ª): מום שעוה ... יועיל מגסות החזה למשוח בה ויעורב עם שמן הויאולי וימנע החלב מן העקודים בשדי המיניקות ([Pers.] *mūm*; [i.e., Hebr.] *sha'awah*: Wax: ... When it is rubbed [on the chest] it is useful for its roughness, [especially] when it is mixed with violet oil. It prevents coagulation of milk in the breast of the wet nurse). Nathan ha-Me'ati translates Arab. تعقّد as קלפות and Anonymous I has התקרש.

---

272 מֻקְל: Ms[1].

273 '*muql*': I.e., bdellium, i.e., the gum resin of plants from the *Burseraceae* family, esp. *Commiphora africana* (A.Rich.) Endl. and *Commiphora mukul* (Hook. ex Stocks) Engl.

274 Trans. and ed. by M. Gaster, in *Studies and Texts in Folklore, Magic, Mediaeval Romance, Hebrew Apocrypha, and Samaritan Archaeology* (Repr., New York 1971), 2:33 (Engl. trans.); 3:264 (Hebr. text).

· II. **nodules**: Arab. عقدة, *Plur.* عقد · Ibn Sīnā, *K. al-Qānūn* II · trans. Zeraḥyah Ḥen, *Sefer ha-Qanun* (Ms Oxford, Bodleian Libaries, Opp. Add. Fol. 12, fol. 203[b]): וַג׳ אַקוֹרוֹן שרשי עשב כמו הבוֹדָא[275] (*הבורדי) ימצא רובו במקואות המימות ובמימות ועל אלו השרשים עקודים נוטין ללובן ויש בהם ריח רע ([Arab.] *wajj*; [i.e., Arab.] *āqūrun* [from Gr. ἄκορον]: Sweet flag [*Acorus calamus* L.]: [It is] the root of a plant resembling papyrus. It is mostly found growing near water reservoirs and [other] waters. These roots bear white nodules and have a bad smell). Nathan ha-Me'ati and Anonymous I both render Arab. عقد as קשרים (see entry קֶשֶׁר).

עֲקִירָה • עקירת השנים · **tooth extraction**: Arab. قلع الأسنان · Ibn Sīnā, *K. al-Qānūn* II · trans. Nathan ha-Me'ati, *Sefer ha-Qanun* (Ms Oxford, Bodleian Libraries, Can. Or. 88, fol. 85[b]): חנטל ... ואם יבושל בשמן זית ויטיפו ממנו באזן יועיל לכאב[276] האזנים וימהר עקירת השנים ([Arab.] *ḥanẓal*: Colocynth [*Citrullus colocynthis* (L.) Schrad.]: ... If it is cooked in olive oil, which is then dripped into the ear, it is useful for tinnitus[277] and for quickly extracting a tooth). Hebr. עקירת השנים does not feature in attestations from medieval Hebr. medical literature in the current dictionaries. Anonymous I renders Arab. قلع الأسنان as עקירת השנים, just like Nathan, and Zeraḥyah Ḥen translates the Arab. term as העתיק השן חוצה (see entry [עתק]).

עֹקֶץ · **burr**: Arab. قمع · Ibn Sīnā, *K. al-Qānūn* II · trans. Nathan ha-Me'ati, *Sefer ha-Qanun* (Ms Oxford, Bodleian Libraries, Can. Or. 88, fol. 118[ש]): קאקלה ... יש בו עם החמום קיבוץ וקל וחומר אשר לו עוקצים והוא הנק׳ קמאע בערבי ויותר העוקץ עצמו ([Arab.] *qāqulla*: Black cardamom [*Amomum subulatum* Roxb.]: ... It is astringent and warming, especially in the variety having burrs, called QM'ʿ [i.e, **qimʿ* or *Plur.* **aqmāʿ*] in Arab. Even more so the burr itself). Hebr. עֹקֶץ or עוֹקֶץ is attested in Rabb. literature as 'peduncle of fruits; stalk' (cf. JD 1057; BM 4681). Zeraḥyah Ḥen translates Arab. قمع as פִּצֹּלֶת (see entry) and Anonymous I renders the Arab. term as פְּטוֹטֶרֶת (see entry).

עָקַץ · **to cause gripes (colic)**: Arab. أمغص · Ibn Sīnā, *K. al-Qānūn* II · trans. Zeraḥyah Ḥen, *Sefer ha-Qanun* (Ms Oxford, Bodleian Libaries, Opp. Add. Fol. 12, fol. 199[b]): דַּנְד הוא קַטַפּוּץ ... הציני הוא יותר טוב ויותר חזק מן ההודיי והסחרי רע ומאוחר המעשה מסער ועוקץ וראוי שיקלף הסיני עם הברזל ([Arab. *dand*; i.e., [Rom.] QaṬaPuWṢ [i.e., *catapucia*]: Purging croton [*Croton tiglium* L.]: ... Chinese [croton] is better and stronger than the Indian [variety]. [The variety] that grows among rocks is inferior, slow in action, causing pain and gripes (colic). The Chinese [variety] should be peeled off with an iron [knife]). Hebr. עָקַץ is not attested in this sense in the current dictionaries. Nathan ha-Me'ati translates Arab. أمغص as עקץ המעים (see next entry) and Anonymous I has הכאיב הבטן (see entry [כאב]).

---

275 הבוֹדָא (*הבורדי): البردي a.
276 כאב האזנים: الدوي a.
277 'tinnitus': Trans. acc. to a.

• עקץ המעים · **to cause gripes (colic)**: Arab. أمغص · Ibn Sīnā, *K. al-Qānūn* II · trans. Nathan ha-Me'ati, *Sefer ha-Qanun* (Ms Oxford, Bodleian Libraries, Can. Or. 88, fol. 78[b]): דנד ... הצני יותר משובח ויותר חזק מההנדי והנולד בסלעים רע מעוכב במפעלו מוליד התלאה עוקץ המעים (Arab. *dand*: Purging croton [*Croton tiglium* L.]: ... Chinese [croton] is better and stronger than the Indian [variety]. [The variety] that grows among rocks is inferior, slow in action, causing pain and gripes (colic)). Hebr. עקץ המעים is not attested in the current dictionaries. Nathan also uses the compound noun עקיצת המעיים in the sense of 'gripes; colic' in his *Sefer ha-Qanun* (cf. NM 6:168). Zeraḥyah Ḥen simply translates Arab. أمغص as עָקַץ (see previous entry) and Anonymous I has הכאיב הבטן (see entry [כאב]).

עָקָר • המורסות אשר בעקר האזן → מֻרְסָה.

[ערב] • *Hitpa'el* **הִתְעָרֵב** • **התערב בזוהמה** · **to become rancid**: Arab. زنخ · Ibn Sīnā, *K. al-Qānūn* II · trans. Nathan ha-Me'ati, *Sefer ha-Qanun* (Ms Oxford, Bodleian Libraries, Can. Or. 88, fol. 99[a]): לוז ... ושמנינותו פחות משמנינות האגוזים אע״פ שבו שמנינות מרובה מתערב בזוהמה ([Arab.] *lawz* / [Hebr.] *luz*: Almond [*Prunus dulcis* (Mill.) D.A. Webb]: ... Although it contains less oil (fat) than walnut, it is yet rich in oil (fat), which becomes rancid). Hebr. התערב בזוהמה is not attested in the current dictionaries. Anonymous I renders Arab. زنخ as *Hif'il* הריח (see entry [ריח]).

עָרֹב · **vermin; noxious insects**: Arab هوامّ · Ibn Sīnā, *K. al-Qānūn* II · trans. Zeraḥyah Ḥen, *Sefer ha-Qanun* (Ms Oxford, Bodleian Libaries, Opp. Add. Fol. 12, fol. 198[a]): דִּפְלֵי לַנְדְּרוּ ... הוא סם והנה יעורב עם יין ורודא וישתנו וינצל מסם הערוב ([Arab.] *diflā*; [i.e., Rom.] LaNəDəRWu: Oleander [*Nerium oleander* L.]: ... It is a poison, but if it is mixed with wine and common rue and ingested, it saves from (neutralises) the poisonous effects of vermin). Hebr. עָרֹב features in the Bible in the sense of a) vermin in general; pests; noxious insects, or b) a particular type of fly, esp. a horse fly (cf. KB 879). Ben Yehuda also quotes the term in an attestation from Abraham ibn Ezra's poetry. In his trans. of Maimonides' *Medical Aphorisms*, Zeraḥyah translates Arab. هوامّ as חיות in XXI.50 (cf. BMMZ 199, l. 15), as החיות והשרצים in XXII.64 (cf. BMMZ 214, ll. 23–24), and as השרצים והחיות הרעות in XXIV.51 (cf. BMMZ 240, l. 20) (cf. also BMMG no. 4595). Nathan ha-Me'ati translates Arab. هوامّ as שרצים, Anonymous I has רמשים, and Anonymous II has זוחלי עפר (see entry זָחַל).

עָרוֹב → עָרֹב.

עֹרֶף • נקב העורף → נֶקֶב.

• הנקרה בעורף → נִקְרָה.

עַרְפִּלִי · **cloud-like**: Lat. *nebulosus* · Guy de Chauliac, *Inventarium sive Chirurgia Magna* (cf. CMM 1:233, ll. 8–9) · trans. Anonymous (Ms Paris, BnF, héb. 1189, fol. 127[a]): אמנם הפוליפוס הוא קשה ומכאיב וערפלי ומאוס ומוסרח ([This type of] polyp [i.e., that, which comes after catarrhal illnesses] is hard, painful, cloud-like, terrible, and fetid). Hebr. עַרְפִּלִי features as עַרְפַּלִי in the sense of 'misty; foggy' in BM 4744 in an attestation from Joseph Caro. It features as עַרְפִּלִי in EM 1380 in the mentioned attestation from Joseph Caro and other attestations from modern Hebr. literature.

עֹרֶק • *Plur.* **עורקים • עורקי הצבעים** · **[lit. 'roots of the dyers']; greater celandine [*Chelidonium majus* L.]**: Arab. عروق الصباغين (cf. IBF no. 1525) · Ibn Sīnā, *K. al-Qānūn* II · trans. Anonymous I, *Sefer ha-Qanun* (Ms Paris, BnF, héb. 1142, fol. 201[a]): ערוק אלצבאג׳ין כלומר עורקי הצבעים ... סחיטתו מועילה מאד לחדד הראות וממרק מה שהוא לפני האישון ממים ולובן ([Arab.] *ʿurūq al-ṣabbāghīn* [lit. 'roots of the dyers']; i.e., [Hebr.] *ʿorqei ha-ṣabbaʿim*: Greater celandine [*Chelidonium majus* L.] (cf. IBF no. 1525): ... Its juice is very good for sharpening the eyesight and for clearing water covering the pupil of the eye and for leucoma). In the sense of 'greater celandine,' Hebr. עורקי הצבעים is a non-attested calque from Arab. عروق الصباغين. Nathan ha-Me'ati renders the Arab. term as ערוק אלצבאגין and Zeraḥyah Ḥen has a mixed Arab.-Hebr. term ערוק הצבעים.

עָשָׂה • **עשה אישפונגי באף** · **to drip (pour) a medicine into the nose**: Arab. سعط · Ibn Sīnā, *K. al-Qānūn* II · trans. Zeraḥyah Ḥen, *Sefer ha-Qanun* (Ms Oxford, Bodleian Libaries, Opp. Add. Fol. 12, fol. 250[b]): סֶלֶק תרדין ... יעשה אישפונגי באף עם מרירת העוף הנקרא כרכי וירפא עוות הפה ויועיל מנגעי האף והמים שלו פושרים יוטף באוזן וישכך הכאב וירחץ עם מימיו הראש ויעביר הסובין ([Arab.] *silq*; [i.e., Hebr. *Plur.*] *teradin*: Beet [*Beta vulgaris* L.]: ... When one drips [its juice] into the nose along with gallbladder of a crane, called [in Arab.] *kurkī*, it cures facial paralysis and is good for nasal ulcers. Its juice dripped into the nose when it is lukewarm relieves earache. When one washes the head with its juice, it removes dandruff). Hebr. עשה אישפונגי באף is a non-attested combination of Hebr. עשה באף and Rom. ʾYŠPWNGY. Synonyms used by Zeraḥyah are עשה שעיטה (see entry below) and *Nifʿal* נִשְׁעַט / *Hofʿal* הָשְׁעַט (see entry שָׁעַט). The Arab. synonym سعط في الأنف is translated by him as חבש באף (see entry חָבַשׁ). Nathan ha-Me'ati translates Arab. سعط as עשה סעוט (see next entry) and Anonymous I renders it as הטיף באף (see entry [נטף]).

• **עשה סעוט** · **to drip (pour) a medicine into the nose**: Arab. سعط · Ibn Sīnā, *K. al-Qānūn* II · trans. Nathan ha-Me'ati, *Sefer ha-Qanun* (Ms Oxford, Bodleian Libraries, Can. Or. 88, fols. 86[a–b]): חנדקוקא ... יכאיב הראש כשעושין ממנו סעוט ויועיל לבעל הכפיון ([Arab.] *ḥandaqūqā*: Lotus:[278] ... It causes headache when one drips its juice as a medicine into the nose; it is beneficial for someone suffering from epilepsy). The term עשה סעוט is not attested in the current dictionaries. The term סעוט is a non-attested loan word from Arab. سعوط 'a medicine that is dripped into the nose' (cf. FAQ 267f.), featuring in BM 4133 in an attestation, a.o., from the *Sefer ha-Qanun*. The Arab. synonym سعط في الأنف is translated by Nathan as עשה תחבשת בחוטם (see entry below). Zeraḥyah Ḥen translates Arab. سعط as שָׁעַט (see entry for *Nifʿal* נִשְׁעַט / *Hofʿal* הָשְׁעַט 'to be dripped (poured) as a medicine into the nose' (for Arab. سُعِطَ)).

---

278 'The Arabic term *ḥandaqūqā* stands for lotos (λωτός) which is a collective name of diverse species of leguminosae, e.g., bird clover/Trigonella caerulea (L.) Ser.; lucerne/Medicago sativa L.; yellow melilot/Melilotus officinalis (L.) Pall.' (MIG no. 341).

• **עשה קרישטיר** · **to apply a clyster, enema**: Arab. حقن · Ibn Sīnā, *K. al-Qānūn* II · trans. Zeraḥyah Ḥen, *Sefer ha-Qanun* (Ms Oxford, Bodleian Libaries, Opp. Add. Fol. 12, fol. 250[b]): סֻמַאק ... עוצר ויעצור הווסת וההגרה מהם וימנע מן הסחג ויעשה בו קרישטיר לדישינטיריאה ולהגרת הרחם ולטחורים ([Arab.] *summāq*: Tanner's sumach [*Rhus coriaria* L.]: ... It causes constipation, stops [excessive] menstrual flow and hemorrhage. It removes abrasions. It is applied as a clyster for dysentery, leukorrhea, and hemorroids). Hebr. עשה קרישטיר is not attested in the current dictionaries. The term קרישטיר (also written as קרישטירי) is a non-attested calque from Rom. (i.e., O. Occ. or O. Cat) *cristeri, crestiri, cresteri*, or *cristiri* (cf. SHS 1:421f. (Pe 36)). Zeraḥyah uses this term for Arab. حقنة throughout in his trans. of Maimonides' *Medical Aphorisms* (i.e., *Sefer ha-Peraqim*) (cf. BMMG no. 1021). Nathan ha-Me'ati translates Arab. حقن as עשה קנקן הנק׳ חקנה (cf. NM 6:171, s.v. עשה קנקן). In the glossary to his *Sefer ha-Qanun*, he explains Hebr. חוקן as: חוקן: ידוע שהוא קרישטירי (ḤWQN (clyster, enema). It is well-known that this [term] is [synonymous with] QRYŚṬYRY) (cf. NM 2:113, 138 (Ḥet 11). Hebr. חוקן is also used by Nathan for Arab. حقنة throughout in his trans. of Maimonides' *Medical Aphorisms* (i.e., *Sefer ha-Peraqim*) (cf. BMMG no. 1021). Anonymous I renders Arab. حقن as עשה חוקן.

• **עשה שעיטה** · **to drip (pour) a medicine into the nose**: Arab. سعوط · Ibn Sīnā, *K. al-Qānūn* II · trans. Zeraḥyah Ḥen, *Sefer ha-Qanun* (Ms Oxford, Bodleian Libaries, Opp. Add. Fol. 12, fol. 190[a]): בַּוְל שתן ... וכן לעשות שעיטה להמשכה ([Arab.] *bawl*; [i.e., Hebr.] *sheten*: Urine: ... It is also [good] for tetanus when it is dripped into the nose). Hebr. עשה שעיטה is not attested in the current dictionaries. Arab. سعط is translated by Zeraḥyah as שָׁעַט (see entry for *Nif'al* נִשְׁעַט / *Hof'al* הָשְׁעַט 'to be dripped (poured) as a medicine into the nose' (for Arab. سُعِطَ)) and עשה אישפונגי באף (see entry above). The Arab. synonym سعط في الأنف is translated by him as חבש באף (see entry חָבַשׁ). Nathan ha-Me'ati translates Arab. سعوط as עשה סעוט (see entry above) and Anonymous I renders it as הטפה באף (see entry הַטָּפָה).

• **עשה תחבשת בחוטם** · **to drip (pour) a medicine into the nose**: Arab. سعط في الأنف · Ibn Sīnā, *K. al-Qānūn* II · trans. Nathan ha-Me'ati, *Sefer ha-Qanun* (Ms Oxford, Bodleian Libraries, Can. Or. 88, fol. 110[a]): סדאב ... יסיר ריח השומים והבצלים ועושים תחבשת ממנו עם סויק לכאב הראש הישן ויש שעושים ממנו תחבשת עם חומץ בחוטם לרעיפת דם הנחירים ([Arab.] *sadhāb*: Common rue [*Ruta graveolens* L.]: ... It removes the smell of garlic and onion. It is used as a plaster with mush for chronic headache. Dripping it into the nose with vinegar stops a nosebleed). Hebr. עשה תחבשת בחוטם is not attested in the current dictionaries. The synonymous Arab. term سعط is translated by Nathan as עשה סעוט (see entry above). Zeraḥyah Ḥen translates Arab. سعط في الأنف as חבש באף (see entry חָבַשׁ).

• *Nif'al* **נַעֲשָׂה** • **נעשה בידים** · **artificial**: Arab. مصنوع · Ibn Sīnā, *K. al-Qānūn* II · trans. Anonymous I, *Sefer ha-Qanun* (Ms Paris, BnF, héb. 1142, fol. 245[b]): תנכר הוא בורגיש[279]

279 בוראייש: תנכר Ms[1].

מהות יש ממנו מחצבי ויש ממנו יעשה בידים ויאמרו לו מתג(?) הזהב ([Arab.] *tinkār*; i.e., [Rom.] BWRGYŠ [read: BWR'YŠ, i.e., O. Occ. *borais* (cf. SHS 1:333 (Mem 63)); from Arab. *bawraq*]: Salt, borax, salmiac, chrysocolla (cf. KM 345–349): What is it? There is [a variety] that is a mineral and another [variety] that is artificial, which is called MTG(?) *ha-zahav*). Hebr. נעשה בידים is not attested in this sense in the current dictionaries. Nathan ha-Me'ati translates Arab. مصنوع as שעושים אותו and Zeraḥyah Ḥen renders it as *Part. Pass.* צָבוּעַ (see entry [צבע]).

עֵשֶׂב • עשב מרים · cyclamen, esp. European cyclamen [*Cyclamen purpurascens* Mill.]: Arab. عرطنيثا · Ibn Sīnā, *K. al-Qānūn* II · trans. Zeraḥyah Ḥen, *Sefer ha-Qanun* (Ms Oxford, Bodleian Libaries, Opp. Add. Fol. 12, fol. 255[a]): עַרְטַנִיתַא ... הנעשה ממנו הוא שרשו והוא עשב[280] מרים ([Arab.] *'arṭanīthā*: Cyclamen, esp. European cyclamen [*Cyclamen purpurascens* Mill.] (cf. MIG no. 711): ... [Only] the root is used; [in Hebr. it is called] *ashan Miryam*). Hebr. עשב מרים is a calque from Arab. شجرة مريم (*shajarat Maryam*, meaning also 'cyclamen'), which features in Zeraḥyah's trans. of Maimonides' *Medical Aphorisms* (i.e., *Sefer ha-Peraqim*) XXIII.99 (cf. BMMZ 230, l. 20; BMMG no. 2597).

עֵת • המורסות אשר יקרו בעת המגפה → מֻרְסָה.
• עורר עת הנשים → [עור].
• שפע עת הנשים → שֶׁפַע.

[עתק] • *Hif'il* הֶעֱתִיק • העתיק השן חוצה · to extract a tooth: Arab. قلع الأسنان · Ibn Sīnā, *K. al-Qānūn* II · trans. Zeraḥyah Ḥen, *Sefer ha-Qanun* (Ms Oxford, Bodleian Libaries, Opp. Add. Fol. 12, fol. 212[b]): חנטל קולוקינְטִידַא ... ויועיל לצלילת האוזן ובנקלה יעתיק השן חוצה ([Arab.] *ḥanẓal*; [i.e., Rom.] QWoLWoQiYNṬYDa' [i.e., *colloquintida*, from Lat. *colocyntis*; Gr. κολοκυνθίς]: Colocynth [*Citrullus colocynthis* (L.) Schrad.]: ... It is useful for tinnitus and for easily extracting a tooth). Hebr. העתיק השן חוצה is not attested in the current dictionaries. Nathan ha-Me'ati and Anonymous I both render Arab. قلع الأسنان as עקירת השנים (see entry עֲקִירָה).

---

280 עשב מרים: Emend. ed. עשן מרים Ms.

[פגג] • *Part. Piʿel* מְפַגֵּג • הסם המפגג → סַם.

• הרפואה המפגגת → רְפוּאָה.

פי הרחם • פֶּה • האסף פי הרחם → [אסף].

• צמחי הפה → צֶמַח.

• קשקוש בפה → קִשְׁקוּשׁ.

• קשקש בפה → קִשְׁקֵשׁ.

• רוחות הפה → רוּחַ.

• שחין הפה → שְׁחִין.

פואה • **פוּאַת הצבעים** · **[lit. 'dyers' madder']; common madder [*Rubia tinctorum* L.]:** Arab. فوة الصباغين · Ibn Sīnā, *K. al-Qānūn* II · trans. Zeraḥyah Ḥen, *Sefer ha-Qanun* (Ms Oxford, Bodleian Libaries, Opp. Add. Fol. 12, fol. 259[a]): פוּאַת הצבעים ... ישתה אותה עם מי הקראטין ויועיל מגיד הנשה והפלג אשר עם חולי בהרגשה ([Arab.-Hebr.] *fuwwat ha-ṣabbaʿim* [lit. 'dyers' madder']: Common madder [*Rubia tinctorum* L.]: ... When taken with honey water (*melikraton*) it is beneficial for sciatica, hemiplegia with a sensory defect). Arab.-Hebr. פוּאַת הצבעים is a non-attested compound term consisting of Arab. *fuwwa* 'madder' and Hebr. *ṣabbaʿim* 'dyers.' Nathan ha-Me'ati renders Arab. فوة الصباغين as פוא אלצבאגין and Anonymous I has פוה הצבעים.

פוֹדַגְרָא · **gout:** Arab. نقرس · Ibn Sīnā, *K. al-Qānūn* II · trans. Zeraḥyah Ḥen, *Sefer ha-Qanun* (Ms Oxford, Bodleian Libraries, Opp. Add. Fol. 12, fol. 248[a]): סוּרַנְגֵ׳אן אַרְמוֹדַקְטִילִי ... יועיל מן הפודגרא וישכך הכאב באותה שעה כשיחבוש בו וכשיתרבה לחבוש בו יקשה המורסה וישיבנה כמו אבן ([Arab.] *sūranjān*; [i.e., Rom] 'aRəMWoDaQəṬiYLiY [i.e., O. Occ./O.Cat. (*h*)*ermodactil* (from Gr. ἑρμοδάκτυλος) (cf. BMZ 56f., 91 (Samekh 1))]: Autumn crocus [*Colchicum autumnale* L.]: ... It is useful in gout. Applied as a plaster, it alleviates the pain instantly but its excessive application as a plaster makes the swellings as hard as a stone). Hebr. פוֹדַגְרָא is a non-attested calque from Lat. *podagra*. The same term features in Zeraḥyah's trans. of Maimonides' *Medical Aphorisms* (i.e., *Sefer ha-Peraqim*) (cf. BMMG no. 5257). Nathan ha-Me'ati translates Arab. نقرس as נכאות הרגלים (cf. NM 6:141) and Anonymous I transcribes the Arab. term as נקרס, just like Nathan in his *Sefer ha-Peraqim* (cf. BMMG no. 5257).

פוּךְ • אבן הפוך → אֶבֶן.

פונטורא · **gripes (colic):** Arab. مغص · Ibn Sīnā, *K. al-Qānūn* II · trans. Zeraḥyah Ḥen, *Sefer ha-Qanun* (Ms Oxford, Bodleian Libaries, Opp. Add. Fol. 12, fol. 251[a–b]): סֶדָאבּ רוּטָא ... ייבש הזרע ויפסיקנו ויפיל תאות התשמיש וישכך הפונטורא ([Arab.] *sadhāb*; [i.e., Lat.] RWuṬ'a [i.e., *ruta*]: Common rue [*Ruta graveolens* L.]: ... It makes the semen dry and stops [its production]. It reduces sexual lust and relieves gripes (colic)). In the sense of 'gripes (colic),' Hebr. פונטורא is a non-attested calque from Lat. *punctura*. Nathan ha-Me'ati translates Arab. مغص as עקיצת המעיים (cf. NM 6:168) and Anonymous I renders it as חבלי הבטן (see NM 6:70).

פּוֹרָא · **warts**: Arab. ثآليل · Ibn Sīnā, *K. al-Qānūn* II · trans. Zeraḥyah Ḥen, *Sefer ha-Qanun* (Ms Oxford, Bodleian Libaries, Opp. Add. Fol. 12, fol. 194b):[281] גְּרָאדְ[282] ארבה ... הרגלים שלהם יתלש הפּוֹרָא לפי מה שאומרים ([Arab.] *jarād*; [i.e., Hebr.] *arbeh*: Locusts: ... It is said that their legs remove warts). Hebr. פּוֹרָא is a non-attested loan word from M. Lat. *porrum*, Plur. *porra* 'wart with root ramifying like the bulb of a leek' (cf. ND 863f., s.v. *porre*: 'Forms: *poris**, *porres**. L. *porrum*, *-us* 'leek' ... recorded in the sense 'wart' in ML ... (Cf. MF *por(re)* (FEW 9, 196b)'). Nathan ha-Me'ati translates Arab. ثآليل as היבלות הנקרא תאליל and Anonymous I renders the Arab. term as יבלות (cf. BCD 115 (NM 4:76f.) for Hebr. *Sing.* יַבֶּלֶת as it features in Moses ibn Tibbon's trans. of Ibn al-Jazzār's *Zād al-musāfir* (i.e., *Sefer Sedat ha-Derakhim*) VII.16.1 (cf. IJZ 7:151, l. 22)).

פורפורי · **purple**: Arab. فُرفُري · Ibn Sīnā, *K. al-Qānūn* II · trans. Zeraḥyah Ḥen, *Sefer ha-Qanun* (Ms Oxford, Bodleian Libaries, Opp. Add. Fol. 12, fols. 180b–181a: ... בַּאבּוּנַגְ' ירבה השתן ויוציא החול וכל שכן הפורפורי ממנו ([Arab.] *bābūnaj*: Camomile [*Matricaria chamomilla* L.]: ... It increases the urine (is diuretic) and expels stones, especially the variety with purple [flowers]). In the sense of 'purple,' Hebr. פורפורי is a non-attested calque from Arab. فرفري. Nathan ha-Me'ati translates the Arab. term as כעין החשמל (cf. NM 6:82f.) and Anonymous I renders the Arab. term as פורפורי, just like Zeraḥyah.

פּוֹתֵחַ (*Part.*) → פָּתַח.

[פזר] • *Pi'el* **פִּזֵּר** • **פיזר הרוחות** · **to be carminative (to expel gases)**: Arab. طرد الرياح · Ibn Sīnā, *K. al-Qānūn* II · trans. Zeraḥyah Ḥen, *Sefer ha-Qanun* (Ms Oxford, Bodleian Libaries, Opp. Add. Fol. 12, fol. 224b): כַּרַוִי ... יפזר הרוחות וייבש ואינו כדקדוק הכמון ([Arab.] *karāwi[yā]*: Caraway [*Carum carvi* L.]: ... It is carminative and desiccant, but not as refining as cumin). Hebr. פיזר הרוחות is not attested in the current dictionaries. In addition to פיזר הרוחות, Zeraḥyah translates Arab. طرد الرياح as השליך הרוחות (see entry [שלך]). The synonymous Arab. term كسر الرياح is translated by Zeraḥyah as שיבר הרוחות (see entry [שבר]). Nathan ha-Me'ati translates Arab. طرد الرياح as הוציא הרוחות and Anonymous I renders the Arab. term as מגרש הרוחות.

• *Part. Pi'el* **מְפַזֵּר** · **1. dispersing; discutient**: Arab. مفشّش (Gr. διαφορητικός; cf. UW 199f.) · Ibn Sīnā, *K. al-Qānūn* II · trans. Zeraḥyah Ḥen, *Sefer ha-Qanun* (Ms Oxford, Bodleian Libaries, Opp. Add. Fol. 12, fol. 210b): חֶנַא ... יש בו התרה וקיבוץ ויבשות בלא הזק מתיר ומפזר ופותח לפיות העורקים ולשמן שלו כח מחמם ומחליק ([Arab.] *ḥinnā'*: Henna [*Lawsonia inermis* L.]: ...: It has dissolving, astringent, and drying power without causing any harm. It is dissolvent, discutient, and widens the opening of the vessels; its oil has heating and laxative power). Hebr. *Part. Pi'el* מְפַזֵּר features in MD 227, s.v.

---

281 The same Hebr. term features (for Arab. ثآليل) on fol. 168b, entry אִשְׁקִיל '[Arab.] *ishqīl*: Sea squill [*Drimia maritima* (L.) Stearn],' and on fol. 182b (vowelized פּוֹרַא), entry בָּצָל 'Onion [*Allium cepa* L.].'

282 גְּרָאדְ ארבה :גַּזַם Ms[1]

'discutient,' in addition to מרתיע. In his trans. of Maimonides' *Medical Aphorisms*, Zeraḥyah renders Arab. فشّ 'to dispel, to disperse' as *Pi'el* פיזר (cf. BMMG no. 3850). Nathan ha-Me'ati and Anonymous I both render Arab. مفشّش as מתיך.

· II. **peeling (exfoliating)**: Arab. مقشّر · Ibn Sīnā, *K. al-Qānūn* II · trans. Zeraḥyah Ḥen, *Sefer ha-Qanun* (Ms Oxford, Bodleian Libaries, Opp. Add. Fol. 12, fol. 236[a]): מֵיזַרְיוֹן לָרִיאוּלָא ... הוא חם[283] ומנקה מפזר וחריפותו חזק ([Arab.] *māzaryūn*; [i.e., Lat./Rom.] LaRiY'WuLa' [i.e., M. Lat. or O. Occ. *laureola*; cf. SHS1:103 (Alef 16)]: February daphne [*Daphne mezereum* L.]: ... It is clearing,[284] purifying, peeling (exfoliating), and very pungent). Hebr. *Part. Pi'el* מְפַזֵּר is not attested in this sense in the current dictionaries. Nathan ha-Me'ati and Anonymous I both render Arab. مقشّر as מְקַלֵּף (see entry קָלַף). The Arab. term الدواء القاشر 'the peeling (exfoliating) drug' is translated by Zeraḥyah as הרפואה הקולפת (see entry רְפוּאָה).

• **מפזר הרוחות** · **carminative (expelling gases, flatulence)**: Arab. مفشّش للرياح · Ibn Sīnā, *K. al-Qānūn* II · trans. Zeraḥyah Ḥen, *Sefer ha-Qanun* (Ms Oxford, Bodleian Libaries, Opp. Add. Fol. 12, fol. 187[b]): בַּנְגַּנְגְ׳סְת אַיְנוּ קַשְׁטוּ ... מתיר ומדקדק מפזר הרוחות ([Arab.] *banjankusht*; [i.e., Rom.] 'aYəNWu QaŠəṬW [from Lat. *agnus castus*]: Chaste tree [*Vitex agnus-castus* L.]: ... It is dissolvent, attenuant, and carminative). Hebr. מפזר הרוחות is not attested in the current dictionaries. Nathan ha-Me'ati translates Arab. مفشّش للرياح as מתיר הרוחות and Anonymous I has מתיר הרוח.

פְּטוֹטֶרֶת · I. **pod; pericarp; seed capsule**: Arab. قمع · Ibn Sīnā, *K. al-Qānūn* II · trans. Anonymous I, *Sefer ha-Qanun* (Ms Paris, BnF, héb. 1142, fol. 244[a]): תודרי מהות אמ' דיאסקורידוס הוא עשב דומה העלים כעלי פראשי מרובע השורש[285] ושרשו שעור חצי אמה ויש לו פטוטרות שיש בהם זרעים ארוכים שחורים ([Arab.] *tūdharī*: Hedge mustard [*Sisymbrium officinale* (L.) Scop.]: What is it? According to Dioscorides, it is a herb bearing leaves like white horehound. Its root is quadrangular and measures half a cubit; its pods have oblong black seeds). Hebr. פְּטוֹטֶרֶת features in BM 4889 in the sense of 'stalk; stem (of a fig).' Nathan ha-Me'ati translates Arab. قمع as קְלִפָּה (see entry) and Zeraḥyah Ḥen has פְּצֹלֶת (see entry).

· II. **burr**: Arab. قمع · Ibn Sīnā, *K. al-Qānūn* II · trans. Anonymous I, *Sefer ha-Qanun* (Ms Paris, BnF, héb. 1142, fol. 218[a–b]): קאקלה הוא קרדמוני ... יש בו עם חמום קביצות וכל שכן אותו שיש לו פטוטרת וכל שכן הפטוטרת עצמה ([Arab.] *qāqulla*; i.e., [Rom.] QRDMWNY [from Gr. καρδάμωμον]: Black cardamom [*Amomum subulatum* Roxb.]: It is astringent and warming, especially in the variety having burrs. Even more so the burr itself). Zeraḥyah Ḥen translates Arab. قمع as פְּצֹלֶת (see entry) and Nathan ha-Me'ati has עֹקֶץ (see entry).

---

283 חם: جال a.

284 'clearing': Trans. acc. to a.

285 השורש: Emend. ed. השורה Ms.

פִּיל • אבן שן הפיל → אֶבֶן.
• **עצם הפיל** → עֶצֶם.
• **שן הפיל** → שֵׁן.

פִּלְפֵּל • פלפל השחורים · (lit. 'pepper of the blacks'); **earth almonds** [*Cyperus esculentus* L.]: Arab. حبّ الزلم (cf. DT 482f. (III.121)) · Ibn Sīnā, *K. al-Qānūn* II · trans. Zeraḥyah Ḥen, *Sefer ha-Qanun* (Ms Oxford, Bodleian Libraries, Opp. Add. Fol. 12, fol. 215[a]): חַבְּ אַלזֹלְם גַרְעִינֵי זֹלְם חבּ אלְעַזִיז המהות יאמרו שהוא פלפל השחורים והוא טוב הריח והטעם מאד ויצמח במקומות סהרון[286] ([Arab.] *ḥabb al-zalam*; [i.e., Hebr.] *gar'inei* ZoLəM; [i.e., Arab.] *ḥabb al-'azīz*: Earth almonds [*Cyperus esculentus* L.]: What is it? They say that it means [Hebr.] *pilpel ha-shaḥorim* [i.e., earth almonds]. They are very fragrant and tasty and grow in the region of Shahrazūr). In the sense of 'earth almonds,' Hebr. פלפל השחורים is a non-attested calque from Arab. *fulful as-Sūdān*, a synonym of *ḥabb al-zalam* and *ḥabb al-'azīz* (cf. MSh no. 161). Nathan ha-Me'ati transcribes/translates Arab. حبّ الزلم as חב אלזלם המהות הוא הנק' פלפל אלסודאן and Anonymous I has חב אלזלם כלומ' גרגיר זלם מהות יאמר לזה פלפל אלסודאן כלו' השחורים.

פְּנִימִי • פרי פנימי → פְּרִי.

[פסל] • *Part. Nif'al* **נִפְסָל** · **adulterated**: Arab. مغشوش · Ibn Sīnā, *K. al-Qānūn* II · trans. Anonymous II, *Sefer ha-Qanun* (Ms Parma, Biblioteca Palatina, Cod. Parm. 3045, fol. 26[b]): אפופונקו ... אבל אותו שצבעו שחור הוא נפסל עם אמוניאקו ([Rom.] 'PWPWNQW: Opopanax [i.e., the resin of the sweet myrrh [*Opopanax chironius* W.D.J. Koch]]: ... The variety that has a black color is adulterated with gum ammoniac). Hebr. *Part. Nif'al* נִפְסָל is not attested in this sense in the current dictionaries. Nathan ha-Me'ati, Zeraḥyah Ḥen, and Anonymous I translate Arab. مغشوش as מְזוּיָף (cf. NM 6:65).

פְּצוֹלֶת → פְּצֹלֶת.

פְּצֹלֶת · I. **pod; pericarp; seed capsule**: Arab. قمع · Ibn Sīnā, *K. al-Qānūn* II · trans. Zeraḥyah Ḥen, *Sefer ha-Qanun* (Ms Oxford, Bodleian Libraries, Opp. Add. Fol. 12, fol. 277[a]): תּוּדְּרִי המהות הוא עשב שדומה בעלים לעלי המרוי לפי דיאסקורידוס מרובע השורש והשורש חצי זרוע יש לו פצולת יש בו זרע ארוך שחור ([Arab.] *tūdharī*: Hedge mustard [*Sisymbrium officinale* (L.) Scop.]: What is it? According to Dioscorides, it is a herb bearing leaves like white horehound. Its root is quadrangular and measures half a cubit; its pods have oblong black seeds). Hebr. פְּצֹלֶת only features as a modern term in EM 1458 in the sense of 'a crack in a wall, ceiling.' Nathan ha-Me'ati translates Arab. قمع as קְלִפָּה (see entry) and Anonymous I has פְּטוֹטֶרֶת (see entry).

· II. **burr**: Arab. قمع · Ibn Sīnā, *K. al-Qānūn* II · trans. Zeraḥyah Ḥen, *Sefer ha-Qanun* (Ms Oxford, Bodleian Libraries, Opp. Add. Fol. 12, fol. 249[a]): קָאקֻלָּה קַרְדְּמוֹנִי ... יש בו עם החימום קיבוץ וכל[287] שכן אשר לו פצולת וכל שכן הפצולת בעצמו ([Arab.] *qāqulla*; i.e.,

---

286 סהרון: شهرزور a.
287 וכל שכן (وخصوصا a): Emend. ed. וכל Ms.

[Rom.] QaRəDəMWoNiY [from Gr. καρδάμωμον]: Black cardamom [*Amomum subulatum* Roxb.]: ... It is astringent and warming, especially in the variety having a burr. Even more so the burr itself). Nathan ha-Me'ati translates Arab. قمع as עֹקֶץ (see entry) and Anonymous I has פְּטוֹטֶרֶת (see entry).

· III. **dross**: Arab. خبث (cf. KM 539f.) · Ibn Sīnā, *K. al-Qānūn* II · trans. Zeraḥyah Ḥen, *Sefer ha-Qanun* (MS Oxford, Bodleian Libraries, Opp. Add. Fol. 12, fol. 258b):[288] פִּצ׳ה כסף ... הפצולת שלו הוא קובץ מאד ([Arab.] *fiḍḍa*; [i.e., Hebr.] *kesef*: Silver: ... Silver dross is very astringent). Anonymous I renders Arab. خبث as סיג and Nathan has *Plur.* סיגים.

[פצץ] • *Polel* פּוֹצֵץ • **פוצץ החול** · **to break up (dissolve) stones**: Arab. فتّت الحصاة · Ibn Sīnā, *K. al-Qānūn* II · trans. Zeraḥyah Ḥen, *Sefer ha-Qanun* (MS Oxford, Bodleian Libraries, Opp. Add. Fol. 12, fol. 176b): אִג׳אץ פרונגי ... והגומא שלהם יפוצץ החול בשלפוחית ([Arab.] *ijjāṣ*; [i.e., Rom.] PəRWNəGeY: Plum [*Prunus domestica* L.]: Their gum breaks up (dissolves) bladder stones). Hebr. פּוֹצֵץ is not attested for medieval medical literature in the current dictionaries. Nathan ha-Me'ati translates Arab. فتّت الحصاة as שבר החצץ and Anonymous I has פיתת חצץ.

• *Part. Polel* מְפוֹצֵץ • **הרפואה המפוצצת** → רְפוּאָה.

• *Part. Hitpolel* מִתְפּוֹצֵץ · **brittle**: Arab. يفتّت · Ibn Sīnā, *K. al-Qānūn* II · trans. Zeraḥyah Ḥen, *Sefer ha-Qanun* (MS Oxford, Bodleian Libaries, Opp. Add. Fol. 12, fol. 253a): סמַךְ דג ... היותר משובח שבדגים הוא מה שאינו גדול מאד ולא יהיה קשה בבשרו ולא יבש בלא שמנונית בו כאלו הוא מתפוצץ ולא דבקות כמותר האף ([Arab.] *samak*; [i.e., Hebr.] *dag*: Fish: ... The best fish is that which is not very big, nor hard of its flesh, or dry or greasy; [neither should it be] brittle nor viscous, like nasal mucus). Hebr. *Part. Hitpolel* מִתְפּוֹצֵץ is not attested in this sense in the current dictionaries. Nathan ha-Me'ati translates Arab. يفتّت as *Part. Nif'al* נִפְרָךְ (see entry [פרך]) and Anonymous I has יתפתת (see entry [פתת] for *Hitpa'el* הִתְפַּתֵּת).

פָּרָה • *Part.* פֹּרֶה • **המורסות הפרים** → מֻרְסָה.

פֹּרֶה (*Part.*) → פָּרָה.

פֶּרַח • **פרח המלח** · **salt efflorescence; salt scum**: Arab. زهر(ة) الملح (Gr. ἄνθος ἁλός; cf. KM 684ff.) · Ibn Sīnā, *K. al-Qānūn* II · trans. Zeraḥyah Ḥen, *Sefer ha-Qanun* (MS Oxford, Bodleian Libraries, Opp. Add. Fol. 12, fol. 242a–b): מלח ... ופרחו יותר דק ממנו (Salt: ... The efflorescence of [salt] is finer (more rarefying) than [the salt itself]). Hebr. פרח המלח is not attested in the current dictionaries. Nathan ha-Me'ati translates Arab. زهر(ة) الملح as קצף המלח (see entry קֶצֶף) and Anonymous I combines both terms as קצף ופרח המלח.

---

288 The same Hebr. term features on fol. 239b, entry מַגְנִיטַס אבן קרמִידא '[Arab.] *maghnīṭis* [from Gr. μαγνήτις]; [Hebr.-Rom.] *even ha-QRMiYD'* [i.e., O. Occ./O. Cat. *caramida*]: Magnetite' as part of the term פצולת הברזל for Arab. خبث الحديد 'iron dross.'

• **פרח הנחושת** · [lit. 'flower of copper']; **copper oxide**: a) Arab. زهرة النحاس (cf. KM 686–691) · Ibn Sīnā, *K. al-Qānūn* II · trans. Zeraḥyah Ḥen, *Sefer ha-Qanun* (Ms Oxford, Bodleian Libraries, Opp. Add. Fol. 12, fol. 245b): נחשת ... פרח הנחושת יותר דק ממנו (Copper: ... [Hebr.] *peraḥ ha-neḥoshet* [lit. 'flower of copper,' i.e., copper oxide] is more attenuant than copper [as such]). In the sense of 'copper oxide,' Hebr. פרח הנחושת features in NM 6:164 in an attestation from *Shinnui ha-Shemot ha-Niqra'im Synonimis*. Anonymous I renders Arab. زهرة النحاس as פרח הנחושת, just like Zeraḥyah, and Nathan ha-Me'ati transcribes the Arab. term as זהרת אלנחאס.

· b) Lat. *flos eris* · Guy de Chauliac, *Inventarium sive Chirurgia Magna* (cf. CMM 1:231, ll. 29–32) · trans. Anonymous (Ms Paris, BnF, héb. 1189, fol. 126b): והעזר הב' שיושם דרך הנקב קילור עשוי מטוטיא וסרקקקולא אילואין דם תנין בלושטיאש אנטימוני אלום חלקים שוים ומפרח נחשת רביע חלק (The second treatment (recipe) is to put through the opening [in the fistula] a collyrium made from equal parts of tutty, sarcocol, aloes, dragon's blood [i.e., the resin of *Dracaena cinnabari* Balf. f.], rose or blossom of the wild pomegranate, antimony, alum, and one fourth of a part of copper oxide).

פְּרִי • **פרי פנימי** · **pulp**: Arab. لبّ · Ibn Sīnā, *K. al-Qānūn* II · trans. Nathan ha-Me'ati, *Sefer ha-Qanun* (Ms Oxford, Bodleian Libraries, Can. Or. 88, fol. 74b): גוז הנדי ... המשובח ממנו הוא הלח חזק הלובן ואשר מימיו מתוקים וכשלא ימצא בו מימיות יורה שהוא ישן ויאות להסתפק ממנו בקלפת הפרי הפנימי ([Arab.] *jawz hindī*: Coconut [*Cocos nucifera* L.]: ... The best is that which is fresh, extremely white, and containing sweet water. Lack of water in it indicates that it is old. In such a case, one should only take the skin of its pulp). Hebr. פרי פנימי is not attested in the current dictionaries. Zeraḥyah Ḥen translates Arab. لبّ as לֵב (cf. NM 5:105 for an attestation from Moses ibn Tibbon's trans. of Ibn al-Jazzār's *Zād al-musāfir* (i.e., *Sefer Sedat ha-Derakhim*) III.6) and Anonymous I has לֵבָב (see entry). The Arab. synonym لحم is translated by Nathan as בָּשָׂר (see entry) and the synonymous جوف is rendered by him as תָּוֶךְ (see entry).

[פרך] • *Part. Nif'al* **נִפְרָךְ** · **brittle**: Arab. يفتّت · Ibn Sīnā, *K. al-Qānūn* II · trans. Nathan ha-Me'ati, *Sefer ha-Qanun* (Ms Oxford, Bodleian Libraries, Can. Or. 88, fol. 111a): סמך והוא דג ... היותר משובח מן הדגים הוא מה שאינו קשה הבשר ולא יבש ואין בו דשנות כאלו נפרך ([Arab.] *samak*; i.e., [Hebr.] *dag*: Fish: ... The best fish is that which is [not big], nor hard of its flesh or dry or greasy; [neither should it be] brittle). Hebr. *Part. Nif'al* נִפְרָךְ is not attested for medieval medical literature. Ben Yehuda quotes the term in an attestation from Maimonides' *Mishneh Torah, Sefer Tohorah, Hilkhot Tum'at Met* III Halakhah 10 (cf. BM 5182): בשר המת שנפרך ונעשה כקמח טהור. Zeraḥyah Ḥen translates Arab. يفتّت as מִתְפּוֹצֵץ (see entry [פצץ]) and Anonymous I renders the Arab. term as יתפתת (see entry [פתת] for *Hitpa'el* הִתְפַּתֵּת).

• *Part. Pi'el* **מְפָרֵךְ** • **הסם המפרך** → סַם.

פֶּרֶק • **פרקי העצמות** · **joints**: Arab. مفاصل · Ibn Sīnā, *K. al-Qānūn* II · trans. Anonymous II, *Sefer ha-Qanun* (Ms Parma, Biblioteca Palatina, Cod. Parm. 3045, fols. 26b–

27[a]): אפופונקו ... ומיצויו יצליח לטורח ויגיעה ויצליח לכאב פרקי העצמות ([Rom.] ʾPWPWNQW: Opopanax [i.e., the resin of the sweet myrrh [*Opopanax chironius* W.D.J. Koch]]: ... Its juice takes away tiredness and fatigue and is beneficial for pain in the joints). Hebr. פרקי העצמות is not attested in the current dictionaries. Nathan ha-Me'ati, Zeraḥyah Ḥen, and Anonymous I simply translate Arab. مفاصل as פרקים.

פִּשּׁוּחַ · **tear [of a muscle]**: Arab. فسخ (Gr. ῥῆγμα; cf. UWS 2:246) · Ibn Sīnā, *K. al-Qānūn* II · trans. Zeraḥyah Ḥen, *Sefer ha-Qanun* (Ms Oxford, Bodleian Libraries, Opp. Add. Fol. 12, fol. 247[b]): סְקוֹרְדִּיוֹן ... טוב לפישוח המושקולי ([Arab.] *squrdiyūn*: Water germander [*Teucrium scordium* L.]: ... It is good for muscle tear). Hebr. פִּשּׁוּחַ features in BM 5262 in an attestation from the *Sefer ha-Qanun*: ונאמר כי לפי שהיה פשוח פרוק חבור עמוק אחורי העור (Since *pisshuaḥ* is a dissolution of continuity deep beneath the skin). A synonymous term used by Zeraḥyah to render Arab. فسخ is הֶפְסֵד (see entry). The Arab. synonym هتك is translated by him as חִתּוּךְ and נִתּוּק (see entries) and the synonymous وهن as חֲלָשָׁה (see entry). Nathan translates Arab. فسخ as פְּתִיחָה (see entry) and Anonymous I renders the Arab. term as פִּשּׁוּחַ, just like Zeraḥyah.

פִּשּׁוּט · **spreading**: Arab. انتشار · Ibn Sīnā, *K. al-Qānūn* II · trans. Zeraḥyah Ḥen, *Sefer ha-Qanun* (Ms Oxford, Bodleian Libraries, Opp. Add. Fol. 12, fol. 222[w]): ... כֻּנְדֻּר אוֹלִיבַנוּ מחייה מאד וכל שכן לחבלות החדשות וימנע הנגע הַפִּירְדוֹלֵינט מן הפישוט ([Arab.] *kundur*; [i.e., Rom.] ʾWuLiYBaNWu: Frankincense [*Boswellia sacra* Flueck.]: ... It has a strong healing force, especially for fresh wounds; it prevents the spread of malignant ulcers). Hebr. פִּשּׁוּט is not attested for medieval Hebr. medical literature. Nathan ha-Me'ati translates Arab. انتشار as הוֹסִיף (see entry [יסף]) and Anonymous I has התפשט.

[פשט] • *Part. Hitpa'el* מִתְפַּשֵּׁט • **המורסות המתפשטות** → מֻרְסָה.

פְּשִׁירָה · **tepidity**: Arab. فتور · Ibn Sīnā, *K. al-Qānūn* II · trans. Anonymous I, *Sefer ha-Qanun* (Ms Paris, BnF, héb. 1142, fols. 105[b]–106[a]): דם ... אמר גאלינוס שהוא לפשירת איכותו לא דבר אחר (Blood: ... Galen said that this [property] is due to its tepid quality, not to anything else). Hebr. פְּשִׁירָה features in EM 1493 in the sense of 'cooling; drop in temperature; abatement [of the fever]' in an attestation from the *Sefer ha-Qanun*. Nathan ha-Me'ati translates Arab. فتور as הֲנָחָה (see entry) and Zeraḥyah Ḥen renders the Arab. term as פְּשִׁירָה, just like Anonymous I.

פִּשְׁפֵּשׁ · **tick**: Arab. قُرَاد · Ibn Sīnā, *K. al-Qānūn* II · trans. Anonymous I, *Sefer ha-Qanun* (Ms Paris, BnF, héb. 1142, fol. 213[b]): פסאפין:[289] הוא בעל חיים כפשפש ([Arab.] PSʾFYN [read: PSʾPYS, i.e., *fasāfis*]: Bed bugs: It is a living creature (insect) similar to a tick). Hebr. פִּשְׁפֵּשׁ features in the current dictionaries in the sense of 'bug; bed bug;' cf. BM 5282, s.v. פִּשְׁפָּשׁ. Nathan ha-Me'ati translates Arab. قُرَاد as כנים עגולים (see entry כִּנָּה) and Zeraḥyah Ḥen has קוֹף (see entry).

פָּתוּחַ (*Part. Pass.*) → פָּתַח.

289 פסאפין: פשפש לע' פונידא Ms[1].

פִּתּוּל · I. **twisting**: Arab. انفتال · Ibn Sīnā, *K. al-Qānūn* II · trans. Zeraḥyah Ḥen, *Sefer ha-Qanun* (Ms Oxford, Bodleian Libraries, Opp. Add. Fol. 12, fol. 265[b]): ... קָצַב קנים ישכך פיתול העצבים ([Arab.] *qaṣab*; [i.e., Hebr. *Plur.*] *qanim*: Cane; reed [e.g., giant cane [*Arundo donax* L.] or common reed [*Phragmites australis* (Cav.) Trin. ex Steud.] (cf. MIG no. 432)]: ... It relieves the twisting of nerves). Hebr. פִּתּוּל is not attested as a medical term in the current dictionaries. Nathan ha-Me'ati renders Arab. انفتال as עִוּוּת (cf. NM 6:157, s.v. עוות העצבים for Arab. التواء العصب) and Anonymous I has פְּתַלְתַּלוּת (see entry).

· II. **tent; roll; pledget [for keeping a wound open]**: Lat. *tenta* · Guy de Chauliac, *Inventarium sive Chirurgia Magna* (cf. CMM 1:420, ll. 15–16) · trans. Anonymous (Ms Paris, BnF, héb. 1189, fol. 229[b]): וישאר פתוח עם הפתולים ובמין[290] קשורה משעוה פשוטה ([The wound]) can be kept open by means of a tent or lint put in ordinary wax). Synonyms for פִּתּוּל in the sense of 'tent; roll; pledget' used by Anonymous are עִגּוּל and פְּתִילָה (see entries).

• **חלי פתול הגידים** → חֳלִי.

פָּתַח • *Part.* **פּוֹתֵחַ** • **הסם הפותח** → סַם.

• **הרפואה הפותחת** → רְפוּאָה.

• *Part. Pass.* **פָּתוּחַ** • **המרסא הפתוחה** → מֻרְסָא.

• *Part. Pi'el* **מְפַתֵּחַ** • **הסם המפתח** → סַם.

פְּתִיחָה · **tear [of a muscle]**: Arab. فسخ (Gr. ῥῆγμα; cf. UWS 2:246) · Ibn Sīnā, *K. al-Qānūn* II · trans. Nathan ha-Me'ati, *Sefer ha-Qanun* (Ms Oxford, Bodleian Libraries, Can. Or. 88, fol. 108[a]): סקורדיון ... הוא משובח לפתיחת העצלים ([Arab.] *sqūrdiyūn*: Water germander [*Teucrium scordium* L.]: ... It is an excellent [remedy] for muscle tear). Hebr. פְּתִיחָה does not feature in this sense in the current dictionaries. Synonymous terms for Arab. فسخ used by Nathan are בִּקּוּעַ and בְּקִיעָה (see entries). The Arab. synonym هتك is translated by Nathan as חִתּוּךְ (see entry) and the synonymous Arab. term وهن also as בִּקּוּעַ (see entry). Zeraḥyah Ḥen translates Arab. فسخ as פִּשּׁוּחַ (see entry) and Anonymous I renders the Arab. term as פשוח העצלים.

פְּתִיל • *Plur.* **פתילים** • **פתילי הגידים** · **varicose veins**: Arab. دالية, *Plur.* دوال · al-Rāzī, *K. fī al-Faṣd* · trans. Anonymous, *Ma'amar ba-Haqqazah* (Ms Parma, Biblioteca Palatina, Cod. Parm. 2283,4, fol. 97[b]): ואמנם אלכאהל תועיל מדפיקת הלב עם חמימות והנעשים המקום הנק' אלמעצמין תועיל מהנגעים אשר בזרועות ואשר בשוקים תועיל מאלסכתה והכפיה אשר הם מהדם או מפתילי[291] הגידים הנק' אלדואלי עם חמימות ([Cupping] the hollow of the neck is beneficial for palpitation accompanied by heat; [cupping] the site of the wrists, called [in Arab.] *al-mi'ṣamayn*, [is beneficial] for pustules on the forearms; [cupping] the legs is beneficial for apoplexy and epilepsy caused by blood

290 ובמין קשורה: *et nodis* L.

291 מפתילי הגידים הנק' אלדואלי: ومن الدوار a.

and for varicose[292] veins, called [in Arab.] *al-dawālī*, accompanied by heat). Hebr. פתילי הגידים is not attested in the current dictionaries. A variant reading, featuring in the *Ma'amar ba-Haqqazah*, is חלי פתול הגידים (see entry חֳלִי).

פְּתִילָה · **tent; roll; pledget [inserted into wound or sore]**: Lat. *tuellum* (cf. ND 1123) · Guy de Chauliac, *Inventarium sive Chirurgia Magna* (cf. CMM 1:235, ll. 9–11) · trans. Anonymous (Ms Paris, BnF, héb. 1189, fol. 128ᵇ): אמנם אם החולה יירא חום הברזל אז צוה רוגייר לעשות עגול או פתילה שרויה במרק[293] (But if the patient is afraid of the heat of the [cautery] iron, Roger[294] orders to apply a tent or pledget steeped in a ruptory[295]). As a medical term, Hebr. פְּתִילָה features in the sense of 'suppository' in BM 5325 (cf. BCD 226 (NM 4:169) for an attestation from Shem Tov ben Isaac's *Sefer ha-Shimmush* XXVII). Synonyms for פְּתִילָה in the sense of 'tent; roll; pledget' used by Anonymous are פִּתּוּל and עִגּוּל (see entries).

פְּתַלְתַּלוּת · **twisting**: Arab. انفتال · Ibn Sīnā, *K. al-Qānūn* II · trans. Anonymous I, *Sefer ha-Qanun* (Ms Paris, BnF, héb. 1142, fol. 219ᵃ): קצב ... ישקיט פתלתלות העצבים ([Arab.] *qaṣab*: Cane; reed [e.g., giant cane [*Arundo donax* L.] or common reed [*Phragmites australis* (Cav.) Trin. ex Steud.] (cf. MIG no. 432)]: ... It relieves the twisting of nerves). Hebr. פְּתַלְתַּלוּת or פְּתַלְתֹּלֶת[296] features in EM 1500 as a modern term in the sense of ערבוביה 'confusion.' Nathan ha-Me'ati renders Arab. انفتال as עִוּוּת (cf. NM 6:157, s.v. עוות העצבים for Arab. التواء العصب) and Zeraḥyah Ḥen has שִׁבּוּךְ (see entry).

[פתת] • *Hitpa'el* **הִתְפַּתֵּת** · **to be brittle**: Arab. فتّت · Ibn Sīnā, *K. al-Qānūn* II · trans. Anonymous I, *Sefer ha-Qanun* (Ms Paris, BnF, héb. 1142, fol. 195ᵃ): סמך הוא דג ... הטוב שבדגים מה שלא יהיה גדול הרבה ולא קשה הבשר ולא היבש שבהם ואין דשנות בו כאלו יתפתת ואין נעיות בו ולא זוהמא וטעמו ערב ([Arab.] *samak*; i.e., [Hebr.] *dag*: Fish: ... The best fish is that which is not very big, nor hard of its flesh or dry or greasy; [neither should it be] brittle, nor viscous, nor fetid; its taste should be pleasant). Hebr. פתת is not attested in the *Hitpa'el* conj. in the current dictionaries. Nathan ha-Me'ati translates Arab. فتّت as *Part. Nif'al* נִפְרָךְ (see entry) and Zeraḥyah Ḥen has מִתְפּוֹצֵץ (see entry [פצץ]).

• *Part. Pi'el* **מְפַתֵּת** • הסם המפתת → סַם.

---

292 'varicose veins': 'vertigo' a.

293 במרק: *in ruptorio* L.

294 'Roger': I.e., Rogerius Frugardi, author of the *Chirurgia* composed in the second half of the twelfth century. It was later greatly expanded by Roland of Parma (completed in 1230). Guy de Chauliac's quotations are sometimes derived from this expanded verison, which was in effect a new book; cf. CMM 2:13f.

295 'ruptory' (i.e., a medicine burning and destroying bodily tissue; cf. ND 941): Trans. acc. to L.

296 Cf. R. Alcalay, *Millon Ivri-Angli Shalem: The Complete Hebrew-English Dictionary* (Ramat Gan 1972), 2142.

צ

צָבַע • *Part. Pass.* **צָבוּעַ** · **artificial:** Arab. مصنوع · Ibn Sīnā, *K. al-Qānūn* II · trans. Zeraḥyah Ḥen, *Sefer ha-Qanun* (Ms Oxford, Bodleian Libaries, Opp. Add. Fol. 12, fol. 278ª): תִּנְכָּאר בּוֹרַשׁ יש ממנו מקורי ויש ממנו שהוא צבוע ונקרא מדבק הזהב ([Arab.] *tinkār*; [i.e., Rom.] BoRaŠ [i.e., O. Occ. *borais* (cf. SHS 1:333 (Mem 63)); from Arab. *bawraq*]: Salt, borax, salmiac, chrysocolla (cf. KM 345–349): There is [a variety] that is a mineral and another [variety] that is artificial, which is called [in Hebr.] *medabbeq ha-zahav* (see entry [דבק])). Hebr. צָבוּעַ is not attested in this sense in the current dictionaries. Nathan ha-Me'ati translates Arab. مصنوع as שעושים אותו and Anonymous I renders the Arab. term as נעשה בידים (see entry עָשָׂה).

צַבָּע • *Plur.* **צבעים** · **dyers:** Arab. صبّاغ, *Plur.* صبّاغون · Ibn Sīnā, *K. al-Qānūn* II · trans. Nathan ha-Me'ati, *Sefer ha-Qanun* (Ms Oxford, Bodleian Libraries, Can. Or. 88, fol. 88ᵇ): חגר ארמיני המהות דומה מעט לאבן לאזורד אלא שאינו כבד כמותו וכן אינו שווה בגוונו אבל יש בו כמו חול ואפשר שמסתפקים ממנו הצבעים והמציירים במקום הלאזורד ([Arab.] *ḥajar armīnī*: Armenian stone: What is it? It is somewhat similar to lapis lazuli but it is not as heavy and does not have the same color; it is sandy and dyers and painters may use it as a substitute for lapis lazuli). Hebr. צַבָּע, *Plur.* צבעים, features in the current dictionaries in attestations from Rabb. literature only; cf. JD 1259; BM 5366. Anonymous I renders Arab. صباغون as צבעים, just like Nathan.

• **עורקי הצבעים** → **עֹרֶק.**

• **פואת הצבעים** → **פּוּאָה.**

צַד • **כאב הצד** → **כְּאֵב.**

צֶדַע • *Dual* **צדעים**: **the lateral parts of the neck**: Arab. أخدعان (cf. DKT 813) · al-Rāzī, *K. fī al-Faṣd* · trans. Anonymous, *Ma'amar ba-Haqqazah* (Ms Parma, Biblioteca Palatina, Cod. Parm. 2283,4, fol. 96ᵇ): זאת ההרקה נחלקת לב׳ חלקים הא׳ עם שריטה והב׳ בלא שריטה והמקומות הנהוגים לעשות שריטה בהם הם נקרת הראש והצדעים הנק׳ אלאחדעין[297] (This [kind of] evacuation (i.e., bloodletting) is divided into two parts: the first with scarification and the second without scarification. The sites that are regulary used for scarification are the hollow of the neck and the lateral parts of the neck, called [in Arab.] *akhda'ayn*). Hebr. צֶדַע, *Dual* צדעים, does not feature in this sense in the current dictionaries.

צָהֹב • **המים הצהובים** → **מַיִם.**

צַהֲבוּת · **redness:** Arab. شقرة · Ibn Sīnā, *K. al-Qānūn* II · trans. Zeraḥyah Ḥen, *Sefer ha-Qanun* (Ms Oxford, Bodleian Libaries, Opp. Add. Fol. 12, fol. 252ª): ... סֻנְבֻּל אֶשְׁפִּיקָא אמר דיאסקורידוס היותר טוב הוא אותו שיהיה לו שערות יותר ויהיה נוטה אל הצהבות ויהיה טוב הריח כמו הציפרו ([Arab.] *sunbul* [lit. 'the ear of corn']; [i.e., Lat.] 'eŠəPiYQa' [i.e.,

297 אלאחדעין: Emend. ed. אל אלארדעין קרא Ms.

espica]: Spikenard [*Nardostachys jatamansi* (D. Don) DC.]: … According to Dioscorides, the best spikenard is the one which is rich in reddish hair. It is fragrant like common galingale). Hebr. צְהָבוּת features in EM 1512 as a modern term only. Nathan ha-Me'ati translates Arab. شقرة as צהיבות and Anonymous I has כרכמות.

צָהוֹב → צָהֹב.

צַוָּאר • צואר הרחם · **neck of the uterus; cervix**: Lat. *collum matricis* · Guy de Chauliac, *Inventarium sive Chirurgia Magna* (cf. CMM 1:239, l. 34) · trans. Anonymous (Ms Paris, BnF, héb. 1189, fol. 131[a]): אמנם אותם הנעשים באברים הנמשכים כמו באמה וצואר הרחם הם גרידות חימומים ונגעים המימיים[298] עם מוגליות ומעופשים ומאוכלים ומסורטנים ([Ulcers] that occur in organs that can have a prolapse, such as penis and neck of the uterus (cervix), are: excoriations, heating ulcers, virulent ulcers, putrid ulcers, corrosive ulcers, and cancerous ulcers). Hebr. צואר הרחם features in BM 5412, a.o., in attestations from Maimonides' *Mishneh Torah, Issurei Bi'ah* (cf. MD 152).

• חולית הצואר → חֻלְיָה.

צוֹפֵד (*Part.*) → צָפַד.

צוֹר • ילפת הצור → יַלֶּפֶת.

ציטרין • המים הציטרין → מַיִם.

צינקופיץ · **palpitation of the heart**: Lat./Rom. *sincopis* (cf. ND 164; Arab. خفقان; Gr. καρδιωγμός[299]) · Ibn Sīnā, *K. al-Qānūn* II · trans. Zeraḥyah Ḥen, *Sefer ha-Qanun* (Ms Oxford, Bodleian Libaries, Opp. Add. Fol. 12, fol. 229[b]): לַכָּא … יועיל מן הצינקופיץ ([Aram.] *lakka'* / [Arab.] *lakka* / [Lat.] *lacca* (cf. JD 710): Lac (shellac): … It is beneficial for palpitation of the heart). Hebr. צינקופיץ is a non-attested loan word from Lat./Rom. *sincopis*. Nathan ha-Me'ati and Anonymous I both render Arab. خفقان as דפיקת הלב (cf. BCD 58 (NM 4:39) for an attestation from Moses ibn Tibbon's trans. of Ibn al-Jazzār's *Zād al-musāfir* (i.e., *Sefer Sedat ha-Derakhim*) I.18.1 (cf. IJZ 1–2:468)). The latter term also features in Zeraḥyah's and Nathan's trans. of Maimonides' *Medical Aphorisms* (i.e., *Sefer ha-Peraqim*) VI.34 (cf. BMMZ 64, l. 7; BMMN 70, l. 5; BMMG no. 1410). The term צינקופיץ also features (written as סינקופיץ) in Zeraḥyah's *Sefer ha-Peraqim* XXI.96 (cf. BMMZ 207, l. 18; BMMG no. 1410).

צִיץ · **pod; pericarp; seed capsule**: Arab. قمع · Ibn Sīnā, *K. al-Qānūn* II · trans. Nathan ha-Me'ati, *Sefer ha-Qanun* (Ms Oxford, Bodleian Libraries, Can. Or. 88, fol. 78[a]): דרדאר המהות הוא הנקרא אילן אלבק ויצאו בו ציצים נפוחים ([Arab.] *dardār*: Elm [*Ulmus glabra* Huds.]. What is it? It is that which is called the *baq* tree [i.e., the bug tree; cf. MIG

298 המימיים עם מוגליות: *virulenta* L.

299 In addition to 'palpitation of the heart,' Gr. καρδιωγμός can also mean 'heartburn.' Galen remarks that—acc. to the ancients—the term καρδία can mean both the heart and the cardia of the stomach, and that the term καρδιωγμός is explained by some in the sense of heartburn and by others in the sense of palpitation of the heart (*In Hippocratis Aphorismos commentarius* IV.65 (ed. Kühn, 17b:745f.; cf. NM 3:27, n. 106)).

no. 991]. It produces inflated seed capsules). As a botanical term, Hebr. צִיץ features in BM 5469f. in the sense of 'blossom' only. In addition to צִיץ, Nathan translates Arab. قمع as קְלִפָּה (see entry). Zeraḥyah Ḥen translates the Arab. term. as פְּצֶלֶת (see entry) and Anonymous I has פטוטרות (see entry פְּטוֹטֶרֶת).

צִיר • *Plur.* **צירים** • **צירי העצבים** · **twisted nerves**: Arab. التواء العصب · Ibn Sīnā, *K. al-Qānūn* II · trans. Anonymous II, *Sefer ha-Qanun* (Ms Parma, Biblioteca Palatina, Cod. Parm. 3045, fol. 27[a]): ייניציאנה ... ושתוי ממנו ב׳ דרה׳[300] יצליח לצירי החבלים ויצליח לנופלים ממקום גבוה ([Lat./Rom.] YYNṢY'NH: Gentian [*Gentiana lutea* L.]: ... Two *dirham*s of it taken with[301] wine is beneficial for twisted nerves. It is also beneficial for someone who has fallen from a high place). Hebr. צירי העצבים is not attested in the current dictionaries. Nathan ha-Me'ati translates Arab. التواء العصب as עוות העצב (cf. NM 6:157, s.v. עוות העצבים), Zeraḥyah Ḥen has לפיתת העצבים (cf. NM 6:110), and Anonymous I has רצוץ העצבים (cf. NM 6:206).

[צלח] • *Hif'il* **הִצְלִיחַ** · **to be beneficial**: Arab. نفع · Ibn Sīnā, *K. al-Qānūn* II · trans. Anonymous II, *Sefer ha-Qanun* (Ms Parma, Biblioteca Palatina, Cod. Parm. 3045, fol. 48[a]): לוטוס ארמיני ... תועלתו לקדחת יצליח לקדחת השדפון הוא איטיקא והחוליים שיקרו בעת המגפה בלבד ([Lat.-Arab.] LWṬWS (*lutus*) *armīnī*: Armenian bole: ... Its usefulness for fevers: It is especially beneficial for hectic fevers and [fevers] occurring during the plague (pestilential fevers)). Hebr. *Hif'il* הִצְלִיחַ does not feature in this sense in the current dictionaries. Nathan ha-Me'ati, Zeraḥyah Ḥen, and Anonymous I translate Arab. نفع as הועיל.

צֵלָע • *Plur.* **צלעות** • **חולי הצלעות** → **חֳלִי**.
• **מורסת הצלעות** → **מֻרְסָה**.

צִמְאָה · **thirst**: Lat. *sitis* (Arab. عطش) · Constantinus Africanus, *Viaticum* V.5 · trans. Do'eg ha-Edomi, *Sefer Ya'ir Netiv*: ואם החום הוא הסבה באשר יהיה אפס כח הבשול יהיה זה נכר מצמאת החולה ומקדחותיו וממהירות הדפק ומכרכמות הגוף יאות להשקותו דבר לקרר החום (If the weakness of the digestive faculty is caused by heat, it is indicated by the fact that the patient suffers from thirst and fever, has a fast pulse and a yellow complexion. In this case, one should give him cold drinks to cool the heat). Hebr. צִמְאָה features in the current dictionaries in attestations from the Bible, Moses ibn Ezra, and Mendele Mocher Sforim only (cf. KB 1032; EM 1532). Moses ibn Tibbon translates Arab. عطش as צמא.

צִמּוּק • *Plur.* **צמוקים** • **הצמוקים ההרריים** · **[lit. 'mountain raisins']; stavesacre [*Delphinium staphisagria* L.]**: Arab. ميويزج (cf. MIG no. 332) · Ibn Sīnā, *K. al-Qānūn* II · trans. Zeraḥyah Ḥen, *Sefer ha-Qanun* (Ms Oxford, Bodleian Libaries, Opp. Add. Fol. 12, fol. 240[a]): מִיוּבְזַג׳ אֶשְׁטַפְזִיזַקְרא הוא הצימוקים ההרריים והוא גרעיני הראש בערבי

---

300 ׳דרה׳: بشراب add. a.
301 'with wine': Trans. acc. to a.

חב אלראס ([Arab.] *mayūbazaj* [from Pers. *mawīzak*]; [i.e., Rom.] 'eŠəṬaPəZiYZaQəR' [i.e., O. Occ. *estafizagra*; cf. SHS 1:429f. (Ṣade 2)]: Stavesacre [*Delphinium staphisagria* L]: I.e., [Hebr.] *ha-ṣimmuqim ha-harariyim* (lit. 'mountain raisins'), i.e., [Hebr.] *garʿinei ha-rosh* [lit. 'head seeds'], in Arab. *ḥabb al-ra's* [lit. 'head seed']). In the sense of 'stavesacre,' Hebr. הצמוקים ההרריים is a variant of צמוקי ההר, which features in BCD 230 (NM 4:173) for the synonymous Arab. term زبيب الجبل (in an attestation from Moses ibn Tibbon's trans. of Ibn al-Jazzār's *Zād al-musāfir* (i.e., *Sefer Sedat ha-Derakhim*) I.1.8 (cf. IJZ 1–2:444)) and in BCD 230 (NM 2:17) for the synonymous Arab. term حبّ الرأس (in an attestation from Shem Tov ben Isaac's *Sefer Almansur* (cf. BMZ 52f. (Mem 14))). Nathan ha-Me'ati translates Arab. ميويزج as צמוקי ההר and Anonymous I has צמוקים הריים.

[צמח] • *Part. Hifʿil* מַצְמִיחַ • **הסם המצמיח הבשר** → **סַם**.

• **הרפואה המצמיחה הבשר** → **רְפוּאָה**.

צֶמַח • **צמח הלילה** · **skin affection (pustules) that occurs at night**: Arab. بنات الليل (Gr. ἐπινυκτίς; cf. LSG 649; MIG no. 166; UW 258) · Ibn Sīnā, *K. al-Qānūn* II · trans. Zeraḥyah Ḥen, *Sefer ha-Qanun* (Ms Oxford, Bodleian Libaries, Opp. Add. Fol. 12, fols. 196b–197a): דבק ... ויועיל מן השרי וצמח הלילה ([Arab.] *dibq*: Mistletoe (birdlime) [*Viscum album* L.]: ... It is also beneficial for *sharan*[302] and the skin affection (pustules) that occurs at night). Hebr. צמח הלילה is not attested in the current dictionaries. Anonymous I renders Arab. بنات الليل as בנות הלילה (see entry בַּת).

• *Plur.* **צמחים** • **צמחי הפה** · **aphthae**: Arab. قلاع · Ibn Sīnā, *K. al-Qānūn* II · trans. Anonymous I, *Sefer ha-Qanun* (Ms Paris, BnF, héb. 1142, fol. 123a–b: טבאשיר הוא אשפודי ... מועיל מצמחי הפה הנקרא קלאנג' (*קלאע) ומההשתותמות ([Arab.] *ṭabāshīr*; i.e., [Rom.] 'ŠPWDY [i.e., O. Occ. *espodi*]: Tabasheer (bamboo manna) [i.e., the siliceous secretions found in the internodes of bamboo stems [*Bambusa bambos* (L.) Voss]: It is beneficial for aphthae, called [in Arab.] **qulāʿ* and for anxiety). Hebr. צמחי הפה is not attested in the current dictionaries. Nathan ha-Me'ati translates Arab. قلاع as נגעי הפה (cf. BCD 171 (NM 3:151) for an attestation from his trans. of Hippocrates' *Aphorisms* III.24) and Zeraḥyah Ḥen transcribes it as קלאע.

[צער] • *Part. Hitpaʿel* מִצְטַעֵר · **turbulent**: Arab. اضطراب · Ibn Sīnā, *K. al-Qānūn* II · trans. Zeraḥyah Ḥen, *Sefer ha-Qanun* (Ms Oxford, Bodleian Libraries, Opp. Add. Fol. 12, fol. 253a–b): סמך דג ... ואותו שיעמוד במימות מצטערות מאד והגלים הוא יותר טוב

302 Cf. MIG no. 166: بنات الليل هو الشرى من الحاوي، وقال جالينوس في المقالة الثانية من كتاب حيلة البرء: سُمّي الشرى بنات الليل من قبل أنّ الشرى يعرض بالليل (*Banāt al-layl* (lit. 'daughters of the night') is a pustule (*sharan*) according to (al-Rāzī's) *Ḥāwī*. Galen said in the second chapter of his book '*On the Method of Healing*' (*Ḥīlat al-bur'*): the pustule is called 'daughters of the night', because the pustule occurs at night). For *sharan*, see also entry רְקוּעַ, *Plur.* רקועים.

ויותר צורך להרגיל מאותו שיעמוד במימות השקטות ([Arab.] *samak*; [i.e., Hebr.] *dag*: Fish: ... Fish living in very turbulent and wavy waters are very good because such fish have to exert themselves more than those living in stagnant waters). Hebr. *Part. Hitpa'el* מִצְטַעֵר is not attested in the sense of 'turbulent' in the current dictionaries. Nathan ha-Me'ati translates the Arab. term as מתגעש and Anonymous I has התגעשות.

צָפַד • *Part.* **צוֹפֵד** · **agglutinant; gluey**: Arab. مغرّ · Ibn Sīnā, *K. al-Qānūn* II · trans. Nathan ha-Me'ati, *Sefer ha-Qanun* (Ms Oxford, Bodleian Libraries, Can. Or. 88, fol. 75[r]): גלנאר ... הוא צופד עוצר כל הגרה ויוליד המרה השחורה ([Arab.] *jullanār*: The flower of the wild pomegranate [*Punicum granatum* L.]: ... It is agglutinant, stops the flow [of all kinds of fluids], and produces black bile). In the sense of 'agglutinant,' Hebr. צוֹפֵד features for Lat. *glutinativus* in BCD 233 (NM 4:175) in a later attestation from Estori ha-Parḥi's trans. of Armengaud Blaise's *Tabula Antidotarii* (i.e., *Shemot ha-Mashqim*). Zeraḥyah Ḥen translates Arab. مغرّ as *Part. Pi'el* מְדַבֵּק (see entry [דבק]) and Anonymous I has טח בדבקות (see entry טוּחַ).

• **הסם הצופד** → **סַם**.

צֶפֶד · **agglutination**: Arab. تغرية · Ibn Sīnā, *K. al-Qānūn* II · trans. Nathan ha-Me'ati, *Sefer ha-Qanun* (Ms Oxford, Bodleian Libraries, Can. Or. 88, fol. 57[b]): והמסגר הוא הסם אשר ייבש ויעבה הרוטבא הנופלת בין שני שטחי הנגע הקרובים זה לזה עד שישוב אל הצפד והדבוק וידבק האחד עם האחר כמו דם אל אכוין והצבר (The healing [drug] is a drug that dries up and thickens the fluid collected between the two layers of a wound that are close to each other. [It does so] to an extent that it [i.e., the fluid] becomes agglutinant and viscous and both the ends [of the wound] adhere to each other; [examples of such a drug are] dragon's blood [i.e., the resin of *Dracaena cinnabari* Balf. f.] and aloes). Hebr. צֶפֶד features in BM 5578 in the sense of 'glue' in an attestation from Tanḥum Yerushalmi's commentary on Lam. Zeraḥyah Ḥen translates Arab. تغرية as דִּבּוּק (cf. NM 6:41 for an attestation from Nathan's *Sefer ha-Qanun* II) and Anonymous I has טיחת דבקות (see entry טִיחָה).

צֳרִי · **antidote; theriac**: Arab. ترياق · Ibn Sīnā, *K. al-Qānūn* II · trans. Anonymous II, *Sefer ha-Qanun* (Ms Parma, Biblioteca Palatina, Cod. Parm. 3045, fol. 29[a]): רוקא ... אם יאכל וישתה אחריו יין טוב[303] וריחני הוא כעין צרי לנשיכת חולדה ([Lat.] RWQ' [i.e., (*e*)*ruca*]: Rocket [*Eruca sativa* Mill.]: ... If one eats it and then drinks some fragrant wine, it acts as an antidote for the bite of a weasel). In the sense of 'antidote; theriac,' Hebr. צֳרִי is attested in BCD 234 (NM 4:176) in an attestation from an anonymous trans. of Ibn Sīnā's *K. al-Adwiya al-qalbiyya* (i.e., *Sefer ha-Refu'ot ha-Libbiyot*). Nathan ha-Me'ati, Zeraḥyah Ḥen, and Anonymous I render Arab. ترياق as תריאק.

צִרְעָה • *Plur.* **צרעות** · **Spanish flies (cantharides)**: Arab. ذراريح · Ibn Sīnā, *K. al-Qānūn* II · trans. Nathan ha-Me'ati, *Sefer ha-Qanun* (Ms Oxford, Bodleian Libraries, Can. Or.

303 טוב וריחני: ريحاني a.

88, fol. 89[a]):[304] טין מכתום ... ואני נסיתי אותו למי ששתה ארנבת הים והצרעות ובער׳ דראריח והקיאם תכף ([Arab.] *ṭīn makhtūm*: Sealed earth (*terra*[305] *sigillata*): ... [Galen said]: I tried it in the case of someone who ingested sea hare and Spanish flies (cantharides), [called] in Arab. *dharārīḥ*, and he vomited them immediately). Hebr. *Sing.* צִרְעָה is only attested in the current dictionaries in the sense of 'wasp; hornet' (cf. BM 5647f.). In this sense, Nathan also uses Hebr. צרעות to render the Arab. parallel term زنابير (cf. entry דְּבוֹרָה). Note, that in his trans. of Ibn Sīnā's entry ذراريح 'Spanish flies (cantharides)' (fol. 79[b]), Nathan does not provide a trans. but merely transcribes the Arab. term as דראריח. Zeraḥyah Ḥen translates Arab. ذراريح as Rom. קנטרילי. The latter term also features in Abraham ben Isaac's trans. of Ibn al-Jazzār's *Zād al-musāfir* (i.e., *Sefer Ṣedah la-Oreḥim*) I.1.7 as explanation for Hebr. דרדיחים 'small flies' (cf. NM 5:55, s.v. דַּרְדִּיחַ; IJZ 1–2:539). Anonymous I renders Arab. ذراريح as Lat. קנטרידש (i.e., *cantharides*).

304 The same Hebr. term recurs on fol. 125[b], entry שחם חלב '[Arab.] *shaḥm*; [i.e., Hebr.] *ḥalav*: Fat'.

305 '*terra sigillata*': I.e., red clay, originally from the Aegean island of Lemnos, formed into tablets and impressed with a seal: a popular remedy in ancient Rome and used in medieval medicine as an antidote and astringent (cf. Wallis, *Medieval Medicine*, 551).

ק

קִבּוּל • **חולשת קבול ההריון** → חֻלְשָׁה.

[קבל] • *Pi'el* **קִבֵּל** • **קיבל העפוש הנקרא *רנציד** · **to become rancid**: Arab. زنخ · Ibn Sīnā, *K. al-Qānūn* II · trans. Anonymous I, *Sefer ha-Qanun* (Ms Paris, BnF, héb. 1142, fols. 194[a–b]): סמסם[306] ... הוא הרב שמניות שבזרעים ולכן מקבל העפוש הנקרא רנציד[307] בנקלה ([Arab.] *simsim*: Sesame [*Sesamum indicum* L.]: ... It contains more oil than other seeds and therefore the oil quickly becomes rancid, called [in Rom.] *rancid*). Hebr. קיבל העפוש הנקרא *רנציד is a non-attested calque from Rom. (O. Occ. ?) *rancid*.[308] In addition to קיבל העפוש הנקרא *רנציד (for Arab. زنخ), Anonymous I renders the Arab. term as *Hitpa'el* הִתְיַשֵּׁן (see entry [ישן]) and *Hif'il* הֵרִיחַ (see entry [ריח]). Nathan ha-Me'ati translates Arab. زنخ as *Hitpa'el* הִתְדַּשֵּׁן (see entry [דשן]).

קָבַץ • *Part.* **קוֹבֵץ** • **הרפואה הקובצת** → רְפוּאָה.

קַדַּחַת • **הקדחות בעלי ההקף** · **intermittent fevers**: Arab. الحمّيات ذوات الأدوار · Ibn Sīnā, *K. al-Qānūn* II · trans. Anonymous I, *Sefer ha-Qanun* (Ms Paris, BnF, héb. 1142, fols. 231[b]–232[a]: ראונד ... מועיל מהקדחות הנושנות ובעלי ההקף ([Arab.] *rāwand*: Rhubarb [*Rheum* sp.]: ... It is beneficial for chronic and intermittent fevers). Hebr. הקדחות בעלי ההקף is not attested in the current dictionaries. Nathan ha-Me'ati translates Arab. الحمّيات ذوات الأدوار as הקדחות אשר להם הקפות (see next entry). For the synonymous terms הקדחות הסובבות and הקדחות המקיפות, see entries below.

• **הקדחות אשר להם הקפות** · **intermittent fevers**: Arab. الحمّيات ذوات الأدوار · Ibn Sīnā, *K. al-Qānūn* II · trans. Nathan ha-Me'ati, *Sefer ha-Qanun* (Ms Oxford, Bodleian Libraries, Can. Or. 88, fol. 122[a]): ראונד ... יועיל מהקדחות הישנות ומאשר להם הקפות ([Arab.] *rāwand*: Rhubarb [*Rheum* sp.]: ... It is beneficial for chronic and intermittent fevers). Hebr. הקדחות אשר להם הקפות is not attested in the current dictionaries. In his trans. of Maimonides' *Medical Aphorisms* (i.e., *Sefer ha-Peraqim*) X.19, Nathan translates the Arab. synonym الحمّيات المفارقة as הקדחות הפוסקות (cf. BMMN 125, l. 11; BMMG no. 1144; BCD 239 (NM 2:80)). Anonymous I renders Arab. الحمّيات ذوات الأدوار as

---

306 סמסם: שומשמין Ms[1].

307 *רנציד: Emend. ed. דאנצר Ms.

308 Variant readings featuring in other Mss are: ראנצי (Ms Jerusalem, The National Library of Israel, Fr. 122, fol. 277[a]) and ראנצד (Ms Parma, Palatina, Cod. Parm. 2920, fol. 105[a]). See also J.A. Argenter and J. Ferrer, 'Jewish Texts in Old Catalan,' in: *Manual of Judaeo-Romance Linguistics and Philology*, ed. by G. Mensching and F. Savelsberg, 99–128 (Berlin 2023), 118: "*ràns yr—ràncir* variant of *ranci* 'rancid' (referring to a fatty substance that becomes chemically altered and acquires a distinctive and unpleasant smell and taste)" (DCVB 9, 131b–132a; this form with final -r is a hapax in Catalan; Ben Adret's text refers to a salted meat that has gone off.' The term *r'nsyr* should probably be corrected as *r'nsyd*, since *resh* and *dalet* are often swapped. I thank my colleague and friend Guido Mensching for this reference.

הקדחות בעלי ההקף (see previous entry). For the synonymous terms הקדחות המקיפות and הקדחות הסובבות, see entries below.

• **הקדחות המקיפות** · **intermittent fevers**: Arab. الحمّيات الدائرة (cf. SN 96 (251): 'Wechselfieber (Febres intermittentes)'; D 320: 'fièvre d'accès'; حمّى دائرة مطردة: 'fièvre périodique reglée'; حمّى دائرة غير مطردة 'fièvre intermittente') · Ibn Sīnā, *K. al-Qānūn* II · trans. Zeraḥyah Ḥen, *Sefer ha-Qanun* (Ms Oxford, Bodleian Libaries, Opp. Add. Fol. 12, fol. 180b):[309] בַּאבּוּנַג' ... ימרח עם השמן שלה בקדחות המקיפות וישתה בקדחות הישנות בסופם ([Arab.] *bābūnaj*: Camomile [*Matricaria chamomilla* L.]: ... [A liniment] of camomile is applied in intermittent fevers. It is ingested at the end of chronic fevers). Hebr. הקדחות המקיפות is not attested in the current dictionaries. Anonymous I renders Arab. الحمّيات الدائرة as הקדחות המקיפות, just like Zeraḥyah. In his trans. of Maimonides' *Medical Aphorisms* (i.e., *Sefer ha-Peraqim*) XIX.37, Zeraḥyah renders the Arab. synonym الحمّيات المقلعة as הקדחות שהם נעתקות (cf. BMMZ 180, l. 23; BMMG no. 1145).[310] The Arab. synonym الحمّيات المفارقة, featuring in Maimonides' *Medical Aphorisms*, is translated by him as הקדחות הנבדלות (X.19; cf. BMMZ 121, l. 20; BMMG no. 1144) and as הקדחות הנפסקות (XXV.23; cf. BMMZ 248, l. 4; BMMG no. 1144). For the synonymous terms הקדחות בעלי ההקף and הקדחות אשר להם הקפות, see entries above, and for הקדחות הסובבות, see next entry.

• **הקדחות הסובבות** · **intermittent fevers**: Arab. الحمّيات الدائرة · Ibn Sīnā, *K. al-Qānūn* II · trans. Anonymous I, *Sefer ha-Qanun* (Ms Paris, BnF, héb. 1142, fol. 188a–b: [311]... סכבינג מועיל מן הקדחות הסובבות ([Arab.] *sakbīnaj*: Sagapenum [i.e., the gum resin of the Persian giant fennel [*Ferula persica* Willd.]]: ... It is beneficial for intermittent fevers). Hebr. הקדחות הסובבות is not attested in the current dictionaries. Zeraḥyah Ḥen translates Arab. الحمّيات الدائرة as הקדחות המקיפות (see entry). For the synonymous terms הקדחות בעלי ההקף and הקדחות אשר להם הקפות, see entries above.

קַדְמוֹן · **chronic**: Arab. مزمن · Ibn Sīnā, *K. al-Qānūn* II · trans. Zeraḥyah Ḥen, *Sefer ha-Qanun* (Ms Oxford, Bodleian Libaries, Opp. Add. Fol. 12, fol. 260b): ... פ'רַאסִיוֹן מַרוּבִּי מיצו לכאב האוזן הארוך וינקה ופותח מעברות השמיעה ויסיר הקדמון מכאבו ([Arab. *farāsiyūn* [from Gr. πράσιον]; [i.e., Rom.] MaRWuBiY [from Lat. *marrubium*]: White horehound [*Marrubium vulgare* L.]: ... Its juice is [beneficial] for chronic earache; it cleanses and opens the auditory channels and relieves chronic pain [in the ear]). Hebr. קַדְמוֹן is not attested in this sense in the current dictionaries. A synonym used by Zeraḥyah

---

309 The same Hebr. term features on fol. 192b, entry אִפַּפּוֹנָאק '[Rom.] 'oPaPWoNa'Q: Opopanax [i.e., the resin of the sweet myrrh [*Opopanax chironius* W.D.J. Koch]],' and on fol. 249b, entry סַכַבִּינַג' סָרַפִּינוּ '[Arab.] *sakbīnaj*; [Rom.] SaRaPiYNWu: Sagapenum [i.e., the gum resin of the Persian giant fennel [*Ferula persica* Willd.]].'

310 Cf. BCD 217 (NM 1:175f.), s.v. עָתַק, *Part.* עוֹתֵק 'intermittent': הקדחות שהם עותקות, corr.: הקדחות שהם נעתקות.

311 הסובבות: מקיפות Ms1.

in the same passage is אֶרֶךְ (see entry). Nathan ha-Me'ati translates Arab. مزمن as יָשָׁן (see entry) and Anonymous I renders the Arab. term as *Part. Nif'al* נוֹשָׁן (see entry [ישן]).

קַדְמוֹנִי · **chronic**: Arab. مزمن · Ibn Sīnā, *K. al-Qānūn* II · trans. Anonymous II, *Sefer ha-Qanun* (Ms Parma, Biblioteca Palatina, Cod. Parm. 3045, fol. 26ᵇ): אפופונקו ... ועם דבש יצליח למורסות קדמוניות ולאש זר ([Rom.] 'PWPWNQW: Opopanax [i.e., the resin of the sweet myrrh [*Opopanax chironius* W.D.J. Koch]]: ... Together with honey it is beneficial for chronic ulcers and for carbuncles). Hebr. קַדְמוֹנִי is not attested in this sense in the current dictionaries. Zeraḥyah Ḥen translates Arab. مزمن as אֶרֶךְ (see entry) and Anonymous I has *Part. Nif'al* נוֹשָׁן (see entry [ישן]).

קוֹבֵץ (*Part.*) → קָבַץ.

קוֹל • נמיכות הקול → נְמִיכוּת.

קוּלִיקָא · *ileus*: Arab. إيلاوس (Gr. εἰλεός; cf. UW 222) · Ibn Sīnā, *K. al-Qānūn* II · trans. Zeraḥyah Ḥen, *Sefer ha-Qanun* (Ms Oxford, Bodleian Libaries, Opp. Add. Fol. 12, fol. 180ᵇ): בַּאבּוּנגִ׳ ... ויועיל מהקוליקא הנקראת אילאוס ([Arab.] *bābūnaj*: Camomile [*Matricaria chamomilla* L.]: ... It is beneficial for *colica*, called *ileus*). Hebr. קוליקא is a non-attested calque from Lat./Rom. *colica/colice* (cf. ND 223: 'a painful affliction in the lower abdomen; in some texts said to originate in the colon and involve pain, constipation, flatulence, nausea'). In addition to קוליקא, Zeraḥyah translates Arab. إيلاوس as חולי הקוליקא (see entry חֹלִי). Nathan ha-Me'ati renders Arab. إيلاوس as איליאוש (see entry איליאוש).

• חולי הקוליקא → חֹלִי.

קוֹלֵף (*Part.*) → קָלַף.

קוֹף · **tick**: Arab. قُراد · Ibn Sīnā, *K. al-Qānūn* II · trans. Zeraḥyah Ḥen, *Sefer ha-Qanun* (Ms Oxford, Bodleian Libaries, Opp. Add. Fol. 12, fol. 262ᵇ): פ׳סאפ׳סן הוא בעל חיים דומה לקוף ([Arab.] P̄Se'P̄YSiN [read: P̄S'P̄YS, i.e., *fasāfis*]: Bed bugs: They are living creatures (insects) similar to ticks). Reading Arab. قُراد 'tick' as قِرْد 'monkey,' Zeraḥyah mistakenly translates the Arab. term as קוֹף 'monkey.' Nathan ha-Me'ati translates Arab. قُراد as כנים עגולים (see entry כִּנָּה) and Anonymous I renders the Arab. term as פִּשְׁפֵּשׁ (see entry).

קוּפְסָא (*Aram.*) · **pod; pericarp; seed capsule**: Arab. قمع · Ibn Sīnā, *K. al-Qānūn* II · trans. Nathan ha-Me'ati, *Sefer ha-Qanun* (Ms Oxford, Bodleian Libraries, Can. Or. 88, fol. 92ᵃ): כרסנה ... אמ׳ דיאסקורידוס שהוא עשב קטן וזרעו נולד כאלו הוא מונח בקופסא ([Arab.] *kirsinna*: Bitter vetch [*Vicia ervilia* (L.) Willd.]: ... According to Dioscorides, it is a small herb with seeds [growing] in pods). Aram. קוּפְסָא is not attested in this sense in the current dictionaries. A synonym used by Nathan is קְלִפָּה (see entry). Zeraḥyah Ḥen translates Arab. قمع as פְּצֶלֶת (see entry) and Anonymous I has נְדָנָה (see entry).

קוֹץ • קוץ יהודי · **[lit. 'Jewish thorn']; eryngo, esp. field eryngo [*Eryngium campestre* L.]**: Arab. شوكة يهودية (a synonym of قرصعنة (cf. IBF no. 1360; MIG no. 821)) · *Gloss-*

ary (Ms Moscow, Russian State Library, Guenzburg 573, fol. 160[a]): שוכה יהודית ר״ל קוץ יהודי ([Arab.-Hebr.] *shawka yehudit*; i.e., [Hebr.] *qoṣ yehudi*). In the sense of 'eryngo,' Hebr. קוץ יהודי is a non-attested calque from Arab. شوكة يهودية (*shawka [al-]Yahūdiyya*).

• **קוץ מצרי · [lit. 'Egyptian thorn']; acacia tree [Acacia nilotica (L.) Delile]**: Arab. شوكة مصرية (cf. IBF no. 1362) · *Glossary* (Ms Moscow, Russian State Library, Guenzburg 573, fol. 160[a]): שוכה מצרית קוץ מצרי ([Arab.-Hebr.] *shawka miṣrit*; [i.e., Hebr.] *qoṣ miṣri*). In the sense of 'acacia tree,' Hebr. קוץ מצרי is a non-attested calque from Arab. شوكة مصرية.

קוֹצֶר → קֹצֶר.

קוֹר → קֹר.

קוּר • *Plur.* **קורים • קורי העכביש · cobweb**: Arab. نسج العنكبوت · Ibn Sīnā, *K. al-Qānūn* II · trans. Anonymous I, *Sefer ha-Qanun* (Ms Paris, BnF, héb. 1142, fol. 202[b]): ענכבות[312] ... אמרו קצתם שקורי העכביש אם יעורבו בקצת מן האיספלניות ויונח על המצח והצדעים יבריא קדחת שלישית ([Arab.] *ʿankabūt*: Spider: ... Some [physicians] said that the cobweb, when mixed with some ointments and applied to the forehead and temples, cures tertian fever). Hebr. קורי העכביש features in the current dictionaries in attestations from the Bible (cf. KB 1090) and modern Hebr. literature (cf. EM 1587). Nathan ha-Me'ati and Zeraḥyah Ḥen both translate the Arab. term as אריגת העכביש (see entry אֲרִיגָה).

[קטר] • *Hifʿil* **הִקְטִיר · to foment; to apply as fomentation**: Lat. *suffumigo* (Arab. سكب) · Constantinus Africanus, *Viaticum* V.5 · trans. Do'eg ha-Edomi, *Sefer Ya'ir Netiv*: ועם הרפואה השנית נטהר המים המכורכמים ונגרש אותם בזיעה ובהתרה וזה נעשה במרחץ ועם הקטרות כמו עם שמן קמומילא ונקח אניט מלילוד אברוטנום שמבוק כל אלה יבושלו במים ובהם נקטיר בטן החולה (With the second [kind] of remedies we cleanse and expel the yellowish fluid [of dropsy] through sweating and dissolution. This should be done by bathing and fomentations, such as with camomile oil. We should also take aneth, melilot, abrotanum, and marjoram; all these ingredients should be cooked in water and applied as a fomentation to the stomach of the patient). Hebr. *Hifʿil* הִקְטִיר features in the current dictionaries in the sense of 'to offer incense' (cf. JD 1352; BM 5895f.; EM 1595). Ben Yehuda also gives an attestation of the term in a medical context, derived from Meir Aldabi's *Shevilei Emunah*: ותשוף פי הרחם ותקטיר במשיחה קרה כמו דהן אל בלק אל בלקיה (cf. BM 5896). However, he does not explain the specific meaning of the term in this context. For the related noun הַקְטָרָה, *Plur.* הקטרות 'fomentations,' which is also used by Do'eg in his *Sefer Ya'ir Netiv* V.5, see NM 6:57. Moses ibn Tibbon translates Arab. سكب as שפך.

קִיא • השלשול והקיא → שִׁלְשׁוּל.

---

312 ענכבות: אַריינַאה עכביש Ms[1].

קִלּוּף · I. **abrasion [of the skin]**: Arab. سحج · Ibn Sīnā, *K. al-Qānūn* II · trans. Nathan ha-Me'ati, *Sefer ha-Qanun* (Ms Oxford, Bodleian Libraries, Can. Or. 88, fol. 123[a]): ... ריה ריאת הגמל תרפא הקלוף הנולד ברגל מלחץ המנעל ([Arab.] *ri'a*: Lung: ... Camel lungs heal foot abrasion caused by the pressure of the shoes). Hebr. קִלּוּף features in Rabb. literature in the sense of 'peeling' (cf. BM 5943). In addition to קִלּוּף, Nathan translates Arab. سحج as בְּקוּעַ (see entry) and Anonymous I renders the Arab. term as הפשט העור (see entry הֶפְשֵׁט).

· II. **peeling [of the skin]**: Arab. تقشير (cf. SN 251 (97), s.v. تقشير الجلد 'Desquamatio cutis') · Ibn Sīnā, *K. al-Qānūn* II · trans. Nathan ha-Me'ati, *Sefer ha-Qanun* (Ms Oxford, Bodleian Libraries, Can. Or. 88, fol. 103[b]): מיובזג' ... מיובזג' מעורב עם זרניך או לבדו יועיל אל הגרב והקלוף ([Arab.] *mayūbazaj* [from Pers. *mawīzak*]: Stavesacre [*Delphinium staphisagria* L]: ... Stavesacre as such or mixed with arsenic is useful for scabies and for peeling [of the skin]). Hebr. קִלּוּף in the sense of 'peeling' features in the current dictionaries in attestations from Rabb. literature only (cf. BM 5943). The synonymous Arab. term تقشّر الجلد, as it features in Maimonides' *Medical Aphorisms* II.25 and IX.98, is translated by Nathan (*Sefer ha-Peraqim*) as התקלפות העור (cf. BMMN 39, l. 5; 117, l. 8; BMMG no. 4111). Zeraḥyah Ḥen and Anonymous I both render Arab. تقشير as קִלּוּף as well.

קָלִי · **mush**: Arab. سويق (cf. WCD 517: 'a kind of mush made of wheat or barley (also with sugar and dates)'[313] · Ibn Sīnā, *K. al-Qānūn* II · trans. Zeraḥyah Ḥen, *Sefer ha-Qanun* (Ms Oxford, Bodleian Libaries, Opp. Add. Fol. 12, fol. 251[a]): סַדַאבְּ ... יחדד הראות וכל שכן מיצו עם מיץ השומר והדבש לכחול בו וגם לאכלו וגם יחובש בו עם הקלי על חבטת העין ([Arab.] *sadhāb*: Common rue [*Ruta graveolens* L.]: ... It strengthens the eyesight, especially when its juice is taken orally or used as a eye powder along with fennel juice and honey. Moreover, it is plastered with mush in cases of throbbing sensation in the eyes). A Hebr. synonym for Arab. سويق, i.e., גריש, *Plur.* גרישים, features in Zeraḥyah's trans. of Maimonides' *Medical Aphorisms* (i.e., *Sefer ha-Peraqim*) V.19 (cf. BMMZ 59, l. 6; BMMG no. 2566; cf. also BCD 50 (NM 4:36) for Hebr. גריסים and BCD 51 (NM 4:36) for Hebr. גריש החטה). Nathan ha-Me'ati transcribes Arab. سويق as סויק and Anonymous I has קמח קלי, a term also featuring in Nathan's *Sefer ha-Peraqim* IX.4 (cf. BMMN 103, l. 16; BMMG no. 2566; BCD 245 (NM 2:82)).

קָלַף • *Part.* קוֹלֵף • הרפואה הקולפת → רְפוּאָה.

• *Part. Pi'el* מְקַלֵּף · **peeling (exfoliating)**: Arab. مقشّر · Ibn Sīnā, *K. al-Qānūn* II · trans. Nathan ha-Me'ati, *Sefer ha-Qanun* (Ms Oxford, Bodleian Libraries, Can. Or. 88, fol. 103[b]): מאזריון לאבריולה ... הוא חד[314] מקלף וחריפותו חזק ([Arab.] *māzaryūn*; [i.e., Lat./Rom.] L'BRYWLH [i.e., M. Lat. or O. Occ. *laureola*]: February daphne [*Daphne*

---

313 See also MSh no. 284 (trans. Rosner): 'Semolina: It is wheat, barley and other similar roasted cereals, agitated with butter and then ground.' See also NA 572f.; NT 477; LFF 68.

314 חד: جال a.

mezereum L.]: … It is clearing,[315] purifying, peeling (exfoliating), and very pungent). Hebr. *Pi'el* קִלֵּף features in the sense of 'to peel' in BM 5968 in attestations from Rabb. literature only. Zeraḥyah Ḥen translates Arab. مقشّر as *Part. Pi'el* מְפַזֵּר (see entry [פזר]) and Anonymous I has מְקַלֵּף, just like Nathan. Arab. الدواء القاشر 'the peeling (exfoliating) drug' is translated by Nathan as הסם המקלף (see entry סַם).

• הסם המקלף → סַם.

קְלִפָּה · **I. pod; pericarp; seed capsule**: Arab. قمع · Ibn Sīnā, *K. al-Qānūn* II · trans. Nathan ha-Me'ati, *Sefer ha-Qanun* (Ms Oxford, Bodleian Libraries, Can. Or. 88, fol. 125[b]): תודרי המהות אמר דיאסקורידוס הוא עשב שדומין עליו לעלי אלפראסיון ושוקו[316] מרובע ובו כמו חצי אמה ויש לו קלפות בהם זרע ארוך ושחור ([Arab.] *tūdharī*: Hedge mustard [*Sisymbrium officinale* (L.) Scop.]: What is it? Dioscorides states that it is a herb bearing leaves like white horehound. Its root[317] is quadrangular and measures nearly half a cubit; its pods have oblong black seeds). Hebr. קְלִפָּה features in Rabb. literature in the sense of 1) 'peeling; scaling;' 2) 'scale; husk; skin' (cf. JD 1377); or 3) 'shell; peel' (cf. BM 5970). For different meanings in medieval medical literature, cf. BCD 244. In addition to קְלִפָּה, Nathan translates Arab. قمع as צִיץ (see entry). Zeraḥyah Ḥen translates Arab. قمع as פְּצֹלֶת (see entry) and Anonymous I has פְּטוֹטֶרֶת (see entry).

· **II. rust**: Arab. صدأ (cf. KM 752f.) · Ibn Sīnā, *K. al-Qānūn* II · trans. Zeraḥyah Ḥen, *Sefer ha-Qanun* (Ms Oxford, Bodleian Libaries, Opp. Add. Fol. 12, fol. 216[a]): חַדִּיד: ברזל … קליפתו עם היין על הפודאגרא יועיל ([Arab.] *ḥadīd*; [i.e., Hebr.] *barzel*: Iron: … [Iron] rust, if taken with wine, is useful in gout). Nathan ha-Me'ati translates Arab. صدأ as חלודה.

· **III. eschar**: Lat. *escar* · Guy de Chauliac, *Inventarium sive Chirurgia Magna* (cf. CMM 1:419, ll. 10–11) · trans. Anonymous (Ms Paris, BnF, héb. 1189, fol. 229[a]): מהכווים בכח התרופות שבהן תעשינה הכויות בכח הם מבקעים כי יש מהם שמניחים אחריהם קליפה (Part of the potential cauteries are medicines that can be used for cauterization; such as medicines that induce rupture, for some of them leave behind eschar). In the sense of 'eschar,' Hebr. קְלִפָּה is attested (for Arab. خشكريشة) in BCD 244 (NM 1:112f.) in an attestation from Shem Tov ben Isaac's *Sefer ha-Shimmush* XXX.1.52.

• **הקלפה היבשה** · **eschar (slough)**: Arab. خشكريشة (Gr. ἐσχάρα; cf. UW 270) · Ibn Sīnā, *K. al-Qānūn* II · trans. Nathan ha-Me'ati, *Sefer ha-Qanun* (Ms Oxford, Bodleian Libraries, Can. Or. 88, fol. 81[b]):[318] זאג … כולם שורפים מולידים הקלפה היבשה הנקרא חשכרישה בערבי והם קובצין ([Arab.] *zāj*: Vitriol: … All kinds of vitriol are caustic, produce eschar

315 'clearing': Trans. acc. to a.

316 ושוקו: وجدره a.

317 'Its root': Trans. acc. to a.

318 The same Hebr. term features on fol. 63[b], entry אקחואן '[Arab.] *uqḥuwān*: Feverfew [*Tanacetum parthenium* (L.) Sch. Bip.].'

(slough), called *khashkarīsha* in Arab., and are astringent). Hebr. הקלפה היבשה does not feature in the current dictionaries. Zeraḥyah Ḥen translates Arab. خشكريشة as Lat. קְרוּשְׁטַא (i.e., *crusta*; cf. ND 264) and Anonymous I renders the Arab. term as צָרֶבֶת (cf. BCD 233 (NM 2:77f.) for an attestation from Nathan's trans. of Maimonides' *Medical Aphorisms* (i.e., *Sefer ha-Peraqim*) XV.9, where Nathan translates Arab. خشكريشة as כשכרישה הוא צרבת (cf. BMMN 155, l. 18; BMMG no. 1356 (corr.))).

• *Plur.* **קלפות • קלפות הברזל** · **iron slag (scoria)**: Lat. *scoria ferri* · Guy de Chauliac, *Inventarium sive Chirurgia Magna* (cf. CMM 1:237, ll. 26–27) · trans. Anonymous (Ms Paris, BnF, héb. 1189, fol. 130[a]): אמנם אם הם נושנים אז יעשה משיחה מקלפות הברזל תעמוד זמן רב בשמש (But if they [i.e., ulcers in the ears] become chronic, one should prepare a salve from iron slag, which should be left in the sun for a long time). Hebr. קלפות הברזל is not attested in the current dictionaries. For the synonymous אבק הברזל (for Lat. *ferrugo*), featuring in Do'eg ha-Edomi's trans. of Constantinus Africanus' *Viaticum* (i.e., *Sefer Ya'ir Netiv*) IV.19, see NM 6:13.

קְלִפִּי · **crusted**: Lat. *crustosus* · Guy de Chauliac, *Inventarium sive Chirurgia Magna* (cf. CMM 1:233, ll. 34–35) · trans. Anonymous (Ms Paris, BnF, héb. 1189, fol. 127[b]): אמנם אם הוא מזוהם וקלפי ירוחץ המקום עם יין ודבש (But if the [ulcer/polyp in the nose] is sordid and crusted, the spot should be washed with wine and honey). Hebr. קְלִפִּי features in the sense of 'scaly' (re: animal) in BM 5971 in an attestation from Simeon ben Zemah Duran.

[קנח] • *Pi'el* **קִנֵּחַ** · **to rub**: Arab. مسح · Ibn Sīnā, *K. al-Qānūn* II · trans. Zeraḥyah Ḥen, *Sefer ha-Qanun* (Ms Oxford, Bodleian Libaries, Opp. Add. Fol. 12, fol. 255[a]): עַאקִר קַרְחָא הוא פִּילְטְרוּ ... עם יעורב עם שמן ויקנח בו ירבה בזיעה ([Arab.] *'āqirqarḥā*; i.e., [Rom.] PiYLəṬəRWu: Pellitory [*Anacyclus pyrethrum* (L.) Lag.]: ... When it is mixed with oil and rubbed [on the body], it increases perspiration). In the sense of 'to rub,' Hebr. *Pi'el* קִנֵּחַ features in BM 6023 in attestations from Rabb. literature. Nathan ha-Me'ati and Anonymous I both render Arab. مسح as משח.

קֶצֶף · **clarified butter**: Arab. زبد (cf. LFF 321) · Ibn Sīnā, *K. al-Qānūn* II · trans. Zeraḥyah Ḥen, *Sefer ha-Qanun* (Ms Oxford, Bodleian Libaries, Opp. Add. Fol. 12, fol. 252[a]): סַמְן חמאה ... הוא פועל פעולת הקצף והוא יותר חזק בבישול וברפיון ובחלקות ובחימום פעולת הקצף ([Arab.] *samn*; [i.e., Hebr.] *ḥem'ah*: (Fresh) butter: ... Its action is similar to that of clarified butter, but it is stronger in maturing, relaxing, loosening, and warming). Hebr. קֶצֶף only features in the current dictionaries in the sense of 'froth,' cf. BM 6105f. Nathan ha-Me'ati and Anonymous I both render Arab. زبد as חמאה.

• **קצף הזהב** · **gold calamine**: Arab. إقليميا الذهب (cf. MIG no. 859) · *Glossary* (Ms Moscow, Russian State Library, Guenzburg 573, fol. 158[b]): קלימיה אלדהב ר"ל קצף הזהב ([Arab.] *qalīmiyā al-dhahab*; i.e., [Hebr.] *qeṣev ha-zahav*). Hebr. קצף הזהב does not feature in the current dictionaries. A synonymous סיג הזהב features in Moses ibn Tibbon's trans. of Ibn al-Jazzār's *Zād al-musāfir* (i.e., *Sefer Ṣedat ha-Derakhim*) II.6.7 (cf. BCD 185 (NM 4:119); IJZ 1–2:493).

• **קצף הכסף** · **silver calamine**: Arab. إقليميا الفضّة (cf. MIG no. 859) · *Glossary* (Ms Moscow, Russian State Library, Guenzburg 573, fol. 158[b]): קלימיה אלפצה ר"ל קצף הכסף ([Arab.] *qalīmiyā al-fiḍḍa*; i.e., [Hebr.] *qeṣev ha-kesef*). Hebr. קצף הכסף does not feature in the current dictionaries. A synonymous סיג הכסף features in Moses ibn Tibbon's trans. of Ibn al-Jazzār's *Zād al-musāfir* (i.e., *Sefer Ṣedat ha-Derakhim*) I.7.1 (cf. BCD 185 (NM 4:119); IJZ 1–2:450).

• **קצף המלח** · **salt efflorescence; salt scum**: Arab. زهر(ة) الملح (Gr. ἄνθος ἁλός; cf. KM 684ff.) · Ibn Sīnā, *K. al-Qānūn* II · trans. Nathan ha-Me'ati, *Sefer ha-Qanun* (Ms Oxford, Bodleian Libraries, Can. Or. 88, fol. 105[a]): מלח ... וקצפו יותר רקיק ממנו (Salt: ... The efflorescence of it [i.e., salt] is finer (more rarefying) than [the salt itself]). Hebr. קצף המלח is not attested in the current dictionaries. Zeraḥyah Ḥen translates Arab. زهر(ة) الملح as פרח המלח (see entry פֶּרַח) and Anonymous I combines both terms as קצף ופרח המלח.

קֹצֶר • **קוצר הנשימה** · **asthma (dyspnea; panting)**: Arab. ربو · Ibn Sīnā, *K. al-Qānūn* II · trans. Nathan ha-Me'ati, *Sefer ha-Qanun* (Ms Oxford, Bodleian Libraries, Can. Or. 88, fol. 77[a–b]): דוד ... התולעים האדומים הרומשים תחת המים מרובי הרגלים כשלוקחים אותם ומחככים אותם בדבש יועילו מהחניקות וכן אם אוכלים מהם ויועילו מקוצר הנשימה והצבת הנשימה ([Arab.] *dūd*: Worms: ... The red multi-legged worms that creep beneath the water, if one takes them and rubs the palate with them together with honey they are beneficial for quinsy; and if one eats them they are good for asthma (dyspnea; panting) and orthopnea). Hebr. קוצר הנשימה features (for Lat. *strictura in flatu*) in NM 5:179 in the sense of 'breathlessness; shortness of breath (orthopnea)' in an attestation from Do'eg ha-Edomi's trans. of Constantinus Africanus' *Viaticum* (i.e., *Sefer Ya'ir Netiv*) III.7. In addition to קוצר הנשימה, Nathan translates Arab. ربو as עוצר הנשימה (see entry עֹצֶר). Zeraḥyah Ḥen translates Arab. ربو as Lat./Rom. אסמו and Anonymous I has גניחה. The latter term also features throughout in Nathan's trans. of Maimonides' *Medical Aphorisms* (i.e., *Sefer ha-Peraqim*) (cf. BCD 47 (NM 2:34f.); BMMG no. 2043).

קֹר · **feverish chill**: Arab. نافض · Ibn Sīnā, *K. al-Qānūn* II · trans. Zeraḥyah Ḥen, *Sefer ha-Qanun* (Ms Oxford, Bodleian Libaries, Opp. Add. Fol. 12, fol. 190[b]): בנאת[319] וורדאן ... מועיל להקור הנקרא ריגור בלעז ([Arab.] *banāt wardān*: Cockroach: ... It is useful for feverish chill, called *rigor* in Rom.). Hebr. קר does not feature in the sense of 'feverish chill' in the current dictionaries. In his trans. of Maimonides' *Medical Aphorisms* (i.e., *Sefer ha-Peraqim*) (cf. BMMG no. 5245), Zeraḥyah renders نافض also as רִיגוֹר (see entry), פַּלָּצוּת (cf. BCD 221 (NM 3:189) for attestations from Moses ibn Tibbon's trans. of Maimonides' *Commentary on Hippocrates'* Aphorisms (i.e., *Perush Aphorismi shel Apuqraṭ*) IV.46, VII.4 (cf. BMCH 1:367, l. 15; 406, l. 11)) and קְרִירוּת (cf. BCD 250

319 בנאת וורדאן: Emend. ed. נַבֵאת וורְדֵאן Ms بنات وردان a.

(NM 1:185); BMMZ 78, l. 20; BMMG no. 5245). Nathan ha-Me'ati translates the Arab. term as נְעִירָה (cf. NM 6:141) and Anonymous I has רֶתֶת (cf. BCD 267 (NM 3:223) for an attestation from Do'eg ha-Edomi's trans. of Hippocrates' *Aphorisms* (i.e., *Sefer Agur*) IV.46; see also Nathan's *Sefer ha-Peraqim* (cf. BMMG no. 5245).

• **בקיעי הקור** → בָּקִיעַ.

• **בקיעות הקור** → בְּקִיעָה.

קראטין • **מי הקראטין** → מַיִם.

קרבונקלי · **nausea**: Arab. غثيان (cf. FL 1:148) · Ibn Sīnā, *K. al-Qānūn* II · trans. Zeraḥyah Ḥen, *Sefer ha-Qanun* (Ms Oxford, Bodleian Libaries, Opp. Add. Fol. 12, fol. 212^{b}): נַאנְכְּוַה[320] אַמֵיאוּשׁ ... יועיל מבלילת האצטומכא וישכך הקרבונקלי והתהפך הנפש ([Arab.] *nānakhwāh*; [i.e., Lat./Rom.] 'aMeY'WŠ [i.e., L. Lat./O. Occ./O. Cat./O. Sp. *ameos*; cf. SHS 1:337 (Nun 3)]: Bisnaga (toothpickweed) [*Ammi visnaga* (L.) Lam.]: ... It is beneficial for [excessive] moisture in the stomach, it alleviates nausea, and it [is good for] a stomach that is upset). Hebr. קרבונקלי is a non-attested calque from Rom. *carbuncle* (cf. ND 165) (for Arab. غثيان), featuring, next to קרבונקל, throughout Zeraḥyah's *Sefer ha-Qanun* and other medical works (e.g., Maimonides' *Medical Aphorisms* (i.e., *Sefer ha-Peraqim*); cf. BMMG nos. 3617/3618).[321] Nathan ha-Me'ati and Anonymous I both render Arab. غثيان as אִסְטְנִסוּת (cf. BCD 24 (NM 2:30), a.o., for, an attestation from Nathan's *Sefer ha-Peraqim* XIII.54 (cf. BMMN 152, l. 18; BMMG no. 3618)).

• **מוריש הקרבונקלי** → [ירש].

קָרָה • **המורסות אשר יקרו בעת המגפה** → מֻרְסָה.

קְרוּם • **בקיעות קרום האשך** → בְּקִיעָה.

קָרוּשׁ • **מיץ קרוש** → מִיץ.

קֶרִי • **החלום בראית קרי** → חֲלוֹם.

קְרִיעָה · **hernia**: Arab. فتق (Gr. ἐντεροκήλη; cf. UW 245) · Ibn Sīnā, *K. al-Qānūn* II · trans. Zeraḥyah Ḥen, *Sefer ha-Qanun* (Ms Oxford, Bodleian Libaries, Opp. Add. Fol. 12, fol. 251^{b}): סַם אַבְרָץ בלע' שְׁגוּמִיל ... והוא מועיל מאד בקריעה ([Arab.] *sāmm*[322] *abraṣ*; i.e., Rom. ŚGWuMiYL: Lizard (gecko): ... They are very beneficial for hernia). Hebr. קְרִיעָה is not attested in this sense in the current dictionaries. Nathan ha-Me'ati translates Arab. فتق as הֶתֶר (see entry) and Anonymous I has בקיעות קרום האשך (see entry בְּקִיעָה).

---

320 נַאנְכְּוַה: Emend. ed. נַאנְכָּה Ms.

321 For the Hebr. term מוריש הקרבונקלי (for Arab. مغث 'causing nausea'), see entry [ירש].

322 *sāmm abraṣ* (سام أبرص) 'lizard (gecko)': Cf. Aristotle, PA660b6–7: οἱ σαῦροι (cf. LSG 1586); idem, *K. al-Ḥayawān* (ed. Kruk, 55: السام أبرص); Lane 188, s.v. سامّ أبرص: 'the species of lizard described above, voce بُرص: A species of the lizard called gecko, of a leprous hue;' FL 2:349: 'lacerta magnae species;' JAD 2:23: 'Lexicologists state that it is one of the large kinds of geckos;' ibid. n. 1: 'A species of gecko. In Egypt gen. Ptyodactylus;' D 1:680: 'salamandre.'

קְרִירוּת • בקיעות הקרירות → בְּקִיעָה.

קרישטיר • עשה קרישטיר → עָשָׂה.

קֶרֶן • בעל הקרן → בַּעַל.

• *Plur.* קרנים • בעל הקרנים → בַּעַל.

קָשֶׁה • מורסות קשות → מֻרְסָה.

קִשּׁוּט · **pain relief; palliative care**: Lat. *pallior* · Guy de Chauliac, *Inventarium sive Chirurgia Magna* (cf. CMM 1: 238, l. 33) · trans. Anonymous (Ms Paris, BnF, héb. 1189, fol. 130[b]): אמנם המפולשים הם תחת סוג הנאצורים שבהם כמו שנאמ׳ לא יועיל להם הרפוי רק יספיק להם הקשוט (But penetrating [ulcers] belong to the categorie of fistulas (*nāsūrim*); as I said before healing is not beneficial in their case, but pain relief is sufficient). Hebr. קִשּׁוּט is not attested in this sense in the current dictionaries.

קִשּׁוּר · **stiffness**: Arab. تعقّد (Gr. ἀγκύλη; cf. UW 67) · Ibn Sīnā, *K. al-Qānūn* II · trans. Nathan ha-Me'ati, *Sefer ha-Qanun* (Ms Oxford, Bodleian Libraries, Can. Or. 88, fol. 102[a]): מקל אליהוד ומקל אלמכי ... יועיל מבקיע העצל ומן הקווץ והוא תשנג׳ בערבי ומקושי העצבים וקשורם ([Arab.] *muql*[323] *al-Yahūd* and [Arab.] *muql Makkī*: Judean and Meccan bdellium: ... It is useful in muscle rupture, spasms, i.e., *tashannuj* in Arab., and hardness and stiffness of the nerves). In the sense of 'stiffness,' Hebr. קִשּׁוּר is a non-attested semantic borrowing from Arab. تعقّد. Zeraḥyah Ḥen translates Arab. تعقّد as עִקּוּד (see entry) and Anonymous I has הִתְקַשְּׁרוּת (see entry). A synonym of Arab. تعقّد, i.e., تحجّر, featuring as تحجّر المفاصل 'stiffness of the joints (ankylosis)' in the *K. al-Qānūn* II, is translated by Nathan as אִבּוּן (cf. NM 6:13, s.v. אבון הפרקים).

[קשט] • *Pi'el* קִשֵּׁט · **to relief pain (to provide palliative care)**: Lat. *pallio* · Guy de Chauliac, *Inventarium sive Chirurgia Magna* (cf. CMM 1:227, ll. 20–22) · trans. Anonymous (Ms Paris, BnF, héb. 1189, fol. 124[b]): כי בכמו אלה הנה הסכמתי יותר לקשט מלרפאת (For in such cases, I agree that it is better to relief pain than to cure). Hebr. *Pi'el* קִשֵּׁט is not attested in this sense in the current dictionaries.

• *Pu'al* קֻשַּׁט · **to be relieved from pain (to be provided with palliative care)**: Lat. *pallior* · Guy de Chauliac, *Inventarium sive Chirurgia Magna* (cf. CMM 1:232, ll. 21–22) · trans. Anonymous (Ms Paris, BnF, héb. 1189, fol. 127[a]): ואם לא יוכל לעשות עוד יקושט המקום כמו שנאמר למעלה ועם זה הקילור משובח מאד מטדריק (If nothing more can be done, [the pain caused by] the spot should be relieved, as I said above; the following collyrium is strongly recommended by Theodoric [Borgognoni]). See previous entry.

קֹשִׁי • קשי הנשימה · **asthma (dyspnea; panting)**: Arab. ربو · al-Rāzī, *K. fī al-Faṣd* · trans. Anonymous, *Ma'amar ba-Haqqazah* (Ms Parma, Biblioteca Palatina, Cod. Parm. 2283,4, fol. 93[b]): וב׳ גידים הנק׳ אלודג׳ין ומקומם בצואר ותועיל הקזתם לנמיכות הקול הנק׳

---

323 '*muql*': I.e., bdellium, i.e., the gum resin of plants from the *Burseraceae* family, esp. *Commiphora africana* (A.Rich.) Endl. and *Commiphora mukul* (Hook. ex Stocks) Engl.

(Two veins called 'jugular veins,' their location is in the neck, bleeding them is beneficial for hoarseness of the voice called [in Arab.] *buḥūḥat al-ṣawt*, lung pain, asthma (dyspnea; panting), called [in Arab.] *al-rabw*, and elephantiasis). ⟨אל⟩בחוחה אלצות ולכאב הריאה ולקשי הנשימה הנק' אלרבו ולחלי הצרעת[324] Hebr. קשי הנשימה is not attested in the current dictionaries. Synonyms featuring in medieval Hebr. medical literature are מצוק הנשימה (cf. NM 6:125) and צרות הניפוש/הנשימה (cf. BMMG no. 3059).

קִשְׁקוּשׁ • קישקוש בפה · rinsing the mouth; mouthwash: Arab. مضمضة (Gr. διάκλυσμα; cf. UW 195) · Ibn Sīnā, *K. al-Qānūn* II · trans. Zeraḥyah Ḥen, *Sefer ha-Qanun* (Ms Oxford, Bodleian Libaries, Opp. Add. Fol. 12, fols. 232ᵇ–233ᵇ: לבן חלב ... ועוד החלב מתרופות נגעי הריאה והטיסיש ויועיל הקישקוש בו בפה והגרגרים מן החנק והזביחה ומורסות האוולא ושתי השקדים ([Arab.] *laban*; [i.e., Hebr.] *ḥalav* Milk: ... Milk is also a [good] medicine for pulmonary ulcers and phthisis. Rinsing the mouth and gargling [with milk] is useful in diphtheria, angina, swollen uvula (uvillitis), and swollen tonsils (tonsillitis)). Hebr. קישקוש בפה is not attested in the current dictionaries. Zeraḥyah also translates Arab. مضمضة as קשקש בפה (see next entry קִשְׁקֵשׁ) and Anonymous I renders Arab. مضمضة as מִצְמוּץ (cf. NM 6:126).

קִשְׁקֵשׁ • קשקש בפה · to rinse one's mouth; to use as a mouthwash: Arab. مضمضة · Ibn Sīnā, *K. al-Qānūn* II · trans. Zeraḥyah Ḥen, *Sefer ha-Qanun* (Ms Oxford, Bodleian Libaries, Opp. Add. Fol. 12, fol. 174ᵃ): אִעַאלוּג׳ ... המקשקש בפיו מבישולו ייטיב ריח הפה ([Arab.] *aghālūjī*: Agarwood [*Aquilaria malaccensis* Lam.]: ... If one rinses one's mouth with a decoction of it, it improves [bad] breath). Hebr. קשקש בפה is not attested in the current dictionaries. Zeraḥyah also translates Arab. مضمضة as קישקוש בפה (see previous entry קִשְׁקוּשׁ). Nathan ha-Me'ati translates Arab. مضمضة as רחץ הפה (see entry רָחַץ) and Anonymous I renders the Arab. term as מִצְמוּץ (cf. NM 6:126). Zeraḥyah translates the verb تمضمض in his trans. of Maimonides' *Medical Aphorisms* (i.e., *Sefer ha-Peraqim*) as רחץ הפה (XXI.10; cf. BMMZ 194, l. 16; BMMG no. 4867) and as העביר בתוך הפה (XXII.68; cf. BMMZ 215, l. 9; BMMG no. 4867).

קֶשֶׁר • *Plur.* **קשרים · nodules**: Arab. عقدة, *Plur.* عقد · Ibn Sīnā, *K. al-Qānūn* II · trans. Nathan ha-Me'ati, *Sefer ha-Qanun* (Ms Paris, BnF, héb. 1136, fol. 76ᵃ): וג המהות הוא שורש צמח צומח על הרוב בשפתות הנהרות על זה השורש יש קשרים לבנים בו ריח נתעב ([Arab.] *wajj*: Sweet flag [*Acorus calamus* L.]: What is it? It is the root of a plant that mostly grows on river banks. It has roots that bear white nodules and it has a bad smell). Hebr. קֶשֶׁר, *Plur.* קשרים, is not attested in this sense in the current dictionaries. For different meanings in a medical context, cf. BCD 253f. Anonymous I renders Arab. عقد as קשרים, just like Nathan, and Zeraḥyah Ḥen translates Arab. عقد as עקודים (see entry עִקּוּד).

---

324 ולחלי הצרעת: و الجذام a.

ראוּת • חולשת הראות ← חֻלְשָׁה.

• כסוי הראות ← כִּסּוּי.

רְאִיָּה • חחלום בראית קרי ← חֲלוֹם.

ראֹשׁ • הזלות הראש ← הֲזָלָה.

• כאב חצי הראש ← כְּאֵב.

• נקרת הראש ← נִקְרָה.

• *Plur.* **ראשים • ראשי הירכים** · **groin**: Arab. أربية · Ibn Sīnā, *K. al-Qānūn* II · trans. Nathan ha-Me'ati, *Sefer ha-Qanun* (Ms Oxford, Bodleian Libraries, Can. Or. 88, fol. 114[a]):[325] ערק הוא זיעה ... זיעת המתאבקים יועיל ממורסת ראשי הירכים ובערבי ארביה ויתיך אותם ([Arab.] *ʿaraq*; i.e., [Hebr.] *ze'ah*: Sweat: ... The sweat of wrestlers is beneficial for swellings in the groin, [called] in Arab. *urbiyah*, and dissolves them). Hebr. ראשי הירכים is not attested in the current dictionaries. In his trans. of Maimonides' *Medical Aphorisms* (i.e., *Sefer ha-Peraqim*) XIX.32, Nathan translates Arab. أربية as אורבים (cf. BMMN 182, l. 19; BMMG no. 34). Zeraḥyah Ḥen translates Arab. أربية as טִיטִילִי and Anonymous I renders the Arab. term as שד.

[רבב] • *Part. Puʿal* **מְרוּבָּב** · **rob [i.e., fruit or vegetable juice boiled down to syrup]**: a) Arab. مربّى or مربّب (cf. FAQ 247ff., also featuring as *murabbab*) · Ibn Sīnā, *K. al-Qānūn* II · trans. Zeraḥyah Ḥen, *Sefer ha-Qanun* (Ms Oxford, Bodleian Libaries, Opp. Add. Fol. 12, fol. 226[a]): כַּרְפַּס ... מתיר לנפיחה פותח לסתימה מזיע משכך לכאב והמדברי מנגע מחליא והמרובב ממנו יותר ניאות למחוממים (Celery [*Apium graveolens* L.]: ... It relieves flatulence. It opens blockages, induces perspiration, and allays pain. The wild variety is ulcerating and causes pain; its rob is more suitable for those who have a hot temperament). In the sense of 'rob,' Hebr. מְרוּבָּב is a non-attested semantic borrowing from Arab. مربّى or مربّب. Nathan translates Arab. مربّى as מָעוֹג (cf. NM 6:121f.). Synonyms used by Zeraḥyah are *Part. Puʿal* מְגֻדָּל (see entry [גדל]) and מרוקח עם דבש (cf. NM 6:122, s.v. מָעוֹג). Anonymous I renders Arab. مربّى as *Part. Puʿal* מְרוּקָּח (see entry [רקח]).

· b) Arab. ربّ · Ibn Sīnā, *K. al-Qānūn* II · trans. Zeraḥyah Ḥen, *Sefer ha-Qanun* (Ms Oxford, Bodleian Libaries, Opp. Add. Fol. 12, fol. 228[a]): כֻּמַּתְּרֵי ... וראוי שישתה אחריהם מי הדבש עם הבשמים ומרבבו מועיל לשילשול הקולירִיקו ([Arab.] *kummathrā*: Pear [*Pyrus communis* L.]: ... After its [consumption,] one should drink honey water with aromatics. Its rob is useful for treating bilious diarrhea). In addition to מְרוּבָּב, Zeraḥyah renders Arab. ربّ as מירבב in his *Sefer ha-Qanun* II (see entry). Nathan ha-Me'ati translates Arab. ربّ as עסיס מבושל (see entry עָסִיס).

325 The same Hebr. term also features on fol. 103[b] (for Arab. أربية), entry מרזנגוש '[Arab.] *marzanjūsh*: Marjoram [*Origanum majorana* L.]'.

[רבה] • *Hif'il* **הִרְבָּה** • **הרבה השתן** · **to cause diuresis:** Arab. أدرّ البول (Gr. διουρητικός; cf. UWS 1:202) · Ibn Sīnā, *K. al-Qānūn* II · trans. Zeraḥyah Ḥen, *Sefer ha-Qanun* (Ms Oxford, Bodleian Libaries, Opp. Add. Fol. 12, fol. 243ᵃ): מַוְז ... יוסיף בזרע והוא ניאות לכליות וירבה השתן ([Arab.] *mawz*: Banana [*Musa paradisiaca* L.]: ... It increases the sperm, is suitable for kidney [ailments] and causes diuresis). Hebr. הרבה השתן is not attested in the current dictionaries. Nathan ha-Me'ati and Anonymous I both render Arab. أدرّ البول as הגיר השתן (see entry [נגר]).

רֶגֶל • **רגל עורב** · **buckhorn plantain [*Plantago coronopus* L.]**: Arab. رجل الغراب (cf. IBF no. 1031) · *Glossary* (Ms Moscow, Russian State Library, Guenzburg 573, fol. 159ᵃ): רג'ל אלג'ראב הוא רגל עורב ([Arab.] *rijl al-ghurāb*; i.e., [Hebr.] *regel 'orev*). In the sense of 'buckhorn plantain,' Hebr. רגל עורב is a non-attested calque from Arab. رجل الغراب.

• *Dual* **רגלים** • **רגלי החגבים** · **Indian plum [*Flacourtia jangomas* (Lour.) Raeusch.] (?)**: Arab. أرجل الجراد (the identification of the term is problematic; it is probably identical with Arab. *zarnab* (cf. MIG no. 923; MSh no. 137); the latter term stands most probably for 'Indian plum [*Flacourtia jangomas* (Lour.) Raeusch.]' (cf. MIG no. 317)) · Ibn Sīnā, *K. al-Qānūn* II · trans. Zeraḥyah Ḥen, *Sefer ha-Qanun* (Ms Oxford, Bodleian Libaries, Opp. Add. Fol. 12, fol. 230ᵇ): לשון השור המהות עשב רחב העלים כמו המרו ועצו[326] חלק וענפים גסים כמו רגלי החגבים ומראהו בין ירקות ואתרוגיות ([Hebr.] *leshon ha-shor* [lit. 'ox tongue']: Borage [*Borago officinalis* L.]: What is it? It is a plant with wide leaves like cat thyme and[327] those are rough in touch, and the wood of its branches is like that of Indian plum (?) and its color is yellowish green). Hebr. רגלי החגבים is a non-attested calque from Arab. أرجل الجراد. Nathan ha-Me'ati translates the Arab. term as חגבים and Anonymous I has רגלי החגב.

• **יתדות הרגלים** → יָתֵד.

• **מכאוב הרגלים** → מַכְאוֹב.

[רדם] • *Part. Hif'il* **מַרְדִּים** • **הסם המרדים החוש** → סַם.

רוּחַ • **הסם המשבר הרוח** → סַם.

• **הרפואה המשברת הרוח** → רְפוּאָה.

• *Plur.* **רוחות** • **רוחות הפה** · **yawning:** Arab. تثاؤب · al-Rāzī, *K. fī al-Faṣd* · trans. Anonymous, *Ma'amar ba-Haqqazah* (Ms Parma, Biblioteca Palatina, Cod. Parm. 2283,4, fol. 92ᵇ): התפשטות[328] האי⟨...⟩ ורוחות הפה הנק' אלתמטא ואלתתאב וכובד הראש וגדל הדפק ועבי השתן ואדמימותו וכובד[329] הרגשת האיברים ורפיון הדעת ומתיקות הפה ונגעיו ויציאת הדם מנחיריו והצמחים הנק' אלדממאל הנפתחים מהרה ([Symptoms of overfilling with blood]: Stretching[330] [...] and yawning, called [in Arab.] *al-tamaṭṭā wa-al-tathā'ub*,

---

326 ועצו חלק וענפים גסים: وخشنه الملمس وقضبان خشبه a.

327 'and those are rough in touch, and the wood of its branches': Trans. acc. to a.

328 התפשטות האי: والتمطي⟨...⟩ a.

329 וכובד˚ הרגשת האיברים: Emend. ed. וכובד הרעשת האיברים Ms وكدر الحواس a.

330 'Stretching (والتمطي)': The Arab. term is possibly synonymous with التثاؤب; cf. DBK 2:1124, s.v. تمطى 'étendre les bras en baillant' (stretching the arms while yawning).

heaviness of the head, magnitude of pulse, thick and red urine, troubled[331] sensations, apathy, sweetness of the mouth, its vesication, nosebleeds, and boils, called [in Arab.] *al-damāmīl*, which burst quickly). Hebr. רוחות הפה is not attested in the current dictionaries. In their trans. of Maimonides' *Medical Aphorisms* (i.e., *Sefer ha-Peraqim*) IX.42, Nathan ha-Me'ati translates Arab. تثاؤب as פיהוק הנקרא בדאלייאר (cf. BMMN 108, ll. 16–17; BMMG no. 4919) and Zeraḥyah Ḥen has גיהוק (cf. BMMZ 103, l. 23; BMMG no. 4919).

- **מפזר הרוחות** → [פזר].
- **שיבר הרוחות** → [שבר].
- **השליך הרוחות** → [שלך].

רוּחִי · **gaseous**: Arab. ريحي · Ibn Sīnā, *K. al-Qānūn* II · trans. Anonymous I, *Sefer ha-Qanun* (Ms Paris, BnF, héb. 1142, fols. 93b–94a: חנטל ... משלשל הלבנה העבה מן הפרקים והעצבים ביחוד ומשלשל גם כן המרות ומועיל מן קולנג' הלח והרוחי מאד) ([Arab.] *ḥanẓal*: Colocynth [*Citrullus colocynthis* (L.) Schrad.]: ... It purges thick phlegm out of the joints and especially the nerves; it also purges the biles and it is beneficial for very moist, gaseous colic). Hebr. רוּחִי features in BM 6494, a.o., in an attestation from the *Sefer ha-Qanun* and is translated by Ben Yehuda as 'windy; airy.' Nathan ha-Me'ati translates Arab. ريحي as אשר[332] בו רוח and Zeraḥyah Ḥen has רֵיחִי (see entry).

רוֹחֵץ (*Part.*) → רָחַץ.

רוטא • **גומא של הרוטא המדברית** → **גּוֹמָא**.

רוּטְבָּה → רֵטְבָּה.

רוֹעַ → רֹעַ.

רוֹעֶה • **זמר הרועה** → **זֶמֶר**.

- **כיס הרועה** → **כִּיס**.
- **מזמר הרועה** → **מזמאר**

[רוץ] • **רָץ** · **to flow, stream**: Arab. جرى · Ibn Sīnā, *K. al-Qānūn* II · trans. Zeraḥyah Ḥen, *Sefer ha-Qanun* (Ms Oxford, Bodleian Libaries, Opp. Add. Fol. 12, fol. 257a): עדשים ... מנפחים מורכבים מכח קובץ מטהר ויראו בשינה חלומות רעות וקליפותיו[333] אינם קובצים ובכלם יש נפיחה מעבה הדם ואינו רץ בעורקים (Lentils: ... They are astringent, consist of astringent and detergent power, induce bad dreams, and their[334] husks are very astringent; all lentils are flatulent, thicken the blood so that it cannot stream through the vessels). In the sense of 'to flow, stream,' Hebr. רָץ is a non-attested semantic borrowing from Arab. جرى. In the same sense, the Hebr. term features as a semantic borrowing from Lat. *discurro* in NM 5:185 in an attestation from Do'eg ha-Edomi's

---

331 'troubled sensations': Trans. acc. to a.

332 אשר בו רוח: Cf. fol. 80a–b, entry חנדקוקא '[Arab.] *ḥandaqūqā*: Lotus': יועיל מכאב האצטו' הקר ואשר בה רוחות.

333 וקליפותיו אינם קובצים: وقبض قشره كثير a.

334 'their husks are very astringent': Trans. acc. to a.

trans. of Constantinus Africanus' *Viaticum* (i.e., *Sefer Ya'ir Netiv*) I.22.1 (cf. IJZ 1–2:624). Nathan ha-Me'ati and Anonymous I both render Arab. جرى as עבר.

רוק → רֹק.

[רחב] • *Part. Hitpa'el* **מִתְרַחֵב** • **המורסות המתרחבות** → מֻרְסָה.

רֵחַיִם • **אבן הרחים** → אֶבֶן.

רֶחֶם • **הרחם החנוק** · **a suffocated womb [by its displacement, by its rising upwards in a disease called 'hysterical suffocation'[335]]**: Arab. الرحم المختنق · Ibn Sīnā, *K. al-Qānūn* II · trans. Nathan ha-Me'ati, *Sefer ha-Qanun* (Ms Oxford, Bodleian Libraries, Can. Or. 88, fol. 76[b]): גאליה ... יועיל מכאב הרחם הקר אם תסבול אותו האשה ומהמורסות הקשות מליחה לבנה וישלשל דם הוסת ויוריד הרחם החנוק וינקהו ויכינהו להריון ([Arab.] *ghāliya* [i.e., a perfume composed of musk, ambergris, camphor, and ben oil, cf. SHS 1:413 (Pe 20)]: ... When a woman applies it as a pessary, it is useful for cold pain and hard phlegmatic swellings of the womb. It stimulates menstrual flow and brings down (returns to its position) a suffocated womb, cleanses it, and prepares it for pregnancy). Hebr. הרחם החנוק is not attested in the current dictionaries. Anonymous I renders Arab. الرحم المختنق as הרחם הנחנק (see next entry).

• **הרחם הנחנק** · **a suffocated womb [by its displacement, by its rising upwards in a disease called 'hysterical suffocation'[336]]**: Arab. الرحم المختنق · Ibn Sīnā, *K. al-Qānūn* II · trans. Anonymous I, *Sefer ha-Qanun* (Ms Paris, BnF, héb. 1142, fol. 272[a]): גאליה ... מועילה מכאיבי הרחם הקרים הנחה למטה וממורסותיו הקרות והלבניות ומגיר הנדות ומוריד הרחם הנחנק ומנקהו ומכינו להריון ([Arab.] *ghāliya* [i.e., a perfume composed of musk, ambergris, camphor, and ben oil, cf. SHS 1:413 (Pe 20)]: ... When a woman applies it as a pessary, it is useful for cold pain and cold phlegmatic swellings of the womb. It stimulates menstrual flow and brings down (returns to its position) a suffocated womb, cleanses it, and prepares it for pregnancy). Hebr. הרחם הנחנק is not attested in the current dictionaries. Nathan ha-Me'ati translates Arab. الرحم المختنق as הרחם החנוק (see previous entry).

• **הגרת לחות הרחם** → הֲגָרָה.

• **הגרת לחויות הרחם** → הֲגָרָה.

• **הגרת רוטבות הרחם** → הֲגָרָה.

• **הגרת הרחם** → הֲגָרָה.

• **חנק הרחם** → חֶנֶק.

• **פי הרחם** → פֶּה.

• **צואר הרחם** → צַוָּאר.

---

335 Cf. Bos (ed. and trans.), *Ibn al-Jazzār on Sexual Diseases* XI ('On Hysterical Suffocation'), 46: 'a displacement of the womb whereby it came into sympathy with the upper parts of the body, casusing suffocation and sensory disturbances.'

336 See the preceding note.

רָחַץ • רחץ הפה · **to rinse one's mouth; to use a mouthwash**: Arab. مضمضة · Ibn Sīnā, *K. al-Qānūn* II · trans. Nathan ha-Me'ati, *Sefer ha-Qanun* (Ms Oxford, Bodleian Libraries, Can. Or. 88, fol. 65[a]): אעאלוג׳י ... כשרוחצין הפה בתבשילו ייטיב הריח ([Arab.] *aghālūjī*: Agarwood [*Aquilaria malaccensis* Lam.]: ... If one rinses one's mouth with a decoction of it, it improves [bad] breath). In addition to רחץ הפה, Nathan translates Arab. مضمضة as שכשך הפה (see entry שִׁכְשֵׁךְ) and in his trans. of Maimonides' *Medical Aphorisms* XXI.10 and XXII.68 as מצמץ (cf. BMMN 196, l. 26; 217, l. 18; BMMG no. 4867). Zeraḥyah Ḥen translates Arab. مضمضة as קשקש בפה (see entry קִשְׁקֵשׁ) and Anonymous I has מִצְמוּץ (cf. NM 6:126).

• *Part.* רוֹחֵץ • הסם הרוחץ → סַם.

• הרפואה הרוחצת → רְפוּאָה.

רְטִבָה • *Plur.* רוטבות • **הרוטבות הנעצרות תחת העור** · **edemas**: Arab. الرطوبات المحتقنة تحت الجلد · Ibn Sīnā, *K. al-Qānūn* II · trans. Nathan ha-Me'ati, *Sefer ha-Qanun* (Ms Oxford, Bodleian Libraries, Can. Or. 88, fol. 103[b]): מרקשיתא ... יועיל כשמושחים בו עם חומץ אל הבהק והצרעת[337] והעדשים ובער׳ נמש ומתיר כמו כן הרוטבות הנעצרות תחת העור והוא מרקיק השער ומחדשו[338] ([Arab.] *marqashīthā*: Marcasite: ... Rubbing it with vinegar is useful in *bahaq*[339] (alphos), *baraṣ*,[340] and freckles, [called] in Arab. *namash*. It dissolves edemas. It makes the hair thin and curly[341]). In the sense of 'edemas,' Hebr. רוטבות הנעצרות תחת העורה is a non-attested calque from Arab. الرطوبات المحتقنة تحت الجلد. Zeraḥyah Ḥen translates the Arab. term as הלחויות הנחבאות תחת העור (see entry לַחוּת) and Anonymous I has הלחויות הנעצרות תחת העור (see also entry לַחוּת).

• הגרת רוטבות הרחם → הֲגָרָה.

רְטִיָּה · **rubbing in; smearing**: Arab. لُطُوخ (cf. WKAS 2.2:692) · Ibn Sīnā, *K. al-Qānūn* II · trans. Anonymous I, *Sefer ha-Qanun* (Ms Paris, BnF, héb. 1142, fol. 92[b]): חלתית ... מועיל מחולי השועל רטיה בחומץ ופלפל ([Arab.] *ḥiltīt* / [Hebr.] *ḥiltit*: Resin of asafetida [*Ferula assa-foetida* L.]: ... It is useful for alopecia [when it is] rubbed in with vinegar and pepper). Hebr. רְטִיָּה features in the current dictionaries and secondary literature in

---

337 והצרעת: البرص a.

338 ומחדשו: ويجعده a.

339 '*bahaq* (alphos)': There are three varieties of the disease called *bahaq* acc. to Ibn al-Jazzār (cf. IJZ 7:108, n. 196): white, black, and dust-colored. The white variety is perhaps identical with *Vitiligo alba*, while the black variety is possibly a sort of melanoderma. Arab. *bahaq* stands for Gr. ἀλφός, cf. UW 97: 'weiße Hautflecken.' Durling, *Dictionary of Medical Terms*, 34, translates the Gr. term as: 'dull-white leprosy.' See entry בַּהַק: הבהק הלבן.

340 '*baraṣ*' (cf. IJZ 7:108, n. 195): This disease has two varieties, namely white and black, which are sometimes summarized under the general term *baraṣ*. The white variety is perhaps identical with *Sklerodermia circumscripta*, while the black variety may be *Psoriasis vulgaris* or *Ichthyosis vulgaris*. The Arab. term *baraṣ* stands for Gr. λέπρα ('leprosy') (cf. UW 97, 387f.). As their is no consensus on the exact meaning of the Arab. term, I have retained the Arab. term in my translation.

341 'curly': Trans. acc. to a.

the sense of 'emollient; plaster; compress.' Moses ibn Tibbon uses it in the sense of 'fomenting; fomentation' (for Arab. تكميد) in his trans. of Maimonides' *Commentary on Hippocrates' Aphorisms* (i.e., *Perush Aphorismi shel Apuqraṭ*) VI.31 (cf. BCD 261 (NM 3:216); BMCH 1:399, l. 4). Nathan ha-Me'ati translates Arab. لطوخ as לִכְלֵךְ (see entry) and Zeraḥyah Ḥen has *Inf. Hif'il* לְהָטִיחַ (see entry טוּחַ).

רִיגוֹר · **feverish chill**: Arab. نافض (Lat. *rigor*; cf. ND 926) · Ibn Sīnā, *K. al-Qānūn* II · trans. Zeraḥyah Ḥen, *Sefer ha-Qanun* (Ms Oxford, Bodleian Libaries, Opp. Add. Fol. 12, fols. 168ᵇ–169ᵃ): אֶשְׁקִיל ... החומץ שלו מועיל מן הריגור הארוך ([Arab.] *ishqīl*: Sea squill [*Drimia maritima* (L.) Stearn]: ... Its vinegar is useful for chronic feverish chill). Hebr. רִיגוֹר is a non-attested calque from Lat. *rigor*. In his trans. of Maimonides' *Medical Aphorisms* (i.e., *Sefer ha-Peraqim*) (cf. BMMG no. 5245), Zeraḥyah Ḥen renders نافض in addition to רִיגוֹר also as פַּלָּצוּת (cf. BCD 221 (NM 3:189) for attestations from Moses ibn Tibbon's trans. of Maimonides' *Commentary on Hippocrates' Aphorisms* (i.e., *Perush Aphorismi shel Apuqraṭ*) IV.46, VII.4 (cf. BMCH 1:367, l. 15; 406, l. 11)) and קְרִירוּת (cf. BCD 250 (NM 1:185); BMMZ 78, l. 20; BMMG no. 5245). Nathan ha-Me'ati translates Arab. نافض as נְעִירָה (cf. NM 6:141) and Anonymous I has רֶתֶת (cf. BCD 267 (NM 3:223) for an attestation from Do'eg ha-Edomi's trans. of Hippocrates' *Aphorisms* (i.e., *Sefer Agur*) IV.46).

[ריח] • *Hif'il* הֵרִיחַ · **to become rancid**: Arab. زنخ · Ibn Sīnā, *K. al-Qānūn* II · trans. Anonymous I, *Sefer ha-Qanun* (Ms Paris, BnF, héb. 1142, fol. 149ᵃ): ... לוז הוא שקד שמניותו פחות משמניות האגוז וגם כי יש בו שמניות רבה בסבתה יריח ([Arab.] *lawz* / [Hebr.] *luz*; i.e., [Hebr.] *shaqed*: Almond [*Prunus dulcis* (Mill.) D.A. Webb]: ... Although it contains less oil (fat) than walnut, it is yet rich in oil (fat) so that it becomes rancid). Hebr. הֵרִיחַ is not attested in the sense of 'to become rancid' in the current dictionaries. In addition to הֵרִיחַ, Anonymous I renders Arab. زنخ as רנציד* קיבל העפוש הנקרא (see entry [קבל]). Nathan ha-Me'ati translates Arab. زنخ as התערב בזוהמה (see entry [ערב]).

רֵיחִי · **gaseous**: Arab. ريحي · Ibn Sīnā, *K. al-Qānūn* II · trans. Zeraḥyah Ḥen, *Sefer ha-Qanun* (Ms Oxford, Bodleian Libaries, Opp. Add. Fol. 12, fol. 212ᵇ): חנטל קוֹלוֹקִינְטִידָא ... ישלשל הלחה הלבנה והגסה מן הפרקים והעצבים בלבד וישלשל גם כן המרות ויועיל מן הקוליקא הלחה והריחיית מאד ([Arab.] *ḥanẓal*; [i.e., Rom.] QWoLWoQiYNṬYDa' (i.e., *colloquintida*, from Lat. *colocyntis*; Gr. κολοκυνθίς): Colocynth [*Citrullus colocynthis* (L.) Schrad.]: ... It purges thick phlegm out of the joints and especially the nerves; it also purges the biles and it is beneficial for very moist, gaseous colic). Hebr. רֵיחִי is not attested in the current dictionaries. Nathan ha-Me'ati translates Arab. ريحي as אשר בו רוח[342] and Anonymous I has רוּחִי (see entry).

---

342 אשר בו רוח: Cf. fol. 80ᵃ⁻ᵇ, entry חנדקוקא '[Arab.] *ḥandaqūqā*: Lotus': יועיל מכאב האצטו' הקר ואשר בה רוחות.

רֵיקָן · **hollow**: Arab. أجوف · Ibn Sīnā, *K. al-Qānūn* II · trans. Zeraḥyah Ḥen, *Sefer ha-Qanun* (Ms Oxford, Bodleian Libaries, Opp. Add. Fol. 12, fol. 226ᵃ): כַּרְפַּס ... וממנו מין הנקרא סמרניון[343] והוא יותר גדול מן הפרדסי ושוקו ריקן נוטה אל הלובן (Celery [*Apium graveolens* L.]: ... Another variety is called [in Arab.] *samarnion*;[344] it is bigger than the garden variety. Its stem is hollow and whitish). Hebr. רֵיקָן is not attested in this sense in the current dictionaries. Nathan ha-Me'ati and Anonymous I both render Arab. أجوف as חלול.

רֵיקָנוּת • על הריקנות · **on an empty stomach**: Arab. على الريق · Ibn Sīnā, *K. al-Qānūn* II · trans. Zeraḥyah Ḥen, *Sefer ha-Qanun* (Ms Oxford, Bodleian Libaries, Opp. Add. Fol. 12, fol. 222ᵃ⁻ᵇ): כֻּנְדֻּר אוּלִיבָּנוּ ... יועיל לשכל ויחזק אותו ויש בני אדם מי שיצוה בשתיית משרתו על הריקנות (Arab.] *kundur*; [i.e., Rom.] 'WuLiYBaNWu: Frankincense [*Boswellia sacra* Flueck.]: ... It is beneficial for the mind and strengthens it. Some order to drink an infusion of it on an empty stomach). Hebr. על הריקנות is not attested in the current dictionaries. The same term is used by Zeraḥyah in his trans. of Maimonides' *Medical Aphorisms* (i.e., *Sefer ha-Peraqim*) XXII.36 (cf. BMMZ 211, l. 12; BMMG no. 2246). For רֵיקָנוּת in the sense of 'emptiness,' see NM 5:186f. for an attestation from Abraham ben Isaac's trans. of Ibn al-Jazzār's *Zād al-musāfir* (i.e., *Sefer Ṣedah la-Oreḥim*) I.24.1 (cf. IJZ 1–2:581). Nathan ha-Me'ati translates Arab. على الريق as על הצום and Anonymous I renders the Arab. term as בריקות נפש (cf. BCD 262 (NM 2:86), s.v. רֵיקוּת) for an attestation from Nathan's *Sefer ha-Peraqim* XXII.36 (cf. BMMN 214, l. 1; BMMG no. 2246)).

רַךְ • סימנים רכים → סִמָּן.

רִכּוּךְ · **softening, mollification, relaxation, slackening**: Arab. استرخاء Ibn Sīnā, *K. al-Qānūn* II · trans. Anonymous II, *Sefer ha-Qanun* (Ms Parma, Biblioteca Palatina, Cod. Parm. 3045, fol. 30ᵃ): דַּרְסִיסֵיאַם ... יצליח לרכוך החבלים ([Arab.] *dārshīsha'ān*: Broom [*Genista acanthoclada* DC. or *Cytisus spinosus* Lam.] (cf. MIG no. 223): ... It is beneficial for relaxation (slackening) of the nerves). Hebr. רִכּוּךְ does not feature in this sense in the current dictionaries. A variant reading רַכּוּת features (for Lat. *mollicies*) in NM 6:200 in an attestation from Do'eg ha-Edomi's trans. of Constantinus Africanus' *Viaticum* (i.e., *Sefer Ya'ir Netiv*) IV.13. Nathan ha-Me'ati, Zeraḥyah Ḥen, and Anonymous I translate Arab. استرخاء as רִפְּיוֹן (cf. NM 6:205 for the Hebr. term רפיון האצטומכה 'atony of the stomach (gastric atony)' featuring in Moses ibn Tibbon's trans. of Ibn al-Jazzār's *Zād al-musāfir* (i.e., *Sefer Ṣedat ha-Derakhim*) IV.13).

[רכך] • *Pi'el* **רִכֵּךְ** · **to soften, relieve**: Arab. ليّن · Ibn Sīnā, *K. al-Qānūn* II · trans. Nathan ha-Me'ati, *Sefer ha-Qanun* (Ms Oxford, Bodleian Libraries, Can. Or. 88, fol. 126ᵃ): תרנגבין ... יועיל מהשעול וירכך החזה ([Arab.] *taranjubīn* [from Pers. *tarangubīn*]: Manna:[345]

343 סמרניון: Emend. ed. סחרינון Ms سمرنيون a.

344 '*samarnion*': Trans. acc. to a.

345 'Manna': I.e., the crystallized honeydew of certain scale insects, in particular the manna

... It is beneficial for cough and for relieving a [congested] chest). Hebr. רִכֵּךְ features in the sense of 'to soften, ease' in BM 6599 in an attestation from Solomon ibn Ayyub's trans. of Ibn Rushd's commentary on Ibn Sīnā's *Urjūza* (i.e., *Perush Ibn Rushd 'al Ḥaruzei Ibn Sina*) (1261). For the Hebr. terms ריכך הבטן 'to soften the stools' (for Arab. ليّن الطبيعة) and רכוך הבטן 'prescribing laxatives' (for Arab. إلانة البطن), featuring in Nathan's trans. of Maimonides' *Medical Aphorisms* (i.e., *Sefer ha-Peraqim*) XVII.33, XII.8, cf. NM 1:150, s.v. החליק הטבע; BMMN 175, l. 4; resp. NM 1:149f., s.v. להחליק הבטן; BMMN 139, l. 21; BMMG no. 4696. Zeraḥyah Ḥen translates Arab. ليّن as *Hif'il* הֶחֱלִיק (see entry [חלק]) and Anonymous I has *Pi'el* רִכֵּךְ, just like Nathan.

רמד · **ophthalmia**: Arab. رمد · Ibn Sīnā, *K. al-Qānūn* II · trans. Zeraḥyah Ḥen, *Sefer ha-Qanun* (Ms Oxford, Bodleian Libaries, Opp. Add. Fol. 12, fol. 192[b]): ג׳נְצְיַאנָה יהיה נעשה ממנו טיחה ללרמד ... ([Lat.-Rom.] ǦiNəṢiY'NaH (cf. Zeraḥyah's trans. of Maimonides' *Medical Aphorisms* (i.e., *Sefer ha-Peraqim*) IX.88, XXII.29: ג(׳)נציאנה (BMMZ 111, l. 15; 210, l. 17; BMMG no. 715)): Great yellow gentian [*Gentiana lutea* L.]: ... A salve is prepared from it to treat ophthalmia). In the sense of 'ophthalmia,' Hebr. רמד is a non-attested loan word from Arab. رمد and also features in Zeraḥyah's and Nathan ha-Me'ati's trans. of Maimonides' *Medical Aphorisms* (i.e., *Sefer ha-Peraqim*) (cf. BMMG no. 2175). Here, Nathan translates Arab. رمد as אפר בערבי רמד (cf. BCD 26 (NM 1:78) for the Hebr. terms אפר and אפר העינים in the sense of 'ophthalmia,' and also NM 5:77, s.v. חלי העינים) and Anonymous I has רמד, just like Zeraḥyah. A synonym featuring in medieval medical literature is חלי העינים (cf. NM 5:77 and further variants in Zeraḥyah's *Sefer ha-Peraqim* (cf. BMMG no. 2175): החולי שבעין הנקרא רמד / חולי העין הנקרא רמד / חולי העינים הנקרא רמד.

רִמּוֹן • **גיד הרמון המדברי** → גִּיד.

• **שרש הרמון המדברי** → שֹׁרֶשׁ.

רנציד* • **קיבל העפוש הנקרא *רנציד** → [קבל].

רִסּוּק • **רסוק האזן** · **tear (puncture) in the ear**: Arab. شدخ الأذن (Arab. شدخ; i.e., Gr. ῥῆγμα 'breakage; fracture; laceration; rupture; rent; tear;' cf. UW 587; LSG 1568) · Ibn Sīnā, *K. al-Qānūn* II · trans. Anonymous I, *Sefer ha-Qanun* (Ms Paris, BnF, héb. 1142, fol. 134[b]): כברית ... עוצר הזכאם בעשון כשיתעשן ויעשה בחומץ ודבש על רסוק האזן ([Arab.] *kibrīt*: Sulphur: ... It stops rheum when it is applied as a fumigation; with vinegar and honey it is used for a tear (puncture) in the ear). Hebr. רסוק האזן does not feature in the current dictionaries. Nathan ha-Me'ati translates Arab. شدخ الأذن as רצוץ האזן (see entry רצוץ) and Zeraḥyah Ḥen has לחיצת האזן (see entry לְחִיצָה). The Hebr. translators probably interpreted Arab. شَدْخ as derived from شَدَخَ in its general meaning of 'to break, crush, press, squeeze' (cf. Lane 1519) and not in the specific meaning listed

mealybug [*Trabutina mannipara* (Hemprich & Ehrenberg, 1829)], that feeds on the tamarisk [*Tamarix* L.]; cf. Lane 306; MSh no. 386.

above. Arab. شدخ, featuring as part of the term شدخ العضل 'muscle tear (rupture)' in the *K. al-Qānūn*, is translated by Anonymous I as גרידת העצלים (cf. NM 6:206, s.v. רצוץ העצלים).

רַע • חולי המים הרעים הבשריי → חֳלִי.

רֹעַ • רוע ברזל · **[lit. 'badness of iron']; iron dross; iron slag**: Arab. خبث الحديد · *Shinnui ha-Shemot ha-Niqra'im Synonimi*, Kaf 61 (Ms Florence, Biblioteca Medicea Laurenziana, Or. 17, fol. 61[a]): כבר חדיד ה׳ רוע ברזל ובלע׳ פירווייני ([Arab.] KBR ḤDYD [read: KBT ḤDYD, i.e., *khabath* [*al-*]*ḥadīd*]; i.e., [Hebr.] *ro'a ha-barzel*, in Rom. PYRWYYNY [i.e., Ital.-Rom. *ferrugine*[346]]). In the sense of 'iron dross; iron slag,' Hebr. רוע ברזל (lit. 'badness of iron') is a non-attested calque from Arab. خبث الحديد, resulting from reading Arab. *khabath* ('dross; slag') as *khubth* ('badness'). A synonym (for Lat. *ferrugo*) featuring in Do'eg ha-Edomi's trans. of Constantinus Africanus' *Viaticum* (i.e., *Sefer Ya'ir Netiv*) IV.19 is אבק הברזל (cf. NM 6:13f.).

רַעַד · **trembling; tremor**: Arab. رعشة (Gr. τρόμος; cf. UW 685) · Ibn Sīnā, *K. al-Qānūn* II · trans. Anonymous II, *Sefer ha-Qanun* (Ms Parma, Biblioteca Palatina, Cod. Parm. 3045, fol. 30[b]): תרנגלים ותרנגלות ... מרק התרנגלים כמו שנאמר יצליח לרעד ולכאב פרקי העצמות וצריך שיתבשלו עם פוליפוגיאו ועם אניטו (Roosters and hens (chicken): ... The [type of] chicken soup mentioned before is beneficial for tremors and pain in the joints, if cooked with polypody and dill). Hebr. רַעַד features in the sense of 'trembling' in the current dictionaries in attestations from the Bible, Rabb., medieval, and modern poetic literature (cf. BM 6641; EM 1727). Nathan ha-Me'ati translates Arab. رعشة as רעישה (cf. BCD 264 for attestations from Shem Tov ben Isaac's *Sefer ha-Shimmush* XXVII (cf. NM 4:196) and the anonymous trans. of Maimonides' *Commentary on Hippocrates' Aphorisms* (i.e., *Perush Aphorismi shel Apuqraṭ*) VI.26 (cf. NM 3:220); BMCH 1:589, l. 3; cf. also NM 6:202, s.v. רַעַשׁ) and Zeraḥyah Ḥen has רַעַשׁ (cf. NM 6:202).

רְעִיפָה • רעיפת דם מהאף · **nosebleed:** Lat. *fluxus sanguinis de naribus* · Guy de Chauliac, *Inventarium sive Chirurgia Magna* (cf. CMM 1:235, l. 14) · trans. Anonymous (Ms Paris, BnF, héb. 1189, fol. 128[b]): מרעיפת דם מהאף (On nosebleed). Hebr. רעיפת דם מהאף is attested in NM 6:201, s.v. רְעִיפָה, as רעיפת הדם מן האף in a reference to Shem Tov Ben Isaac's *Sefer Almansur*. Synonymous terms featuring in medieval medical literature are רעיפת דם מן החוטם and רעיפת דם מן הנחירים (cf. ibid.; BCD 264 (NM 3:219)).

[רפא] • *Part. Hitpa'el* **מִתְרַפֵּא** · **paralyzed**: Arab. مسترخ (Gr. παραλύομαι; cf. UW 497) · Ibn Sīnā, *K. al-Qānūn* II · trans. Zeraḥyah Ḥen, *Sefer ha-Qanun* (Ms Oxford, Bodleian Libaries, Opp. Add. Fol. 12, fol. 201[b]): הַלִילַגְ׳ מִירַבַּלֹנִי ... הציתרינו ללעין המתרפא ויועיל ([Arab.] *halīlaj* [from Pers. *halīlah*]; [Rom.] MiYRaBaLoNiY: (Chebulic) myrobalan:

346 I thank Sebastian Lauschus and Luca Refrigeri for this explanation.

… When the yellow [variety is applied] to paralyzed eyes, it is useful). In the sense of 'paralyzed' Hebr. *Part. Hitpa'el* מִתְרַפֵּא, a variant reading of מִתְרַפֶּה, is a non-attested semantic borrowing from Arab. مسترخ. Nathan ha-Me'ati translates Arab. مسترخ as רָפֶה (see entry) and Anonymous I has נִרְפֶּה (see next entry).

[רפה] • *Part. Nif'al* **נִרְפֶּה** · **paralyzed**: Arab. مسترخ (Gr. παραλύομαι; cf. UW 497) · Ibn Sīnā, *K. al-Qānūn* II · trans. Anonymous I, *Sefer ha-Qanun* (Ms Paris, BnF, héb. 1142, fols. 108ᵇ–109ᵃ): הלילג כרכומי הנקר' שיטרין … הכרכומי לעין הנרפית ויועיל ([Arab.-Hebr.] *halīlaj* [from Pers. *halīlah*] *karkummi*; called [in Rom.] ŠYṬRYN: Yellow myrobalan: … When the yellow [variety is applied] to paralyzed eyes, it is useful). In the sense of 'paralyzed,' Hebr. *Part. Nif'al* נִרְפֶּה is a non-attested semantic borrowing from Arab. مسترخ. Nathan ha-Me'ati translates Arab. مسترخ as רָפֶה (see next entry) and Zeraḥyah Ḥen has *Part. Hitpa'el* מִתְרַפֵּא (see previous entry).

• *Part. Pi'el* **מְרַפֶּה** • **הרפואה המרפה** → רְפוּאָה.

רָפֶה · **paralyzed**: Arab. مسترخ · Ibn Sīnā, *K. al-Qānūn* II · trans. Nathan ha-Me'ati, *Sefer ha-Qanun* (Ms Oxford, Bodleian Libraries, Can. Or. 88, fol. 79ᵇ): הלילג … המכורכם יועיל לעין הרפה ([Arab.] *halīlaj* [from Pers. *halīlah*]: (Chebulic) myrobalan: … The yellow [variety] is useful for paralyzed eyes). In the sense of 'paralyzed,' Hebr. רָפֶה is a non-attested semantic borrowing from Arab. مسترخ. Zeraḥyah Ḥen renders Arab. مسترخ as *Part. Hitpa'el* מִתְרַפֵּא (see entry) and Anonymous I has *Part. Nif'al* נִרְפֶּה (see previous entry).

רְפוּאָה • **הרפואה המאדימה** · **the rubefacient drug**: Arab. الدواء المحمر · Ibn Sīnā, *K. al-Qānūn* II · trans. Zeraḥyah Ḥen, *Sefer ha-Qanun* (Ms Oxford, Bodleian Libaries, Opp. Add. Fol. 12, fol. 160ᵃ): והמאדימה היא הרפואה אשר מטבעה שתחמם האבר אשר היא פוגשת חימום חזק עד שימשוך הדם משיכה חזקה תגיע עד שטחה ויאדימנה (A rubefacient [drug] is a drug that—by its nature—intensely warms an organ, which it touches [i.e., comes in contact with], so that the blood is strongly attracted towards it [i.e., the organ], reaches its outside, and turns it red). Hebr. הרפואה המאדימה is not attested in the current dictionaries. Nathan ha-Me'ati translates Arab. الدواء المحمر as הסם המאדים and Anonymous I renders it as הסם המאדם (for both terms, see entry סַם).

• **הרפואה האוכלת** · **the corrosive drug**: Arab. الدواء الأكّال · Ibn Sīnā, *K. al-Qānūn* II · trans. Zeraḥyah Ḥen, *Sefer ha-Qanun* (Ms Oxford, Bodleian Libaries, Opp. Add. Fol. 12, fol. 160ᵃ): והאוכלת היא שטבעה להפליג בהתרתו וחבלתו שתפחות מעצם הבשר כמו הזינגאר (A corrosive [drug] is—by its nature—[a drug] with strong solvent and ulcerative properties, which reduce the substance of the flesh [of the organ]; [an example of such a drug is] verdigris). Hebr. הרפואה האוכלת is not attested in the current dictionaries. Nathan ha-Me'ati translates Arab. الدواء الأكّال as הסם האוכל and Anonymous I has הסם המאכל (for both terms, see entry סַם).

• **הרפואה המבטלת** · **the anesthetic (benumbing, narcotic; soporific) drug**: Arab. الدواء المخدر · Ibn Sīnā, *K. al-Qānūn* II · trans. Zeraḥyah Ḥen, *Sefer ha-Qanun* (Ms

Oxford, Bodleian Libaries, Opp. Add. Fol. 12, fols. 160b–161a):[347] והמבטלת היא הרפואה אשר תפליג מקרירותו לאבר שישים עצם הרוח הנושא אותו כח התנועה וההרגשה קרה במזגו עבה בעצמותו ולא יעשנו הכח הנפשי (An anesthetic (benumbing; narcotic; soporific) [drug] is a drug that has such a strong cooling effect on an organ that it makes the substance of the pneuma of an organ—which is carried to the organ by the faculty of movement and sensation—cold in temperament and dense in substance. Consequently, the psychical faculty does not have an effect on it anymore). Hebr. הרפואה המבטלת is not attested in the current dictionaries. Nathan ha-Me'ati translates Arab. الدواء المخدر as הסם המבטל ההרגש and Anonymous I has הסם המרדים הרגש (for both terms, see entry סַם).

• **הרפואה המבשלת** · **the ripening (coctive) drug**: Arab. الدواء المنضج · Ibn Sīnā, *K. al-Qānūn* II · trans. Zeraḥyah Ḥen, *Sefer ha-Qanun* (Ms Oxford, Bodleian Libaries, Opp. Add. Fol. 12, fol. 160a): והמבשלת היא הרפואה אשר מטבעה שתקנה לליחה בישול כי היא מחממת במיצוע וביושר ויש בו כח מקבץ עוצר הליחה עד שתתבשל ולא תתיך בעוצם (A ripening (coctive) [drug] is a drug that—by its nature—ripens (concocts) the humor because of its moderate heat; it has an astringent property that retains the humor until it is ripe and does not dissolve it forcefully). Hebr. הרפואה המבשלת features as *Plur.* הרפואות המבשלות in BM 641 in an attestation from the *Sefer ha-Qanun*. Nathan ha-Me'ati and Anonymous I both render Arab. الدواء المنضج as הסם המבשל (cf. BCD 187 (NM 4:124), where it features in an attestation from an anonymous trans. of Ibn Sīnā's *K. al-Adwiya al-qalbiyya* (i.e., *Sammim Libbiyim*).

• **הרפואה המדקדקת** · **the attenuant drug**: Arab. الدواء الملطّف · Ibn Sīnā, *K. al-Qānūn* II · trans. Zeraḥyah Ḥen, *Sefer ha-Qanun* (Ms Oxford, Bodleian Libaries, Opp. Add. Fol. 12, fol. 159b): הרפואה המדקדקת היא אשר מטבעה שתשים עצמות הליחה יותר רקיקה עם חמימות ממוצעת כמו האיספו והשדוּרֵאיֵנֵי והקמומילא (An attenuant drug is—by its nature—[a drug] that, through its moderate heat, attenuates the substance of the humor; [examples of such drugs are] hyssop, thyme, and camomile). In the sense of 'the attenuant drug,' Hebr. הרפואה המדקדקת features in BM 985f., s.v. דִקְדֵק, in an attestation from, a.o., the *Sefer ha-Qanun*. It also features in Zeraḥyah's trans. of Maimonides' *Medical Aphorisms* (i.e., *Sefer ha-Peraqim*) IX.87 (cf. BMMZ, 111, ll. 6–7; BMMG no. 1898). Nathan ha-Me'ati translates Arab. الدواء الملطّف as הסם המרקיק (cf. NM 6:149) and Anonymous I renders the Arab. term as הסם המדקדק (cf. BCD 188 (NM 4:125) for an attestation from an anonymous trans. of Ibn Sīnā's *K. al-Adwiya al-qalbiyya* (i.e., *Sammim Libbiyim*)).

• **הרפואה[348] המזירה** · **the repellent drug**: Arab. الدواء الرادع · Ibn Sīnā, *K. al-Qānūn* II · trans. Zeraḥyah Ḥen, *Sefer ha-Qanun* (Ms Oxford, Bodleian Libaries, Opp. Add.

347 In his trans. of Maimonides' *Medical Aphorisms* (i.e., *Sefer ha-Peraqim*) IX.38, Zeraḥyah translates Arab. *Plur.* أدوية مخدرة 'soporific drugs' as רפואה מבטלת החוש (cf. BMMZ 103, l. 12; BMMG no. 1884).

348 הרפואה המזירה: Emend. ed. והמזיר Ms.

Fol. 12, fol. 160b): והמזירה[349] היא הפך למושך והיא הרפואה אשר מטבעה בעבור קרירותה שתחדש באבר קרירות ויעצרנו בו ויעצור נקביו וישבר חמימותו המושך ויקפיא הנגר אליו ויעצרנו וימנענו מן ההגרה אל האבר וימנע האבר מן לקבלו כמו ענבי[350] הדוב במורסות (A repellent [drug] is the reverse of the attracting one; it is a drug that—by its nature—, because of its coldness, produces coldness in an organ, condenses it, constricts its pores, breaks its attracting heat and condenses the fluid flowing towards it, stops it, and prevents it from reaching the organ. Thus the organ cannot absorp it. [An example of a drug with this effect is] black nightshade [in the case of] swellings). Hebr. הרפואה המזירה is not attested in the current dictionaries. Nathan ha-Me'ati and Anonymous I both render Arab. الدواء الرادع as הסם המרתיע (cf. BCD 189 (NM 4:131) for an attestation from an anonymous trans. of Ibn Sīnā's *K. al-Adwiya al-qalbiyya* (i.e., *Sammim Libbiyim*)).; for *Part. Hif'il* מַרְתִּיעַ, see also entry [רתע]).

• **הרפואה המחבלת · the ulcerative drug**: Arab. الدواء المقرح · Ibn Sīnā, *K. al-Qānūn* II · trans. Zeraḥyah Ḥen, *Sefer ha-Qanun* (Ms Oxford, Bodleian Libaries, Opp. Add. Fol. 12, fol. 160a–b): והמחבלת היא אשר מטבעה שתכלה ותתיך הליחות המגיעות בין חלקי העור ומושכת החומר הרע אליה עד שובו חבלה כמו האנקרדי (An ulcerative [drug] is [a drug] that—by its nature—destroys and dissolves the humors, which come between the parts of the skin and attracts the [harmful] matter towards it until it forms an ulcer; [an example of such a drug is] marking nut). Hebr. הרפואה המחבלת is not attested in the current dictionaries. For the verb [חבל], *Pi'el* חִבֵּל, in the sense of 'to ulcerate,' cf. BCD 88 (NM 1:145) for an attestation from Zeraḥyah's trans. of Maimonides' *Medical Aphorisms* (i.e., *Sefer ha-Peraqim*) XXIII.46 (cf. BMMZ 223, l. 5; BMMG no. 4047). Nathan ha-Me'ati translates Arab. الدواء المقرح as הסם המנגע (see entry) and Anonymous I has הסם המשחין.

• **הרפואה המחזקת · the tonic drug**: Arab. الدواء المقوي · Ibn Sīnā, *K. al-Qānūn* II · trans. Zeraḥyah Ḥen, *Sefer ha-Qanun* (Ms Oxford, Bodleian Libaries, Opp. Add. Fol. 12, fol. 160b): והמחזקת היא הרפואה אשר מדרכה שתמצע עצמות האבר ומזגו עד שימנע מקבלת המותרות והחליים (A tonic [drug] is a drug that—by its nature—balances the consistency and temperament of an organ to an extent that it prevents the absorption of superfluous matters and disorders). Hebr. הרפואה המחזקת is not attested in the current dictionaries. Nathan ha-Me'ati translates Arab. الدواء المقوي as הסם המחזיק and Anonymous I has הסם המחזק (see entry סַם).

• **הרפואה המחיה · the healing drug (a drug that promotes cicatrization)**: Arab. الدواء المدمل · Ibn Sīnā, *K. al-Qānūn* II · trans. Zeraḥyah Ḥen, *Sefer ha-Qanun* (Ms Oxford, Bodleian Libaries, Opp. Add. Fol. 12, fol. 161b): והמחיה היא הרפואה אשר תנגב ותעצור[351] הלחות הנופל בין שני שטחים של החבלה השכנים עד שישוב אל הדיבוק והחיבור וידבק האחד

349 והמזירה היא: Emend. ed. והמזיר הוא Ms.
350 ענבי הדוב: عنب الثعلب a.
351 ותעצור: ويكثف a.

באחר כמו דם תנין והאלואין (The healing [drug] is a drug that dries up and thickens[352] the fluid collected between the two layers of a wound that are close to each other. [It does so] to an extent that it [i.e., the fluid] becomes agglutinant and viscous and both the ends of the wound adhere to each other; [examples of such a drug are] dragon's blood [i.e., the resin of *Dracaena cinnabari* Balf. f.], and aloes). Hebr. הרפואה המחיה is not attested in the current dictionaries. For the verb [חיה], *Pi'el* חִיָּה, in the sense of 'to heal; to promote cicatrization,' see entry [חיה]. Nathan ha-Me'ati translates Arab. الدواء المدمل as הסם המסגר and Anonymous I renders the Arab. term as הסם המבריא (for both terms, see entry סַם).

• **הרפואה המחככת · the pruritic drug**: Arab. الدواء المحكك · Ibn Sīnā, *K. al-Qānūn* II · trans. Zeraḥyah Ḥen, *Sefer ha-Qanun* (Ms Oxford, Bodleian Libaries, Opp. Add. Fol. 12, fol. 160[a]): והמחככת היא אשר מטבעה בחממה וחימומה שתמשוך אל הנקבים ליחות נושכות מחככות לא תפליג לעשות חבלה (A pruritic [drug] is [a drug] that—by its nature—has such a strong heating power that it attracts the irritant pruritic humor towards the pores, but not to the extent of producing ulcers). Hebr. הרפואה המחככת is not attested in the current dictionaries. Nathan ha-Me'ati and Anonymous I both render Arab. الدواء المحكك as הסם המחכך (see entry סַם).

• **הרפואה המחליקה · the smoothing drug**: Arab. الدواء المملس · Ibn Sīnā, *K. al-Qānūn* II · trans. Zeraḥyah Ḥen, *Sefer ha-Qanun* (Ms Oxford, Bodleian Libaries, Opp. Add. Fol. 12, fol. 161[a]):[353] והמחליקה היא הרפואה הדבקה אשר מדרכה שתתפשט על אבר גס פישוט יחליק השטח וישוב נראה אותו בו יותר חלק (A smoothing [drug] is a viscous drug, which—by its nature—spreads over the surface of a rough organ and smoothens it. The external surface of that body becomes smoother). Hebr. הרפואה המחליקה features in BCD 265 (NM 1:26) for Lat. *medicina abstertiva* 'detergent remedy' in an attestation from Hillel ben Samuel's trans. of Bruno Longobucco's *Cyrurgia Magna* (i.e., *Sefer Keritut*); it also features in NM 5:190 for Arab. الدواء الملين 'the softening remedy' in an attestation from Zeraḥyah's trans. of Maimonides' *Medical Aphorisms* (i.e., *Sefer ha-Peraqim*) XXI.64 (cf. BMMZ 201, l. 24; BMMG no. 1873). Nathan ha-Me'ati translates Arab. الدواء المملس as הסם המחליק (see entry סַם).

• **הרפואה המחתכת · the cutting, biting, pungent drug**: Arab. الدواء المقطّع · Ibn Sīnā, *K. al-Qānūn* II · trans. Zeraḥyah Ḥen, *Sefer ha-Qanun* (Ms Oxford, Bodleian Libaries, Opp. Add. Fol. 12, fol. 160[r]): והמחתכת היא הרפואה אשר מטבעה שתעבור בדקותה בין שטח האבר[354] ובין הליחה הדבקה הנדבק בה ויפריד אותה (A cutting (biting, pungent) [drug] is a drug that—by its nature—penetrates because of its tenuity between the sur-

352 'thickens': Trans. acc. to a.

353 For the Hebr. parallel term דברים מחליקים (for Arab. الأشياء المزلقة 'laxatives'), cf. NM 6:43f. and entry הרפואה הממעידה below.

354 האבר ובין הליחה הדבקה ובין הליחה הדבקה הנדבק בה: Emend. ed. הליחה הדבקה ובין השטח הנדבק בה Ms العضو والخلط اللزج الذي التزق به a.

face of an organ and the attached viscous humor, and separates the latter from the former). Hebr. הרפואה המחתכת is not attested in the current dictionaries. Nathan ha-Me'ati and Anonymous I both render Arab. الدواء مقطّع as הסם המחתך (see entry סַם).

• **הרפואה החותמת** · **the cicatrizing drug**: Arab. الدواء الخاتم · Ibn Sīnā, *K. al-Qānūn* II · trans. Zeraḥyah Ḥen, *Sefer ha-Qanun* (Ms Oxford, Bodleian Libaries, Opp. Add. Fol. 12, fol. 161[b]): והחותמת היא הרפואה המיבשת אשר תייבש שטח החבלה עד שובה קְרוּשְׁטָה מעליה נקיה[355] מן החולי עד שיצמח העור הטבעי (A cicatrizing [drug] is a desiccant drug that dries up the surface of a wound until it forms a scab (crust). This scab provides[356] protection against injuries until the natural skin regenerates). Hebr. הרפואה החותמת is not attested in the current dictionaries. For the verb חָתַם in the sense of 'to cicatrize,' cf. BCD 109 (NM 1:152f.) for an attestation from Zeraḥyah's trans. of Maimonides' *Medical Aphorisms* (i.e., *Sefer ha-Peraqim*) IX.95 (cf. BMMZ 112, l. 19; BMMG no. 1289). Nathan ha-Me'ati translates Arab. الدواء الخاتم as הסם החותם (see entry סַם).

• **הרפואה הכווה** · **the cauterizing drug**: Arab. الدواء الكاوي · Ibn Sīnā, *K. al-Qānūn* II · trans. Zeraḥyah Ḥen, *Sefer ha-Qanun* (Ms Oxford, Bodleian Libaries, Opp. Add. Fol. 12, fol. 160[b]):[357] והכווה היא תאכל הבשר וישרוף העור שרפה מייבשת (A cauterizing [drug] is [a drug] that corrodes the flesh and burns and dries the skin). Hebr. הרפואה הכווה is not attested in the current dictionaries. Nathan ha-Me'ati and Anonymous I both render Arab. الدواء الكاوي as הסם הכווה (see entry סַם).

• **הרפואה המלכלכת** · **the drug that infects (contaminates)**: Arab. الدواء الموسّخ · Ibn Sīnā, *K. al-Qānūn* II · trans. Zeraḥyah Ḥen, *Sefer ha-Qanun* (Ms Oxford, Bodleian Libaries, Opp. Add. Fol. 12, fol. 161[a]): והמלכלכת הנגעים היא הרפואה הלחה אשר תתערב עם לחות הנגעים וישימה הרבה וימנע הניגוב והחיות (A [drug] that infects (contaminates) a wound is a moist drug that mixes with the moisture (secretion) of the wound and increases it, and [thus] prevents the wound from drying and from forming a scar (cicatrization)). Hebr. הרפואה המלכלכת is not attested in the current dictionaries. Nathan ha-Me'ati and Anonymous I both render Arab. الدواء الموسّخ as הסם המטנף (see entry סַם).

• **הרפואה הממעידה** · **the lubricant drug**: Arab. الدواء المزلق · Ibn Sīnā, *K. al-Qānūn* II · trans. Zeraḥyah Ḥen, *Sefer ha-Qanun* (Ms Oxford, Bodleian Libaries, Opp. Add. Fol. 12, fol. 161[a]): והממעידה היא הרפואה אשר מדרכה שימלא שטח גוף פוגש לדרך עצור בו

355 نقية מן החולי: تكنه من الآفات a.

356 'provides protection against': Trans. acc. to a.

357 In his trans. of Maimonides' *Medical Aphorisms* (i.e., *Sefer ha-Peraqim*) XV.6, Zeraḥyah translates Arab. الأدوية التي تحرق وتكوي 'the caustic remedies' as רפואה שורפת ומכווה (cf. BMMZ 153, l. 12; BMMG no. 1913).

והוא[358] חוץ ממנו ויהיו חלקיו מקבלים להגרה בשילשולו (A lubricant [drug] is a drug that—by its nature—moistens the surface of a substance that is blocked in a passage, when it [i.e., the drug] encounters it. It[359] [i.e., the drug] releases it [i.e., the substance] and makes its parts more capable of flowing [by its moistening effect]). Hebr. הרפואה הממעידה is not attested in the current dictionaries. Anonymous I renders Arab. الدواء المزلق as הסם הממעיד (see entry סַם).

• **הרפואה המנגבת · the desiccant drug**: Arab. الدواء المجفف · Ibn Sīnā, *K. al-Qānūn* II · trans. Zeraḥyah Ḥen, *Sefer ha-Qanun* (Ms Oxford, Bodleian Libaries, Opp. Add. Fol. 12, fol. 161[a]): והמנגבת היא הרפואה אשר תכלה הלחויות בהתרתה ויבשה ודיקדוקה (A desiccant [drug] is a drug that destroys fluids through its dissolving, drying, and refining [quality]). Hebr. הרפואה ההמנגבת is not attested in the current dictionaries. Nathan ha-Me'ati translates Arab. الدواء المجفف as הסם המיבש and Anonymous I has הסם המנגב (for both terms, see entry סַם).

• **הרפואה המנפחת · the flatulent drug**: Arab. الدواء المنفخ · Ibn Sīnā, *K. al-Qānūn* II · trans. Zeraḥyah Ḥen, Sefer ha-Qanun (Ms Oxford, Bodleian Libaries, Opp. Add. Fol. 12, fol. 161[r]: והמנפחת היא הרפואה אשר בעצמותה לחות זר ועב כשתפעל בה החום הטבעי לא יהיה נתך מהרה אבל ישתנה אל רוח כמו הפִּישׁוֹלִי (A flatulent [drug] is a drug whose substance has foreign and dense moisture. When innate heat acts on it, it does not dissolve swiftly but is transformed into wind; [an example of such a drug is the] black-eyed pea). Hebr. הרפואה המנפחת is not attested in the current dictionaries. Nathan ha-Me'ati and Anonymous I both render Arab. الدواء المنفّخ as הסם הנופח (see entry סַם).

• **הרפואה המסתמת · the obstruent drug**: Arab. الدواء المسدّد · Ibn Sīnā, *K. al-Qānūn* II · trans. Zeraḥyah Ḥen, *Sefer ha-Qanun* (Ms Oxford, Bodleian Libaries, Opp. Add. Fol. 12, fol. 161[a]): והמסתמת היא הרפואה היבשה אשר בה לחות מועט ודבק יתדבקו בו הפיות ויסתמום ותעצור הנגר (An obstruant [drug] is a dry drug with a small quantity of viscous fluid with which it adheres to the openings [in the body] and clogs them and blocks the flow [of the substance]). Hebr. הרפואה המסתמת is not attested in the current dictionaries. Nathan ha-Me'ati translates Arab. الدواء المسدّد as הסם האוטם and Anonymous I renders the Arab. term as הסם הסותם (for both terms, see entry סַם).

• **הרפואה המעבה · 1. the roughening drug**: Arab. الدواء المخشن · Ibn Sīnā, *K. al-Qānūn* II · trans. Zeraḥyah Ḥen, *Sefer ha-Qanun* (Ms Oxford, Bodleian Libaries, Opp. Add. Fol. 12, fol. 159[b]): והמעבה היא הרפואה אשר תשים שטח האבר משתנה החלקים בהרמה ובנמוך (A roughening [drug] is a drug that makes the surface of an organ uneven in height and depth). Hebr. הרפואה המעבה is not attested in the current dictionaries. Nathan ha-Me'ati translates Arab. الدواء المخشن as הסם המעבה and Anonymous I renders the Arab. term as הסם המנחיר (for both terms, see entry סַם).

---

358 והוא חוץ ממנו: حتى يبرئه عنه a.

359 'It [i.e., the drug] releases it [i.e., the substance]': Trans. acc. to a.

· II. the thickening (inspissating) drug: Arab. الدواء المغلظ · Ibn Sīnā, *K. al-Qānūn* II · trans. Zeraḥyah Ḥen, *Sefer ha-Qanun* (Ms Oxford, Bodleian Libaries, Opp. Add. Fol. 12, fol. 160r: והמעבה היא הפך המדקדקת זאת היא רפואה אשר דרכה שתשים עצמות הלחות יותר גס או בהיותו מקפיא או בעיבויו או לעירובו (A thickening (inspissating) [drug] is the opposite of an attenuant one. It is a drug that—by its nature—makes the consistency of humors more dense either by its coagulating or thickening property, or by merging with them). Nathan ha-Me'ati translates Arab. الدواء المغلظ as הסם המוליד הגסות and Anonymous I renders the Arab. term as הסם המעבה (for both terms, see entry סַם).

• **הרפואה המעכלת** · **the digestive drug**: Arab. الدواء الهاضم · Ibn Sīnā, *K. al-Qānūn* II · trans. Zeraḥyah Ḥen, *Sefer ha-Qanun* (Ms Oxford, Bodleian Libaries, Opp. Add. Fol. 12, fol. 160a): והמעכלת היא אשר מטבעה להקנות[360] עיכול וכבר ידעת זה במה שקדם (A digestive [drug] is [a drug] that—by its nature—helps[361] the digestion [of food]. This is already known from what I said before). Hebr. הרפואה המעכלת is not attested in the current dictionaries. Nathan ha-Me'ati and Anonymous I both render Arab. الدواء الهاضم as הסם המעכל (see entry סַם).

• **הרפואה המעפשת** · **the putrefactive drug**: Arab. الدواء المعفن · Ibn Sīnā, K. *al-Qānūn* II · trans. Zeraḥyah Ḥen, *Sefer ha-Qanun* (Ms Oxford, Bodleian Libaries, Opp. Add. Fol. 12, fol. 160b): והמעפשת היא שטבעה להפסיד מזג הרוח ההולך אל האבר ומזג לחות בהתרה עד שלא יהיה ראוי שיהיה חלק לאותו האבר ולא יגיע לשרפו ולאכלו (A putrefactive [drug] is [a drug] that—by its nature—corrupts the temperament of the pneuma that flows to an organ and also the temperament of the humor through dissolution, to such an extent that they are not suitable to be parts of the organ, but not to an extent where these are burnt or corroded).[362] Hebr. הרפואה המעפשת is not attested in the current dictionaries. Nathan ha-Me'ati and Anonymous I both render Arab. الدواء المعفن as הסם המעפש (see entry סַם).

• **הרפואה המפגגת** · **the drug that makes crude (unripe)**: Arab. الدواء المفجّج · Ibn Sīnā, *K. al-Qānūn* II · trans. Zeraḥyah Ḥen, *Sefer ha-Qanun* (Ms Oxford, Bodleian Libaries, Opp. Add. Fol. 12, fol. 160b): והמפגגת הוא הפך המעכלת וגם כן למבשלת והיא אשר תבטל בקרירותה פעולת החום היסודי והזר גם כן במזון[363] עד שישאר בלתי מעוכל ולא מבושל (A [drug] that makes unripe (crude) is the opposite of a digestive and ripening [drug]. It is [a drug] that—by its cold [nature]—makes the action of innate and extraneous

360 להקנות: يفيد a.
361 'helps': Trans. acc. to a.
362 In his trans. of Maimonides' *Medical Aphorisms* (i.e., *Sefer ha-Peraqim*) XXIII.101, Zeraḥyah translates Arab. *Plur.* أدوية معفنة 'putrefying remedies' as רפואה מעפשת (cf. BMMZ, 231, l. 1; BMMG no. 1892).
363 במזון: والخلط add. a.

heat on both food and[364] humors ineffective). Hebr. *Pi'el* פִּגֵּג features in BM 4810 in the sense of 'to clot.' Our paragraph is quoted by Ben Yehuda (ibid.) as והמפגג הוא אשר בקרירותו יבטל פועל החום במזון או הליחה in an attestation from Joseph Vidal Benveniste's *Sefer Gerem ha-Maʿalot*. Nathan ha-Me'ati and Anonymous I both render Arab. الدواء المفجّج as הסם המפגג (see entry סַם).

• **הרפואה הפותחת · the deobstruent drug**: Arab. الدواء المفتّح · Ibn Sīnā, *K. al-Qānūn* II · trans. Zeraḥyah Ḥen, *Sefer ha-Qanun* (Ms Oxford, Bodleian Libaries, Opp. Add. Fol. 12, fol. 159ᵇ):[365] והפותחת היא אשר מטבעה שתניע החומר העומד בתוך חללי הדרכים אל חוצה למען השאיר הסמפונות פתוחות וזה הוא יותר חזק מן המטהר כמו הפֵּיטְרוּצִינוֹלוֹ (A deobstruent [drug] is [a drug] that—by its nature—moves the [humoral] matter lying in the cavities of the passages to the outside so that they stay open. These drugs are stronger than the detergent ones; [an example of such a drug is] parsley). Hebr. הרפואה הפותחת is not attested in the current dictionaries. Nathan ha-Me'ati translates Arab. الدواء المفتّح as הסם המפתח and Anonymous I renders the Arab. term as הסם הפותח (cf. BCD 191 (NM 4:134–135) for an attestation from an anonymous trans. of Ibn Sīnā's *K. al-Adwiya al-qalbiyya* (i.e., *Sammim Libbiyim*)). For both terms, see entry סַם.

• **הרפואה המפוצצת · the [stone-]crushing (lithontriptic) drug**: Arab. الدواء المفتّت · Ibn Sīnā, *K. al-Qānūn* II · trans. Zeraḥyah Ḥen, *Sefer ha-Qanun* (Ms Oxford, Bodleian Libaries, Opp. Add. Fol. 12, fol. 160ᵇ):[366] והמפוצצת היא שטבעה במצאה ליחה דומה לאבן תקטין חלקיה ותדק אותם כמו המפוצצת החול וכמו אבן היהודית ודומה לה (A [stone-]crushing (lithontriptic) [drug] is [a drug] that—by its nature—, when it comes across a humor similar to stone (petrified humor), reduces it into small pieces and crushes it like [a drug] that breaks up stones; [an example of such a drug is] the Jews' stone and similar [stones]). Hebr. הרפואה המפוצצת is not attested in the current dictionaries. Nathan ha-Me'ati translates Arab. الدواء المفتّت as הסם המפרך and Anonymous I has הסם המפתת (for both terms, see entry סַם).

• **הרפואה המצמיחה הבשר · the drug that makes the flesh grow**: Arab. الدواء المنبت للحم · Ibn Sīnā, *K. al-Qānūn* II · trans. Zeraḥyah Ḥen, *Sefer ha-Qanun* (Ms Oxford, Bodleian Libaries, Opp. Add. Fol. 12, 161ᵇ):[367] והמצמיחה הבשר היא הרפואה אשר מדרכה שתשנה הדם היורד על החבלה לבשר לישר מזגו והקפיאו בניגוב (A [drug] that makes the flesh

364 'and humors': Add. acc. to a.

365 In his trans. of Maimonides' *Medical Aphorisms* (i.e., *Sefer ha-Peraqim*) IX.3, Zeraḥyah translates Arab. *Plur.* الأدوية المفتّحة 'the opening medications' as הרפואה הפותחת as well (cf. BMMZ 98, ll. 14–15; BMMG no. 1931).

366 In his trans. of Maimonides' *Medical Aphorisms* (i.e., *Sefer ha-Peraqim*) XXI.65, Zeraḥyah translates Arab. الأدوية المفتّتة للحصى 'the stone-crushing remedies' as הרפואה המשברת לחול (cf. BMMZ 202, l. 4; BMMG no. 1930).

367 The Hebr. term also features in Zeraḥyah's trans. of Maimonides' *Medical Aphorisms* (i.e., *Sefer ha-Peraqim*) XV.55, 56 (cf. BMMZ 161, ll. 16, 20; BMMG no. 1874).

grow is a drug that—by its nature—changes the blood, which streams to a wound, into flesh by moderating the temperament of the blood and coagulating it through desiccation). Hebr. הרפואה המצמיחה הבשר is not attested in the current dictionaries. Nathan ha-Me'ati and Anonymous I both render Arab. الدواء المنبت للحم as הסם המצמיח הבשר (see entry סַם).

• **הרפואה הקובצת · the astringent drug**: Arab. الدواء القابض · Ibn Sīnā, *K. al-Qānūn* II · trans. Zeraḥyah Ḥen, *Sefer ha-Qanun* (Ms Oxford, Bodleian Libaries, Opp. Add. Fol. 12, fol. 161[a]): והקובצת[368] היא הרפואה אשר תחדש באבר ריבוי תנועה אל הקיבוץ לעצור[369] מקומם ותסתום הדרכים (An astringent [drug] is a drug that produces in an organ excessive movement towards contraction [in its parts], so that they draw together in their site; it also closes the channels). Hebr. הרפואה הקובצת is not attested in the current dictionaries. For the verb קָבֵץ 'to be astringent' and *Part.* קוֹבֵץ 'astringent,' cf. BCD 236f. (NM 1:183, corr. 2:198; 2:79, 81) for attestations from Zeraḥyah's and Nathan ha-Me'ati's trans. of Maimonides' *Medical Aphorisms* (i.e., *Sefer ha-Peraqim*)). In his *Sefer ha-Peraqim* III.112 though, Zeraḥyah translates Arab. الدواء القابض as הרפואה המקבצת (cf. BMMZ 49, l. 11; BMMG no. 1856). Nathan and Anonymous I both render the Arab. term as הסם הקובץ (cf. BCD 191 (NM 4:135) for an attestation from an anonymous trans. of Ibn Sīnā's *K. al-Adwiya al-qalbiyya* (i.e., *Sammim Libbiyim*)).

• **הרפואה הקולפת · the peeling drug**: Arab. الدواء القاشر · Ibn Sīnā, *K. al-Qānūn* II · trans. Zeraḥyah Ḥen, *Sefer ha-Qanun* (Ms Oxford, Bodleian Libaries, Opp. Add. Fol. 12, fol. 160[b]): והקולפת[370] כמו כן היא הרפואה אשר מדרכה מריבוי נקיונה שתטהר חלקי העור הנפסדים כמו הקושט (A peeling [drug] is also a drug that—by its nature [and] its intense cleansing property—cleans the decayed parts of the skin; [an example of such a drug is] costus). Hebr. הרפואה הקולפת is not attested in the current dictionaries. Nathan ha-Me'ati and Anonymous I both render Arab. الدواء القاشر as הסם המקלף (see entry סַם). Arab. مقشر in the sense of 'peeling (exfoliating)' is translated by Zeraḥyah as *Part. Pi'el* מְפַזֵּר (see entry [פזר]).

• **הרפואה הרוחצת · the abluent drug**: Arab. الدواء الغسّال · Ibn Sīnā, *K. al-Qānūn* II · trans. Zeraḥyah Ḥen, *Sefer ha-Qanun* (Ms Oxford, Bodleian Libaries, Opp. Add. Fol. 12, fol. 161[a]):[371] והרוחצת היא כל רפואה אשר מדרכה שתטהר לא בכח פועל בו אבל בכח מתפעל (An abluent [drug] is any drug that—by its nature—cleanses not through its active power but through its passive power). Hebr. הרפואה הרוחצת is not attested in the current-

368 והקובצת: Emend. ed. והעוצרת Ms והקובץ Ms[1].

369 לעצור מקומם: لتتكاثف في موضعها a.

370 והקולפת: Emend. ed. והקולף Ms.

371 In his trans. of Maimonides' *Medical Aphorisms* (i.e., *Sefer ha-Peraqim*) XXIII.100, Zeraḥyah translates Arab. الدواء الغسّال 'the cleansing medicine' as הרפואה המכבסת (cf. BMMZ 230, l. 22; BMMG no. 1870; NM 5:190).

rent dictionaries. Nathan ha-Me'ati and Anonymous I both render Arab. الدواء الغسّال as הסם הרוחץ (see entry סַם).

• **הרפואה המרפה** · **the relaxing (slackening) drug**: Arab. الدواء المرخي · Ibn Sīnā, *K. al-Qānūn* II · trans. Zeraḥyah Ḥen, *Sefer ha-Qanun* (Ms Oxford, Bodleian Libaries, Opp. Add. Fol. 12, fol. 159^b):[372] והמרפה היא אשר מטבעה שתשים עצמות האיברים המתקשים בנקביהם לחים בחמימותו ולחותו ויקרה מזה שהנקבים ישובו יותר רחבים וידחה מה שבו מן המותרות יותר נקל כמו תחבושת האניט וזרע הפשתן (A relaxing [drug] is—by its nature—[a drug] that, through its heat and moisture, softens the substance of organs, having dense pores. Consequently, the pores become wider and the expulsion of superfluous matter deposited there becomes easier; [an example of such a drug is] the plaster of dill and linseed). Hebr. הרפואה המרפה is not attested in the current dictionaries. Nathan ha-Me'ati and Anonymous I both render Arab. الدواء المرخي as הסם המרפה (cf. BCD 189; NM 4:130 for an attestation from an anonymous trans. of Ibn Sīnā's *K. al-Adwiya al-qalbiyya* (i.e., *Sammim Libbiyim*)).

• **הרפואה המשברת הרוח** · **the carminative drug**: Arab. الدواء الكاسر الرياح · Ibn Sīnā, *K. al-Qānūn* II · trans. Zeraḥyah Ḥen, *Sefer ha-Qanun* (Ms Oxford, Bodleian Libaries, Opp. Add. Fol. 12, fol. 160^a): והרפואה המשברת הרוח היא מטבעה שתשים עצמות הרוח דק אוירי בחמימותו ויבשותו (A carminative drug is [a drug] that—by its nature—dilutes the substance of the gas and makes it airy through its heat and dryness). Hebr. הרפואה המשברת הרוח is not attested in the current dictionaries. Nathan ha-Me'ati renders الدواء الكاسر الرياح as הסם המשבר הרוחות and Anonymous I renders the Arab. term as הסם המשבר הרוח (see entry סַם).

• **הרפואה השוחטת** · **the constricting drug**: Arab. الدواء العاصر · Ibn Sīnā, *K. al-Qānūn* II · trans. Zeraḥyah Ḥen, *Sefer ha-Qanun* (Ms Oxford, Bodleian Libaries, Opp. Add. Fol. 12, fol. 161^a): והשוחטת הוא אשר יבליג בקבוצו והיותו מאסף החלקים עד שיהיו הלחויות הרקיקות העומדות בחלליהם אל הלחיצה וההפרדה (A constricting [drug] is [a drug] whose astringency and condensing [quality] on the organs is so strong that the thin fluids, which have collected in their interstices, are compressed and removed). Hebr. הרפואה השוחטת is not attested in the current dictionaries. Nathan ha-Me'ati translates Arab. الدواء العاصر as הסם העוצר and Anonymous I has הסם המעסה (for both terms, see entry סַם).

• **הרפואה השורפת** · **the caustic drug**: Arab. الدواء المحرق · Ibn Sīnā, *K. al-Qānūn* II · trans. Zeraḥyah Ḥen, *Sefer ha-Qanun* (Ms Oxford, Bodleian Libaries, Opp. Add. Fol. 12, fol. 160^b):[373] והשורפת היא הרפואה אשר יהיה מטבעה שתתיר הדק מן הליחות והאיברים ותשאר הדבר הדומה לדשן כמו הפורביו (A caustic [drug] is a drug that—by its nature—

372 In his trans. of Maimonides' *Medical Aphorisms* (i.e., *Sefer ha-Peraqim*) XV.26, Zeraḥyah translates Arab. *Plur.* الأدوية المرخية 'the slackening medicines' as רפואות מרפות (cf. BMMZ 156, l. 22; BMMG no. 1919).

373 In his trans. of Maimonides' *Medical Aphorisms* (i.e., *Sefer ha-Peraqim*) XV.6, Zeraḥyah

dissolves the tenuous humors of the organs leaving behind the ashy matter; [an example of such a drug is] resin spurge). Hebr. הרפואה השורפת is not attested in the current dictionaries. Nathan ha-Me'ati and Anonymous I both render Arab. الدواء المحرق as הסם השורף (see entry סַם).

רִפּוּי · **cure; healing**: Lat. *curatio* · Guy de Chauliac, *Inventarium sive Chirurgia Magna* (cf. CMM 1:419, ll. 36–38) · trans. Anonymous (Ms Paris, BnF, héb. 1189, fol. 229b): ואחר נפילת הקליפה ינוקה ברפוי הנגעים אם לא שירצה הוא שיעמוד פתוח להריק הליחות ועשנים אידיים (Once the eschar has fallen off, the [cauterized spot] should be cleaned and healed like ulcers unless he wants the [spot] to stay open so that the humors and vaporous fumes can be evacuated). Hebr. רִפּוּי features in the current dictionaries in attestations from Rabb. literature only (cf. BM 6682; JD 1476).

רְפִידָה • *Plur.* **רפידות** · **plug; tampon; pledget**: Lat. *tentae* · Guy de Chauliac, *Inventarium sive Chirurgia Magna* (cf. CMM 1:232, ll. 4–5) · trans. Anonymous (Ms Paris, BnF, héb. 1189, fol. 126b): ואז תמלא החבורה ברפידות שרויות בחלבון ביצה ולמחרתו ישנהו (Then one should fill the wound with a pledget steeped in egg white and repeat this the next day). Hebr. רְפִידָה, *Plur.* רפידות, features in BCD 266 (NM 1:188; 2:86f.) (for Arab. رفائد) in the sense of 'pads' in attestations from Zeraḥyah Ḥen's (XV.65) and Nathan ha-Me'ati's (XV.69) trans. of Maimonides' *Medical Aphorisms* (i.e., *Sefer ha-Peraqim*) (cf. BMMZ 162, l. 23; BMMN 165, l. 1; BMMG no. 2142).

רִפְיוֹן · **lining [of the stomach]**: Arab. خَمْل · Ibn Sīnā, *K. al-Qānūn* II · trans. Zeraḥyah Ḥen, *Sefer ha-Qanun* (Ms Oxford, Bodleian Libaries, Opp. Add. Fol. 12, fol. 201b): הַלִילַג׳ מִירַבַּלֹנִי ... מועיל לכאב הטחול ויועיל לכלי המזון כלם וכל שכן השחורים כי הם יחזקו האצטומ׳ וכל שכן המגודלים ויחזקו רפיון האצטומ׳ עם העיבוד והנקיון והנישוף ([Arab.] *halīlaj* [from Pers. *halīlah*]; [Rom.] MiYRaBaLoNiY: (Chebulic) myrobalan: ... They are useful for pain in the spleen and for all nutritive organs, especially the black variety, because they strengthen the stomach, above all the preserved ones. They strengthen the lining of the stomach through their astringent, cleansing, and absorbing effect). In the sense of 'lining,' Hebr. רִפְיוֹן is a non-attested semantic borrowing from Arab. خَمْل. Nathan ha-Me'ati and Anonymous I, reading Arab. خَمْل as جمل, translate the term as כלל and כל resp.

• **רפיון הדעת** · **want of intellect (reason); amentia**: Arab. بلادة الذهن (cf. Lane 248, s.v. بلادة: 'stupefaction, dullness; want of intellect') · al-Rāzī, *K. fī al-Faṣd* · trans. Anonymous, *Ma'amar ba-Haqqazah* (Ms Parma, Biblioteca Palatina, Cod. Parm. 2283,4, fol. 92b): התפשטות[374] האי׳⟨...⟩ ורוחות הפה הנק׳ אלתמטא ואלתתאב וכובד הראש וגדל הדפק ועבי השתן ואדמימותו וכובד[375] הרגשת האיברים ורפיון הדעת ומתיקות הפה ונגעיו

translates Arab. *Plur.* الأدوية المحرقة 'the caustic remedies' as Hebr. *Sing.* הרפואה השורפת (cf. BMMZ 153, l. 12; BMMG no. 1914).

374 התפשטות האי׳: والتمطي⟨...⟩ a.

375 וכובד הרגשת האיברים: Emend. ed. וכובד הרעשת האיברים Ms وكدر الحواس a.

ויציאת הדם מנחיריו והצמחים הנק׳ אלדממאל הנפתחים מהרה ([Symptoms of overfilling with blood]: Stretching[376] [...] and yawning, called [in Arab.] *al-tamaṭṭā wa-al-tathā'ub*, heaviness of the head, magnitude of the pulse, thick and red urine, troubled[377] sensations, want of intellect (reason), sweetness of mouth, its vesication, nosebleeds, and boils, called [in Arab.] *al-damāmīl*, that burst quickly). Hebr. רפיון הדעת is not attested in the current dictionaries. In his trans. of Maimonides' *On Asthma* (i.e., *Ma'amar 'al ha-Qaṣeret*) XIII.3, Samuel Benveniste translates the synonymous Arab. term بلادة فهم 'dullness of understanding' as אֱטִימוּת (cf. NM 6:16; BMA 2:297, l. 17). The Arab. term بلادة on its own is rendered in an anonymous trans. of Ibn Sīnā's *K. al-Adwiya al-qalbiyya* (i.e., *Sammim Libbiyim*) as עַצְלָה (cf. BCD 208 (NM 4:153f.)).

רְצוּץ • רצוץ האזן · **tear (puncture) in the ear**: Arab. شدخ الأذن (Arab. شدخ = Gr. ῥῆγμα ('breakage, fracture; laceration, rupture, rent, tear'); cf. UW 587; LSG 1568) · Ibn Sīnā, *K. al-Qānūn* II · trans. Nathan ha-Me'ati, *Sefer ha-Qanun* (Ms Oxford, Bodleian Libraries, Can. Or. 88, fol. 91[b]): כברית ... יעצור הנזילה הנק׳ זכאם[378] וראוי לעשותו עם חומץ ודבש ויועיל לרצוץ האזן ([Arab.] *kibrīt*: Sulphur: ... It stops rheum, called [in Arab.] *zukām*, when[379] it is applied as a fumigation; prepared with vinegar and honey it is beneficial for a tear (puncture) in the ear). Hebr. רצוץ האזן is not attested in the current dictionaries. Hebr. רְצוּץ features as part of the term רצוץ העצלים 'muscle tear (rupture)' in NM 6:206 in an attestation from Nathan's *Sefer ha-Qanun* II. Zeraḥyah Ḥen translates Arab. شدخ الأذن as לחיצת האזן (see entry לְחִיצָה) and Anonymous I has רסוק האזן (see entry רִסּוּק). The Hebr. translators probably interpreted the term شَدْخ as derived from شَدَخَ in its general meaning of 'to break, crush, press, squeeze' (cf. Lane 1519) and not in the specific meaning listed above.

רַק · **unless; except when**: Arab. ما لم · al-Rāzī, *K. fī al-Faṣd* · trans. Anonymous, *Ma'amar ba-Haqqazah* (Ms Parma, Biblioteca Palatina, Cod. Parm. 2283,4, fol. 93[a]): צריך להרחיק העטוף בעת ההקזה הרחקה רבה רק מה שצריך אליו בהכרח (Avoid by all means bloodletting until unconsciousness, unless it is necessary). In the sense of 'unless; except when,' Hebr. רַק is not attested in the current dictionaries. It features in the Bible, a.o., in the sense of 'only' after the negating אין (cf. KB 1286), and in medieval philosophical literature in the sense of 'except; but.'[380]

---

376 'Stretching (والتمطي)': The Arab. term is possibly synonymous with التثاؤب; cf. DBK 2:1124, s.v. تمطّى 'étendre les bras en baillant' (stretching the arms while yawning).

377 'troubled sensations': Trans. acc. to a.

378 זכאם: بحورا add. a.

379 'when it is applied as a fumigation': Add. acc. to a.

380 Cf. M. Goshen-Gottstein, *Syntax and Vocabulary of Mediaeval Hebrew as Influenced by Arabic*, rev. by S. Assif and U. Melammed (Jerusalem 2006) (Hebr.), § 152.

רֹק • רוק הדם · **hemoptysis:** Arab. نفث دم · al-Rāzī, *K. fī al-Faṣd* · trans. Anonymous, *Ma'amar ba-Haqqazah* (Ms Parma, Biblioteca Palatina, Cod. Parm. 2283,4, fols. 92[b]–93[a]): ומי שיקרה לו רוק הדם והרפא צריך שיקדים להקיזו בתחלת תקופת ניסן ואם לא יהיה בגופו מעט מלוי (If someone suffered from hemoptysis and he has healed from it, one may proceed to bleed him in the beginning of spring, even if there is no indication of some overfilling in his body). Hebr. רוק הדם is not attested in the current dictionaries. For the more common variant רקיקת הדם, cf. BCD 267 (NM 3:222f.) for an attestation from Moses ibn Tibbons trans. of Maimonides' *Commentary on Hippocrates' Aphorisms* (i.e., *Perush Aphorismi shel Apuqraṭ*) III.29 (cf. BMCH 1:356, l. 14); cf. also BMMG no. 5200 for Nathan ha-Me'ati's and Zeraḥyah Ḥen's trans. of Maimonides' *Medical Aphorisms* (i.e., *Sefer ha-Peraqim*).

רַקָּה • *Plur.* רקות · **cheeks:** Lat. *genae* (cf. DMLBS 1331) · Guy de Chauliac, *Inventarium sive Chirurgia Magna* (cf. CMM 1: 413, l. 33) · trans. Anonymous (Ms Paris, BnF, héb. 1189, fol. 124[a]): הנה הפנים אחר שהם מחזקים אברים רבים ומתחלפים ויש להם מינים ברקותיהם מהנגעים (Since the face contains many different organs and [different] kinds of ulcers in the cheeks ...). Hebr. רַקָּה, *Plur.* רקות, features in the current dictionaries in the sense of 'temple; parietal bones of the head' only (cf. BM 6728f.; Low LXXX).

רְקוּעַ · **plate:** a) Lat. *plata* · Guy de Chauliac, *Inventarium sive Chirurgia Magna* (cf. CMM 1:420, ll. 19–21) · trans. Anonymous (Ms Paris, BnF, héb. 1189, fol. 229[b]): ועליו יונח עלי הכרוב או האידרא תחת הבגדים או על הגדים בג' כפלים או בכפלים יותרא ברקוע מה מעור או מנחשת או מכסף נקשר (On it should be put leaves of cabbage or ivy beneath or on top of pieces of cloth, folded three times or more, and a plate (piece) of leather or copper or silver should be bound on it). In the sense of 'plate,' Hebr. רְקוּעַ features (for Arab. صفيحة) in NM 6:206 in an attestation from Abraham ben Isaac's trans. Ibn al-Jazzār's *Zād al-musāfir* (i.e., *Sefer Ṣedah la-Oreḥim*) VI.2.

· b) Lat. *lamina* · Guy de Chauliac, *Inventarium sive Chirurgia Magna* (cf. CMM 1:230, ll. 24–25) · trans. Anonymous (Ms Paris, BnF, héb. 1189, fol. 229[b]): וכשיצטרך שהבליטה תהיה גדולה עם רקוע עופרת (And when it is necessary, namely when the protrusion [of the cornea] is large [one should bind upon it] a leaden plate).

• *Plur.* רקועים · **itchy skin affection (skin rash; urticaria?):**[381] Arab. شرى · Ibn Sīnā, *K. al-Qānūn* II · trans. Nathan ha-Me'ati, *Sefer ha-Qanun* (Ms Oxford, Bodleian Librar-

381 Cf. P. Richter, 'Über die spezielle Dermatologie des 'Alī ibn al-'Abbās (Haly Abbas) aus dem 10. Jahrhundert unserer Zeitrechnung,' *Archiv für Dermatologie und Syphilis* 113, no. 1 (1912), 861 Repr. in *Beiträge zur Geschichte der arabisch-islamischen Medizin: Aufsätze*, vol. 3: *Aus den Jahren 1909–1913*, ed. by F. Sezgin, in collaboration with M. Amawi, D. Bischoff, and E. Neubauer (Frankfurt am Main 1987), 477: 'ist wohl das entzündliche rote Bläschen der akuten Hautentzündung und entspricht dem ἔκζεμα Aetii. sowie der miliaria rubra (heat rash) der späteren Autoren.' See also Adams' commentary in *The Seven Books of Paulus Ægineta* IV.9: 'It would appear to have been some peculiar species of eczema, now extinct. It must have been a more formidable disease than the nettle-rash, which certain modern

ies, Can. Or. 88, fol. 83[b]): זיתון וזית ... יועיל אל האודם הנקר׳ חמרה ואל הנמלה ואל הרקועים הנק׳ שרי בער׳ ([Arab.] *zaytūn* and [Arab.] *zayt*: Olive [*Olea europaea* L.] and olive oil: ... It is beneficial for erysipelas, called *ḥumrah* [in Arab.], for herpes, and for itchy skin affection (skin rash; urticaria?), called *sharan* in Arab.). Hebr. רְקוּעַ, *Plur.* רקועים, is not attested in this sense in the current dictionaries. Zeraḥyah Ḥen and Anonymous I both transcribe Arab. شرى as שרא.

[רקח] • *Part. Puʿal* **מְרוּקָּח** · **rob [i.e., fruit or vegetable juice boiled down to syrup]**: Arab. مربّى (cf. FAQ 247ff.) · Ibn Sīnā, *K. al-Qānūn* II · trans. Anonymous I, *Sefer ha-Qanun* (Ms Paris, BnF, héb. 1142, fol. 140[a]): כרפס ... מתיך הנפח פותח הסתימה מזיע משקיט הכאבים והמדברי משחין מכאיב והמקורח ממנו נאות למחוממים (Celery [*Apium graveolens* L.]: ... It relieves flatulence. It opens blockages, induces perspiration and allays pain. The wild variety is ulcerating, and causes pain; its preserve is suitable for those who have a hot temperament). Hebr. *Part. Puʿal* מְרוּקָּח is not attested in this sense in the current dictionaries. It features in the Bible in the sense of 'prepared; mixed' (cf. KB 1289). Nathan translates Arab. مربّى as מָעוֹג (cf. NM 6:121f.) and Zeraḥyah Ḥen has *Part. Puʿal* מְרוּבָּב (see entry [רבב]).

רֶשֶׁם · **effect**: Arab. أثر · Ibn Sīnā, *K. al-Qānūn* II · trans. Anonymous I, *Sefer ha-Qanun* (Ms Paris, BnF, héb. 1142, fol. 201[a]): עناב הוא גוגובש ... והמאמר הנכון בו מה שאמר בו גאלי׳: לא מצאתי לגוגובש בשמירת הבריאות והסרת[382] החולי רושם גדול ([Arab.] *ʿunnāb*; i.e., [Rom.] GWGWBŠ: Jujube [*Ziziphus* sp.]: ... The best statement regarding jujube is that by Galen: I did not find that jujube has a significant effect on preserving the health of healthy people and [restoring the health of sick people]). Hebr. רֶשֶׁם features in medieval medical literature (for Arab. آثار) in the sense of 'spots [on the body]; scars' (cf. next entry). For its different meanings in medieval philosophical literature, cf. PESHAT.[383] Nathan ha-Me'ati translates Arab. أثر as סימן (see entry), and Zeraḥyah Ḥen as מעשה (see entry).

• *Plur.* **רשמים** · **scars**: Lat. *cicatrices* · Guy de Chauliac, *Inventarium sive Chirurgia Magna* (cf. CMM 1:229, ll. 11–12) · trans. Anonymous (Ms Paris, BnF, héb. 1189, fol. 125[a]): רשמים לבנים (White scars). In the sense of 'scar,' Hebr. *Sing.* רֶשֶׁם features (for Arab. آثار) in NM 6:207 in an attestation from Anonymous I's trans. of Ibn Sīnā's *K. al-Qānūn* (i.e., *Sefer ha-Qanun*) II.

[רתע] • *Part. Hifʿil* **מַרְתִּיעַ** • *Plur.* **מרתיעים** · **repelling remedies**: Lat. *repercussiva* (cf. ND 916) · Guy de Chauliac, *Inventarium sive Chirurgia Magna* (cf. CMM 1:230, ll. 17–18) · trans. Anonymous (Ms Paris, BnF, héb. 1189, fol. 125[b]): שאז ... יצטרך מרתיעים (For

---

authorities have taken for the epinyctis of the ancients' (2:41); cf. also IJZ 7:122, n. 268; MIG no. 166. For the synonymous term בנות הלילה, see entry בַּת.

382 והסרת החולי: استرداد الصحة المفقودة a.

383 https://peshat.org/display/peshat_lemmas_00022412 (accessed February 1, 2023).

then ... one needs [to apply] repelling remedies). Hebr. *Part. Hif'il* מַרְתִּיעַ features as part of the term הסם המרתיע in the sense of 'the repellent remedy' (for Arab. الدواء الرادع) in BCD 189 (NM 4:131) in an attestation from an anonymous trans. of Ibn Sīnā's *K. al-Adwiya al-qalbiyya* (i.e., *Sammim Libbiyim*).

ש

שִׁבּוּךְ · **twisting; cramp; spasm**: Arab. تشبّك (cf. D 722) · Ibn Sīnā, *K. al-Qānūn* II · trans. Zeraḥyah Ḥen, *Sefer ha-Qanun* (Ms Oxford, Bodleian Libaries, Opp. Add. Fol. 12, fol. 229$^{a–b}$): לֻבְנֵי ... יחזק האיברים וימנע שבוך האיברים לשתות ולמשוח ויכנס במשיחות העיפות ([Arab.] *lubnā*: Styrax: ... It strengthens the organs and prevents twisting of joints, both when taken orally or applied as a salve. It is incorporated in oils [used] for fatigue). Hebr. שִׁבּוּךְ features in BM 7513 as a synonym of סִבּוּךְ 'intertwining' (cf. BM 3914). Nathan ha-Me'ati translates Arab. تشبّك as חִבּוּךְ (see entry) and Anonymous I renders the Arab. term as הִסְתַּבְּכוּת (cf. BCD 68 (NM 4:45) for an attestation from Shem Tov ben Isaac's *Sefer ha-Shimmush* XXVII).

[שבך] • *Part. Pu'al* מְשֻׁבָּךְ · **interlaced; entangled**: Arab. مشتبك · Ibn Sīnā, *K. al-Qānūn* II · trans. Zeraḥyah Ḥen, *Sefer ha-Qanun* (Ms Oxford, Bodleian Libaries, Opp. Add. Fol. 12, fol. 210^{b}): חֲמֵאמֶא הוא עשב כמו אשכול מעצים משובך ([Arab.] *ḥamāmā*:[384] It is a plant with a cluster of branches interlaced with each other). Hebr. *Part. Pu'al* מְשֻׁבָּךְ features in Samuel ibn Tibbon's trans. of Maimonides' *Guide of the Perplexed* (i.e., *Moreh Nevukhim*) I.0 in an explanation of the Bibl. term משכיות (Prov 25:11): כי המשכיות הם הגופות המפתחים בפתוחים משבכים (The term *maskiyyoth* denotes filigree traceries).[385] Nathan ha-Me'ati translates Arab. مشتبك as מסתבך and Anonymous I as מצטבך.

[שבר] • *Pi'el* שִׁבֵּר • שיבר הרוחות · **to be carminative (to relieve flatulence, gas)**: Arab. كسر الرياح · Ibn Sīnā, *K. al-Qānūn* II · trans. Zeraḥyah Ḥen, *Sefer ha-Qanun* (Ms Oxford, Bodleian Libaries, Opp. Add. Fol. 12, fol. 212^{a}): חלתית אַשָׁא פֵ׳דֵידָא ... ישבר הרוחות וישליכם בהתרתו ([Arab.] *ḥiltīt* / [Hebr.] *ḥiltit*; [i.e., Rom.] 'aŠa' FeDeYDa': Resin of asafetida [*Ferula assa-foetida* L.]: ... It is carminative and expels gases by dissolving them). In the sense of 'to be carminative,' Hebr. שיבר הרוחות is a non-attested calque from Arab. كسر الرياح. The synonymous Arab. term فشّش الرياح, *Part.* مفشّش للرياح, is translated by Zeraḥyah as מפזר הרוחות (see entry [פזר]). Nathan ha-Me'ati and Anonymous I both render Arab. كسر الرياح as שיבר הרוחות, just like Zeraḥyah.

• *Part. Pi'el* מְשַׁבֵּר • הסם המשבר הרוח → סַם.

• הרפואה המשברת הרוח → רְפוּאָה.

שַׁד • *Plur.* שדים • ענבי השדים → עֵנָב.

---

384 An identification of the Arab. term is hardly possible. It may refer to 1) a plant species in the *Vitaceae* family—perh. *Cissus vitiginea* L.; 2) 'melegueta pepper,' i.e., the seeds of *Aframomum melegueta* K. Schum.; or 3) two species of *Bryonia* sp., namely *Bryonia alba* L. ('white bryony') and *Bryonia dioica* Jacq. ('Cretan bryony'); cf. DT 98f. (I.12).

385 Cf. BM 7514; Maimonides, *Moreh Nevukhim*, ed. by J.E. Shemuel (Jerusalem, 1984), 10; *The Guide of the Perplexed*, trans. by Shl. Pines (Chicago, 1963), 1:11.

שׁוּב • **שב כדבק** · **to become mouldy**: Arab. تكرّج (cf. WKAS 1:120) · Ibn Sīnā, *K. al-Qānūn* II · trans. Nathan ha-Me'ati, *Sefer ha-Qanun* (Ms Oxford, Bodleian Libraries, Can. Or. 88, fol. 82[a]): אס והוא ההדס ... ציציו הוא הלבן ומיץ הפרי שלו הוא יותר משובח ומיצו כשיתישן יחלש וישוב כדבק ויאות לעשותו עוגות ([Arab.] *ās*; i.e., [Hebr.] *ha-hadas*: Myrtle [*Myrtus communis* L.]: ... The flower of the white [variety] is the best and so is the extract of its fruit. But if the extract becomes old, it grows weak and becomes mouldy. Therefore, one should make pastilles of them). Hebr. שב כדבק is not attested in the current dictionaries. Anonymous I renders Arab. تكرّج as *Hitpa'el* הִתְדַּבֵּק (see entry [דבק]).
• *Hif'il* **הֵשִׁיב** • **השיב עכור** · **to make [something] thick; to thicken**: Arab. إخثار · Ibn Sīnā, *K. al-Qānūn* II · trans. Nathan ha-Me'ati, *Sefer ha-Qanun* (Ms Oxford, Bodleian Libraries, Can. Or. 88, fol. 57[a]): והמוליד הגסות הוא בהפך המרקיק והוא הסם מדרכו שישים תכונת הרוטבה יותר גסה אמנם בקפיאתו ואמנם שישיבנו עכור (A thickening (inspissating) [drug] is the opposite of an attenuant one. It is a drug that—by its nature—makes the consistency of humors more dense either by its coagulating or thickening property). Hebr. עָכוּר features in the current dictionaries in the sense of 'turbid' only. Zeraḥyah Ḥen translates Arab. إخثار as עבוי and Anonymous I (interpreting Arab. إخثار as deriving from the root خار) has דעיכה.

[שוה] • *Hif'il* **הִשְׁוָה** · **to balance**: Arab. عدّل · Ibn Sīnā, *K. al-Qānūn* II · trans. Anonymous I, *Sefer ha-Qanun* (Ms Paris, BnF, héb. 1142, fol. 13[A]): והמחזק הוא הסם שדרכו להשוות עצם האבר ומזגו עד שימנע מלקבל המותרים הנהפכים אליו והפגעים (A tonic [drug] is a drug that—by its nature—balances the consistency and temperament of an organ to the extent that it prevents the absorption of superfluous matters and disorders that move towards it). Hebr. *Hif'il* הִשְׁוָה is not attested for medieval medical literature. Nathan ha-Me'ati translates Arab. عدّل as *Pi'el* יִשֵּׁר (see entry [ישר]) and Zeraḥyah Ḥen has *Pi'el* מִצַּע (see entry [מצע]).

שׁוֹחֵט (*Part.*) → **שָׁחַט**.

שׁוּם • **שום מדברי** · **[lit. 'wild garlic']; water germander [*Teucrium scordium* L.]**: Arab. سقورديون (cf. MIG no. 45) · Ibn Sīnā, *K. al-Qānūn* II · trans. Nathan ha-Me'ati, *Sefer ha-Qanun* (Ms Oxford, Bodleian Libraries, Can. Or. 88, fol. 108[r]): סקורדיון המהות הוא השום המדברי ([Arab.] *sqūrdiyūn*. What is it? It is [Hebr.] *ha-shum ha-midbari*). In the sense of 'water germander,' Hebr. שום מדברי is a non-attested calque from Arab. ثوم بريّ, a synonym of سقورديون (cf. MIG no. 45). Zeraḥyah Ḥen renders Arab. سقورديون as השומים המדברי⟨ם⟩ and Anonymous I has שום מדברי, just like Nathan.

שׁוֹרֵף (*Part.*) → **שָׂרַף**.

שׁוֹרֶשׁ → **שֹׁרֶשׁ**.

שָׁחוֹר • *Plur.* **שחורים** • **פלפל השחורים** → **פִּלְפֵּל**.

שָׁחַט • *Part.* **שׁוֹחֵט** • **הרפואה השוחטת** → **רְפוּאָה**.

שְׁחִי • **בית השחי** → **בַּיִת**.

שְׁחִין • **שחין אדום** · **heat rash; miliaria rubra**: Arab. حصف (Gr. ἵδρωα; cf. UW 306) · Ibn Sīnā, *K. al-Qānūn* II · trans. Nathan ha-Me'ati, *Sefer ha-Qanun* (Ms Oxford, Bodleian

Libraries, Can. Or. 88, fol. 82[r]: זנג׳פור ... מסגר הנגעים ויצמיח הבשר בנגעים וימנע שרפת האש וימנע השחין האדום הנקרא חצף ([Arab.] *zunjufūr*: Cinnabar: ... It closes wounds and heals ulcers, prevents burns and heat rash, called *ḥaṣaf* [in Arab.]). Hebr. שחין אדום does not feature in the current dictionaries. Zeraḥyah Ḥen translates Arab. حصف as קורשטא and Anonymous I simply transcribes the Arab. term as חצף. A synonym featuring in medieval medical literature is Aram. חַסְפְּנִיתָא, featuring in Moses ibn Tibbon's trans. of Ibn al-Jazzār's *Zād al-musāfir* (i.e., *Sefer Ṣedat ha-Derakhim*) VII.24.3 (cf. BCD 105 (NM 1:57); IJZ 7:164, l. 18).

• **שחין הפה** · **aphtha**: Arab. قلاع (Gr. ἄφθα, *Plur.* ἄφθαι; cf. UW 151) · Ibn Sīnā, *K. al-Qānūn* II · trans. Nathan ha-Me'ati, *Sefer ha-Qanun* (Ms Oxford, Bodleian Libraries, Can. Or. 88, fol. 103[a]): מיוזבג׳ ... ויבשלוהו בחומץ וישכשכו בו הפה ויועיל לכאב השנים ורוטבת בשר השנים ועם דבש ירפא שחין הפה ובער׳ קלאע ([Arab.] *maywīzaj*: Stavesacre [*Delphinium staphisagria* L.]: ... When it is cooked with vinegar and used as a gargle, it is good for toothache and mucous secretion from the gums. With honey it cures aphthae, [called] in Arab. *qulāʿ*). In the sense of 'aphtha,' Hebr. שחין הפה features as *Plur.* שחיני הפה in BCD 272 (NM 3:226) in an attestation from Judah Shalom's trans. of Hippocrates' *Aphorisms* III.24, and ibid. (NM 3:225) as השחין אשר בפה in an attestation from Moses ibn Tibbon's trans. of Maimonides' *Commentary on Hippocrates'* Aphorisms (i.e., *Perush Aphorismi shel Apuqraṭ*) III.24 (cf. BMCH 1:355, l. 4). Zeraḥyah Ḥen simply transcribes Arab. قلاع as קלאע and Anonymous I renders the Arab. term as שחיני הפה הרעים (see next entry).

• *Plur.* **שחינים** • **שחיני הפה הרעים** · **aphthae**: Arab. قلاع (Gr. ἄφθα, *Plur.* ἄφθαι; cf. UW 151) · Ibn Sīnā, *K. al-Qānūn* II · trans. Anonymous I (Ms Paris, BnF, héb. 1142, fol. 168[a]): מיובזג ... ויבושל בחומץ וימצמץ בו לכאב השנים ולחות הלסתות ומבריא עם דבש לשחיני הפה הרעים הנקרא קלאע ([Arab.] *maywīzaj*: Stavesacre [*Delphinium staphisagria* L.]: ... When it is cooked with vinegar and used as a gargle, [it is good] for toothache and mucous secretion from the gums. With honey it cures aphthae, called *qulāʿ* [in Arab.]). Hebr. שחיני הפה הרעים is not attested in the current dictionaries. Nathan ha-Me'ati translates Arab. قلاع as שחין הפה (see previous entry) and Zeraḥyah Ḥen simply transcribes the Arab. term as קלאע.

[שחן] • *Part. Hitpaʿel* **מִשְׁתַּחֵן** • **הגרב המשתחן** → **גָּרָב**.

שַׁחֲרוּת • **שחרות העין** · **black eye**: Arab. كمودة العين (Gr. ὑπώπιον;[386] cf. UW2:561f.; LSG 1904) · Ibn Sīnā, *K. al-Qānūn* II · trans. Zeraḥyah Ḥen, *Sefer ha-Qanun* (Ms Oxford, Bodleian Libaries, Opp. Add. Fol. 12, fol. 180[a–b]): בַּאקְלֵי הוא עם הדבש והפיניגרג חובש לשחרות העין ולטרפה ועם אוליבנו וורדים ולובן ביצה חובש להסתרה[387] ([Arab.] *bāqillā*: Broad bean

---

386 Cf. the parallel entry on 'broad bean' [*Vicia faba* L.] in the Arab. trans. of Dioscorides' *De materia medica* (Ms Paris, BnF, arabe 2849, fol. 43[a]): كمودة لون الموضع ويسمى باليونانية اوقوفيا. The term اوقوفيا (read: اوفوفيا) is Gr. ὑπώπιον, *Plur.* ὑπώπια.

387 להסתרה: للجحوز a.

[*Vicia faba* L.]: As a plaster with fenugreek, it is [useful] for a black eye and a blood spot in the eye, and as a plaster with frankincense, egg white, and roses, it is [useful] for protrusion[388] of the eye). Hebr. שחרות העין is not attested in the current dictionaries. Nathan ha-Me'ati translates Arab. كمودة العين as חשכת העין (see entry חֲשֵׁכָה) and Anonymous I has כהות העין (see entry כֵּהוּת).

שִׁילּוּחַ → שִׁלּוּחַ.

שְׁכוּנָה · **sympathetic affection**: Lat. *societas* (Arab. شركة (Gr. συνπάθεια; cf. UWS 2:368)) · Constantinus Africanus, *Viaticum* V.5 · trans. Do'eg ha-Edomi, *Sefer Ya'ir Netiv*: אם כן אינדרופישים הוא מאפיסת המחליף לבדו כי השחתת הדם יחול מחלישות זה הכח. ואנו אמרנו בתחלת הספר כי תחלואי הכבד הם או מעצמו לבדו או משכונת אבר אחר כמו מן האסטומכא מהטחול מהמעים מהכליות או מן האם (Consequently, dropsy only results from the weakness of the transforming [faculty] because the blood gets corrupted when it is weak. I said in the beginning of the book that the illnesses of the liver either originate from the liver itself or because it is sympathetically affected by another organ, such as the stomach, spleen, intestines, kidneys, or the uterus). Hebr. שְׁכוּנָה is not attested for medieval medical literature. It features in the sense of 'contiguity' in medieval philosophical literature; cf. PESHAT.[389] Moses ibn Tibbon translates Arab. شركة as שִׁתּוּף (see entry).

שְׁכִיכָה · **soothing [of pain]**: Arab. تسكين · Ibn Sīnā, *K. al-Qānūn* II · trans. Zeraḥyah Ḥen, *Sefer ha-Qanun* (Ms Oxford, Bodleian Libaries, Opp. Add. Fol. 12, fols. 246ᵇ–247ᵃ):[390] סנדרוס ... ימנע עישונו הרֵיומִי ותועלתו בשכיכת כאב השנים גדולה וחזקה מאד אין כמותו בזה ([Arab.] *sandarūs*: Sandarac [i.e., resin from the sandarac gum tree [*Tetraclinis articulate* (Vahl) Mast.]]: ... A fumigation with sandarac stops catarrh. It is very beneficial for soothing toothache. Nothing is as effective). Hebr. שְׁכִיכָה is attested in Rabb. literature in the sense of 'appeasement' (cf. JD 1573; BM 7095). Nathan ha-Me'ati and Anonymous I both render Arab. تسكين as השקיט.

[שכך] • *Part. Pi'el* מְשַׁכֵּךְ · **relieving, quenching [the thirst]**: Arab. سكّن · Ibn Sīnā, *K. al-Qānūn* II · trans. Zeraḥyah Ḥen, *Sefer ha-Qanun* (Ms Oxford, Bodleian Libaries, Opp. Add. Fol. 12, fol. 277ᵇ): תַּרוּנְגְּבִין מַנְנַא ... משכך הצמא ([Arab.] *taranjubīn* [from Pers. *tarangubīn*]; [Aram.] *manna'*: Manna:[391] ... It relieves (quenches) the thirst). Hebr. *Part. Pi'el* מְשַׁכֵּךְ is not attested in a medical context in the current dictionaries. In the sense of 'to repel,' it features in NM 5:194 in an attestation from Moses

388 'protrusion of the eye': Trans. acc. to a.

389 https://peshat.org/display/peshat_lemmas_00003943 (accessed May 10, 2022).

390 The same Hebr. term features (for Arab. تسكين) on fol. 186ᵃ, entry בַּט אַנְטְרַא '[Arab.] *baṭṭ*; [i.e., Rom.] 'aNəṬəRa' [i.e., Ital.-Rom. *anatra*]: Duck'.

391 'Manna': I.e., the crystallized honeydew of certain scale insects, in particular the manna mealybug [*Trabutina mannipara* (Hemprich & Ehrenberg, 1829)], that feeds on the tamarisk [*Tamarix* L.]; cf. Lane 306; MSh no. 386.

ibn Tibbon's trans. of Ibn al-Jazzār's *Zād al-musāfir* (i.e., *Sefer Ṣedat ha-Derakhim*) II.24.4 (cf. IJZ 1–2:517). Nathan ha-Me'ati and Anonymous I both render Arab. سكّن as השקיט.

שֶׂכֶל • השתוממות השכל → הִשְׁתּוֹמְמוּת.

שִׁכְשֵׁךְ • שכשך הפה · **to rinse one's mouth; to use a mouthwash**: Arab. مضمض · Ibn Sīnā, *K. al-Qānūn* II · trans. Nathan ha-Me'ati, *Sefer ha-Qanun* (Ms Oxford, Bodleian Libraries, Can. Or. 88, fol. 77[a]): דארשישעאן ... יועיל לבאישות הנחירים ועושים ממנו פתילה ויועיל לזה אם ישכשכו הפה בתבשילו יועיל לנגעי הפה הנקרא קלאע בערבי וישמר השנים מאד ([Arab.] *dārshīshaʿān*: Broom [*Genista acanthoclada* DC. or *Cytisus spinosus* Lam.] (cf. MIG no. 223): ... It is beneficial for ozena when it is used as a wick. If its decoction is used as a mouthwash, it is good for aphthae, called *qulāʿ* in Arab., and for preserving the teeth). Hebr. שִׁכְשֵׁךְ features in BM 7113f. in the sense of 'to rinse' and is not attested for medieval medical literature. In addition to שכשך הפה, Nathan translates Arab. مضمض as רחץ הפה, just like Zeraḥyah Ḥen (see entry רָחַץ). Anonymous I renders Arab. مضمض as מצמץ, a term featuring also in Nathan's trans. of Maimonides' *Medical Aphorisms* (i.e., *Sefer ha-Peraqim*) XXI.10 and XXII.68 (cf. BMMN 196, l. 26; 217, l. 18; BMMG no. 4867).

שְׂלָו · **quail**: Arab. سمّان · *Glossary* (Ms Moscow, Russian State Library, Guenzburg 573, fol. 156[b]): סמאן הוא שלו ([Arab.] *summān*; i.e., [Hebr.] *śelav*). Hebr. שְׂלָו is attested in the Bible in the sense of 'quail' (cf. KB 1331; BM 7576). For the identication of Hebr. שְׂלָו as Arab. سمّان, cf. Ibn Janāḥ's *K. al-Uṣūl*.[392] Subsequently, the Hebr. term features (for Arab. سمّان 'quails') in Nathan ha-Me'ati's and Zeraḥyah Ḥen's trans. of Maimonides' *Medical Aphorisms* (i.e., *Sefer ha-Peraqim*) XIII.32 and XX.69 (cf. BMMG no. 2488).

שִׁלּוּחַ • שילוח השתן · **enuresis; strangury**: Arab. تقطير البول (Gr. ἐνουρεω, στραγγουρία; cf. UW 244, 642) · Ibn Sīnā, *K. al-Qānūn* II · trans. Zeraḥyah Ḥen, *Sefer ha-Qanun* (Ms Oxford, Bodleian Libaries, Opp. Add. Fol. 12, fol. 216[a]): חדיד ... והיין המכובה בו הברזל יעצור השלשול הארוך והדושנטאריא ויועיל מרפיון פי הטבעת ושילוח השתן והגרת הנשים ויחזק בתשמיש ([Arab.] *ḥadīd*: Iron: ... Wine in which [hot] iron is extinguished stops chronic diarrhea and dysentery; it is good for the paralysis of the anus, enuresis (strangury), and menstrual bleeding. It also strengthens the sexual desire). Hebr. שילוח השתן is not attested in the current dictionaries. Nathan ha-Me'ati translates Arab. تقطير البول as הטפת השתן (see entry הַטָּפָה).

[שלך] • *Hifʿil* **הִשְׁלִיךְ • השליך הרוחות** · **to be carminative (to expel gases)**: Arab. طرد الرياح · Ibn Sīnā, *K. al-Qānūn* II · trans. Zeraḥyah Ḥen, *Sefer ha-Qanun* (Ms Oxford, Bodleian Libaries, Opp. Add. Fol. 12, fol. 224[b]): כַּמּוֹן ... ישליך הרוחות ויתיר ויש בו חיתוך וניגוב ויש בו קיבוץ (Cumin [*Cuminum cyminum* L.]: ... It expels gases and dissolves; it is also attenuating, drying, and astringent). Hebr. השליך הרוחות is not attested in

---

392 Col. 726.

the current dictionaries. In addition to השליך הרוחות, Zeraḥyah translates Arab. طرد الرياح as פיזור הרוחות (see entry [פזר]). Nathan ha-Me'ati translates Arab. طرد الرياح as הוציא הרוחות and Anonymous I renders the Arab. term as מגרש הרוחות.

שַׁלְפּוּחִית • **אבן השלפוחית** → אֶבֶן.

שִׁלְשׁוּל • **שלשול הגוף** · **dysentery**: Arab. دوسنطاريا (Gr. δυσεντερία; cf. UW 210f.) · Ibn Sīnā, *K. al-Qānūn* II · trans. Nathan ha-Me'ati, *Sefer ha-Qanun* (Ms Oxford, Bodleian Libraries, Can. Or. 88, fol. 126ᵇ):[393] תפאח ... והצלוי בעסה יועיל מהתולעים וכן שלשול הגוף הנקרא דשינטיריאה ([Arab.] *tuffāḥ*: Apple [*Malus domestica* Borkh.]: ... Roasted apple with flour is useful for worms and likewise for dysentery, called [in Arab.] *dūsanṭāriyā*). Hebr. שלשול הגוף is not attested in the current dictionaries. The term שִׁלְשׁוּל on its own features in the sense of 'diarrhea' in BM 7196f. In his trans. of Maimonides' *Medical Aphorisms* XXII.20, 60; XXIII.89, Nathan transcribes Arab. دوسنطاريا as דישנטריא (cf. BMMN 212, l. 6; 216, l. 17; 230, l. 10; BMMG no. 1833). Anonymous I transcribes Arab. دوسنطاريا as דישנטריאה. Synonyms for 'dysentery' featuring in medieval medical literature are שלשול הדם (cf. BCD 276 (NM 3:228) and שלשול עם דם (cf. ibid. (NM 3:229f.)).

• **השלשול והקיא** · **cholera**: Arab. هيضة · Ibn Sīnā, *K. al-Qānūn* II · trans. Nathan ha-Me'ati, *Sefer ha-Qanun* (Ms Oxford, Bodleian Libraries, Can. Or. 88, fol. 116ᵃ): פטר הוא פטריות המין הנקרא קלאעי לא הרג אדם אך יארע ממנו השלשול והקיא הנק' היצה בערבי ([Arab.] *fuṭr*; i.e., [Hebr.] *piṭriyot*: Mushrooms: The variety called QL'ʿY is not fatal but causes cholera, called *hayḍa* in Arab.). In the sense of 'cholera,' Hebr. השלשול והקיא features in BCD 277 (NM 4:206) as שלשול וקיא in an attestation from Shem Tov ben Isaac's *Sefer ha-Shimmush* XXVII. Zeraḥyah Ḥen translates Arab. هيضة as איניישטיאון and Anonymous I has שלשול וקיא.

שִׁלְשֵׁל · **to ease**: Arab. أسهل · Ibn Sīnā, *K. al-Qānūn* II · trans. Zeraḥyah Ḥen, *Sefer ha-Qanun* (Ms Oxford, Bodleian Libaries, Opp. Add. Fol. 12, fol. 249ᵃ): ... סַסָאלִיוּס יתיר הפונטורא הרוחיית וישלשל הלידה ([Arab.] *sasāliyūs*: Massilian hartwort [*Seseli tortuosum* L.]: ... It relieves gaseous gripes and eases childbirth). In the sense of 'to ease,' Hebr. שִׁלְשֵׁל is a non-attested semantic borrowing from Arab. أسهل. Nathan ha-Me'ati translates the Arab. term as מיהר and Anonymous I has מקל.

• **שלשל הדם** · **to cause dysentery**: Arab. أسهل الدم · Ibn Sīnā, *K. al-Qānūn* II · trans. Zeraḥyah Ḥen, *Sefer ha-Qanun* (Ms Oxford, Bodleian Libaries, Opp. Add. Fol. 12, fol. 232ᵃ⁻ᵇ): לַבְלָב לוֹפּוּלוּ מימיו ישלשלו המרה האדומה השרופה וכשלא יהיה מבושלת יהיה יותר חזקה ומין מן הקורייולא רע ישלשל הדם ([Arab.] *lablāb*; [i.e., Rom.] LWoPWLWu: Field bindweed [*Convolvulus arvensis* L.]: Its juice purges out the burnt yellow bile. When it is uncooked it is stronger. Another kind of QWRYYWL' [i.e., Ital. *coreola*[394]] is bad,

393 Ms Paris, BnF, héb. 1136, fol. 105ᵇ, reads: שלשול.

394 I.e., field bindweed; cf. O. Penzig, *Flora Popolare Italiana*, 2 vols. (Genoa 1924), 1:134.

[since] it causes dysentery). Hebr. שלשל הדם is not attested in the current dictionaries. Nathan ha-Me'ati and Anonymous I both render Arab. أسهل الدم as שלשל הדם, just like Zeraḥyah.

שְׁמִירָה · **memory**: Arab. حفظ · Ibn Sīnā, *K. al-Qānūn* II · trans. Zeraḥyah Ḥen, *Sefer ha-Qanun* (Ms Oxford, Bodleian Libaries, Opp. Add. Fol. 12, fol. 201[b]): ... הַלִילַג׳ מִירַבַּלֹנִי הכאבולי יועיל מן החושים והשמירה והדעת ([Arab.] *halīlaj* [from Pers. *halīlah*]; [Rom.] MiYRaBaLoNiY: (Chebulic) myrobalan: ... Chebulic [myrobalan] is good for the senses, memory, and intellect). In the sense of 'memory,' Hebr. שְׁמִירָה features in medieval philosophical literature; cf. BM 7249; KT 4:131; PESHAT.[395] Nathan ha-Me'ati and Anonymous I both render Arab. حفظ as זכרון.

[שמן] • *Part. Hif'il* **מַשְׁמִין** · **fattening**: Arab. مسمن · Ibn Sīnā, *K. al-Qānūn* II · trans. Zeraḥyah Ḥen, *Sefer ha-Qanun* (Ms Oxford, Bodleian Libaries, Opp. Add. Fol. 12, fol. 215[b]): חַבּ אַלְצָּנַוְבַּר גרעִינֵי פִּינְיִי ... היפוי משמין ([Arab.] *ḥabb al-ṣanawbar*; i.e., [Hebr.-Lat./Rom.] *gar'inei* PiYNəYiY: Pine nuts [*Pinus* L.]: Cosmetics: They fatten). Hebr. *Hif'il* הִשְׁמִין is not attested for medieval medical literature in the current dictionaries; cf. BM 7255; EM 1854. Nathan ha-Me'ati translates Arab. مسمن as ישמין and Anonymous I has מַשְׁמִין, just like Zeraḥyah.

שֶׁמֶן • **שמן ההוצאה** · **oil extracted from unripe olives**: Arab. (زيت) الإنفاق (Gr. ὀμφάκινον or ὀμφάκιον; cf. MIG no. 319) · Ibn Sīnā, *K. al-Qānūn* II · trans. Zeraḥyah Ḥen, *Sefer ha-Qanun* (Ms Oxford, Bodleian Libaries, Opp. Add. Fol. 12, fol. 208[a]): ... זיתון זיתים והשמן הנקרא שמן ההוצאה והוא העצור מן הפג: ([Arab.] *zaytūn*; [i.e., Hebr. *Plur.*] *zetim*: Olives [*Olea europaea* L.]: ... The oil called *shemen ha-hoṣa'ah* is that which is extracted from unripe olives). Hebr. שמן ההוצאה is not attested in the current dictionaries. Nathan ha-Me'ati translates Arab. زيت الإنفاق as שמן זית המסתפקים ממנו (cf. next entry) and Anonymous I has שמן אנפקנון (cf. Maimonides on mMen 8.3, where he explains אנפקנון as: הו אלזית אלד׳י יסמיה אלאטבא זית אלאנפאק (That is, the oil which the physicians call: *zayt al-infāq*) (cf. SHS 1:507 (Shin 19)).

• **שמן זית המסתפקים ממנו** · **oil extracted from unripe olives**: Arab. زيت الإنفاق or زيت الأنفاق (Gr. ὀμφάκινον or ὀμφάκιον; cf. MIG no. 319) · Ibn Sīnā, *K. al-Qānūn* II · trans. Nathan ha-Me'ati, *Sefer ha-Qanun* (Ms Oxford, Bodleian Libraries, Can. Or. 88, fol. 83[b]): זיתון וזית ... ושמן זית המסתפקים ממנו והוא המעוצר מן הזיתים הפגים ([Arab.] *zaytūn* and [Arab.] *zayt*: Olive [*Olea europaea* L.] and olive oil: ... The olive oil [called] *ha-mistappeqim*[396] *mimennu* [lit. 'which is used'] is that which is extracted from unripe olives). Hebr. שמן זית המסתפקים ממנו is not attested in the current dictionaries. Zeraḥyah Ḥen translates Arab. زيت الإنفاق as שמן ההוצאה and Anonymous I has שמן אנפקנון (for both terms, see previous entry).

• **אבן יכבה בשמן** → **אֶבֶן**.

---

395 https://peshat.org/display/peshat_lemmas_00004093 (accessed June 23, 2022).
396 For Hebr. *Hitpa'el* הִסְתַּפֵּק, cf. entry [ספק].

שַׁמְנוּנִית · **fat; grease:** Arab. دسومة · Ibn Sīnā, *K. al-Qānūn* II · trans. Zeraḥyah Ḥen, *Sefer ha-Qanun* (Ms Oxford, Bodleian Libaries, Opp. Add. Fol. 12, fol. 253[a]): סַמַךְ דג ... היותר משובח שבדגים הוא מה שאינו גדול מאד ולא יהיה קשה בבשרו ולא יבש בלא שמנונית בו כאלו הוא מתפוצץ ולא דבקות כמותר האף ([Arab.] *samak*; [i.e., Hebr.] *dag*: Fish: ... The best fish is that which is not very big, nor hard of its flesh or dry or greasy; [neither should it be] brittle, nor viscous, like nasal mucus). Hebr. שַׁמְנוּנִית is not attested for medieval Hebr. medical literature; cf. BM 7261. Nathan ha-Me'ati and Anonymous I both render Arab. دسومة as דשנות.

שַׁמְנִיּוּת · **oily quality (oil):** Arab. دهنية · Ibn Sīnā, *K. al-Qānūn* II · trans. Anonymous I, *Sefer ha-Qanun* (Ms Paris, BnF, héb. 1142, fol. 194[a–b]): סמסם[397] ... הוא הרב שמניות שבזרעים ולכן מקבל העפוש הנקרא רנציד[398] בנקלה ([Arab.] *simsim*: Sesame [*Sesamum indicum* L.]: ... It contains more oil than other seeds and therefore the oil quickly becomes rancid). Hebr. שַׁמְנִיּוּת is not attested in the current dictionaries. Nathan ha-Me'ati renders Arab. دهنية as דשן.

שֵׁן • **שן הפיל** · **ivory:** Arab. عاج · Ibn Sīnā, *K. al-Qānūn* II · trans. Anonymous I, *Sefer ha-Qanun* (Ms Paris, BnF, héb. 1142, fol. 128[b]): יברוח ... ונאמר שהשורש ממנו אם יבושל בו שן הפיל שש שעות ירככהו ויקל הפעלו ויענה לְהִפָּעֵל ([Arab.] *yabrūḥ*: Mandrake [*Mandragora officinarum* L.]: ... It is said that ivory, if it is cooked with the root of mandrake for six hours, will become soft and manageable). Hebr. שֵׁן on its own is attested in the sense of 'ivory' in Rabb. literature (cf. JD 1603). For the Aram. counterpart שנא דפיל, cf. LW 4:584. Nathan ha-Me'ati translates Arab. عاج as עצם הפיל and Zeraḥyah Ḥen has השן הנקרא אוֹרִיפַנְט.

- • **אבן שן הפיל** → **אֶבֶן**.
- • **העתיק השן חוצה** → [**עתק**].
- • *Dual* **שִׁנַּיִם** • **זוהמת השנים** → **זהמה**.
- • **טנופת השנים** → **טִנּוֹפֶת**.
- • **ליכלוך השנים** → **לִכְלוּךְ**.
- • **עקירת השנים** → **עֲקִירָה**.

שְׁעוּל · **asthma (dyspnea; panting):** Arab. ربو (cf. UWS 1:180, s.v. ἄσθμα: 'Atemnot, Keuchen') · Ibn Sīnā, *K. al-Qānūn* II · trans. Zeraḥyah Ḥen, *Sefer ha-Qanun* (Ms Oxford, Bodleian Libaries, Opp. Add. Fol. 12, fol. 253[a]): סֶמְסֶם שומשמין ... טוב לצרות הנשימה ולשעול הנקרא רבו ([Arab.] *simsim*; [i.e., Hebr.] *shumshemin*: Sesame [*Sesamum indicum* L.]: ... It is beneficial for orthopnea and asthma (dyspnea; panting).) Hebr. שְׁעוּל features in BM 7348 in the sense of 'cough' only. Zeraḥyah uses the same Hebr. term in his trans. of Maimonides' *Medical Aphorisms* (i.e., *Sefer ha-Peraqim*) VIII.19 and XX.83: השעול הנקרא רבו (cf. BMMZ 89, l. 13; 192, l. 8; BMMG no. 2043). Syn-

---

397 סמסם: שומשמין Ms[1].

398 רנציד: Emend. ed. דאנצר Ms.

onyms employed by Zeraḥyah are Rom. אִזְמוֹ (see entry עֹצֶר: עוצר הנשימה) or אסמו (see entry קֹצֶר: קוצר הנשימה); see also his *Sefer ha-Peraqim* XXIII.79: אלרבו בלעז אסמו (cf. BMMZ 227, l. 19; BMMG no. 2043). Nathan ha-Me'ati, reading Arab. ربو (*rabw*) as *rubūw*, translates the term as גודל and Anonymous I renders the Arab. term as גְּנִיחָה (cf. BCD 47 (NM 2:34f.) for an attestation from Nathan's *Sefer ha-Peraqim* VIII.19).

שַׁעֲוָנִי · **serous:** Lat. *serosus* · Guy de Chauliac, *Inventarium sive Chirurgia Magna* (cf. CMM 1:231, l. 2) · trans. Anonymous (Ms Paris, BnF, héb. 1189, fol. 126ᵃ): ומהמוגלא השעוונית והדבקיית (And from the serous, glutinous pus). Hebr. שַׁעֲוָנִי features in EM 1668 as a modern term in the sense of 'wax-like.'

[שעט] • *Nif'al* **נִשְׁעַט** / *Hof'al* **הָשְׁעַט** · **to be dripped (poured) as a medicine into the nose:** Arab. سعط · Ibn Sīnā, *K. al-Qānūn* II · trans. Zeraḥyah Ḥen, *Sefer ha-Qanun* (Ms Oxford, Bodleian Libaries, Opp. Add. Fol. 12, fol. 214ᵃ): חַנְדַּקוּקָה ... יכאיב כשישעט במיצו ויועיל למי שיפול מחולי איפילינשיאה ([Arab.] *ḥandaqūqā*: Lotus: ... It causes [headache] when its juice is dripped as a medicine into the nose; it is beneficial for someone suffering from epilepsy). In the sense of 'to be dripped as a medicine into the nose,' Hebr. *Nif'al* נִשְׁעַט / *Hof'al* הָשְׁעַט is a non-attested calque from Arab. سُعِطَ. Hebr. *Qal* שָׁעַט features in Zeraḥyah's trans. of Maimonides' *Medical Aphorisms* (i.e., *Sefer ha-Peraqim*) XV.58 (cf. BMMZ 162, l. 1; BMMG no. 2389). A variant reading of the *Qal* conj., סָעַט, features in BM 4134 in an attestation from the *Sefer ha-Qanun* and is translated by Ben Yehuda as 'to inject (into the nose).' A synonym used by Zeraḥyah is עשה אישפונגי באף (see entry עָשָׂה) and the synonymous Arab. term سعط في الأنف is translated by him as חבש באף (see entry חָבַשׁ). Nathan, reading Arab. سعط as سَعَط, translates עשה סעוט (see entry עָשָׂה).

שְׂעִיטָה • **עשה שעיטה** → עָשָׂה.

שֵׂעָר · **stigma [of a flower]:** Arab. شعر · Ibn Sīnā, *K. al-Qānūn* II · trans. Nathan ha-Me'ati, *Sefer ha-Qanun* (Ms Oxford, Bodleian Libraries, Can. Or. 88, fol. 82ᵇ): זעפראן המבחר המשובח ממנו החדש גוונו נאה זך הריח ועל שעריו מעט לובן ([Arab. *za'farān*: Saffron [*Crocus sativus* L.]: Choice: The best [saffron] is that which is fresh, has a nice color, is fragrant, and the upper part of its stigmas is somewhat white). In the sense of 'stigma,' Hebr. שֵׂעָר is a non-attested semantic borrowing from Arab. شعر. Anonymous I renders Arab. شعر as שֵׂעָר, just like Nathan.

• **השער הנוסף** · **ingrown eyelashes (trichiasis):** Arab. شعر العين · Ibn Sīnā, *K. al-Qānūn* II · trans. Nathan ha-Me'ati, *Sefer ha-Qanun* (Ms Oxford, Bodleian Libraries, Can. Or. 88, fol. 92ᵃ): כמון ... כמו כן מועיל בכויה[399] הנולדת בעד מריטת השער הנוסף ([Arab.] *kammūn* / [Hebr.] *kammon*: Cumin [*Cuminum cyminum* L.]: ... [The extract of wild cumin] is also beneficial as[400] an ingredient of caustic drugs used for removing ingrown eyelashes). Hebr. השער הנוסף, which is actually a calque from the Arab. syn-

399 בכויה הנולדת: يقع أيضا في كاويات a.
400 'as an ingredient of caustic drugs': Trans. acc. to a.

onym شعر زائد (cf. HLA 191 (249)), is not attested in the current dictionaries. Zeraḥyah Ḥen translates Arab. شعر العين as שער בעין (see next entry) and Anonymous I renders the Arab. term as השער שבעין.

• **שער בעין · ingrown eyelashes (trichiasis)**: Arab. شعر العين · Ibn Sīnā, *K. al-Qānūn* II · trans. Zeraḥyah Ḥen, *Sefer ha-Qanun* (Ms Oxford, Bodleian Libaries, Opp. Add. Fol. 12, fol. 224[b]): כַּמּוֹן ... והוא כמו כן יכנס בכויות המריטה לשער בעין (Cumin [*Cuminum cyminum* L.]: ... [The extract of wild cumin] is also applied as an ingredient of caustic drugs used for removing ingrown eyelashes). Hebr. שער בעין is not attested in the current dictionaries. Nathan ha-Me'ati translates Arab. شعر العين as השער הנוסף (see previous entry) and Anonymous I has השער שבעין.

• **השרת השער** → הֲשָׁרָה.

• **נפילת השער** → נְפִילָה.

• **סמור השער** → סִמּוּר.

שָׂפָה • *Plur.* **שפתות · seashores**: Arab. شطوط · Ibn Sīnā, *K. al-Qānūn* II · trans. Zeraḥyah Ḥen, *Sefer ha-Qanun* (Ms Oxford, Bodleian Libaries, Opp. Add. Fol. 12, fol. 253[a–b]): סמַךְ דג ... והדג הימיי משובח ודק הבשר כל שכן כשהוא רועה בשפתות סלעות או חול ([Arab.] *samak*; [i.e., Hebr.] *dag*: Fish: ... Sea fish has better and softer meat; especially that which lives in rocky or sandy seashores). In the sense of 'seashore,' Hebr. שָׂפָה is attested as שפת הים in Bibl. literature (cf. KB 1348). Nathan ha-Me'ati translates Arab. شطوط as סלעים אשר על הים.

• *Dual* **שפתים • סדוק השפתים** → סִדּוּק.

שֶׁפַע • **שפע הדם מן הנחירים · nosebleed**: Arab. النزف الرعافي · Ibn Sīnā, *K. al-Qānūn* II · trans. Anonymous II, *Sefer ha-Qanun* (Ms Parma, Biblioteca Palatina, Cod. Parm. 3045, fol. 30[b]): תרנגלים ותרנגלות ... בשר תרנוגלות קטנות מגדל הדעת ומוח תרנגלות מונע שפע הדם מן הנחירים (Roosters and hens (chickens): ... The meat of young hens increases the intellect. The brain of hens stops a nosebleed). Hebr. שפע הדם מן הנחירים is not attested in the current dictionaries. Nathan ha-Me'ati translates Arab. النزف الرعافي as רעיפת דם הנחירים (cf. BMMG no. 2137 for his trans. of Arab. رعاف 'nosebleed(s)' in his trans. of Maimonides' *Medical Aphorisms* (i.e., *Sefer ha-Peraqim*)) and Zeraḥyah Ḥen has הגרת הדם מן האף and הגרת הדם מן הנחירים (cf. BCD 62 (NM 1:138; 3:56) for attestations from his trans. of Maimonides' *Medical Aphorisms* (i.e., *Sefer ha-Peraqim*) IX.2 (cf. BMMN 98, l. 8; BMMG no. 2137) and his *Commentary on Hippocrates' Aphorisms* (i.e., *Perush Aphorismi shel Apuqraṭ*) III.27, V.33 (cf. BMCH 1:453, l. 10; 479, l. 7). Synonymous terms featuring in medieval medical literature are הזלת דם הנחירים (cf. BCD 65 (NM 3:62)); הטפת דם מהנחירים (cf. BCD 66 (NM 1:138f.)); נזלת דם הנחירים (cf. NM 5:131); and רְעִיפָה (cf. NM 6:201).

• **שפע עת הנשים · uterine (menstrual) bleeding**: Arab. نزف الرحم · Ibn Sīnā, *K. al-Qānūn* II · trans. Anonymous II, Sefer ha-Qanun (Ms Parma, Biblioteca Palatina, Cod. Parm. 3045, fol. 48[a]): לוטוס ארמיני ... תועלתו לאברים הדוחים יועיל למורסות המעים ולשלשול ולשפע עת הנשים ([Lat.-Arab.] LWṬWS (*lutus*) *armīnī*: Armenian bole: ... Its usefulness for excretory organs; it is good for intestinal ulcers, diarrhea and uterine (menstrual) bleeding). Hebr. שפע עת הנשים is not attested in the current dictionaries. Nathan ha-Me'ati translates Arab. نزف الرحم as הגרת הרחם, Zeraḥyah Ḥen has רקיקת הדם, and Anonymous I has הזלת הרחם. In their trans. of Ibn al-Jazzār's *Zād al-musāfir* VI.10, Moses ibn Tibbon (*Sefer Ṣedat ha-Derakhim*) translates Arab. نزف as שפעת הדם and Abraham ben Isaac (*Sefer Ṣedah la-Oreḥim*) has שופע נידות (cf. NM 6:214).

שָׂרוּף (*Part. Pass.*) → **שָׂרַף**.

[שרט] • *Nif'al* **נִשְׂרַט** · **to be scarified**: Arab. شُرِطَ · Ibn Sīnā, *K. al-Qānūn* II · trans. Nathan ha-Me'ati, *Sefer ha-Qanun* (Ms Oxford, Bodleian Libraries, Can. Or. 88, fol. 85[a]): חלתית ... אם ישרטו המורסות הרעות הבאושות וישים החלתית עליהם יועיל ([Arab.] *ḥiltīt* / [Hebr.] *ḥiltit*: Resin of asafetida [*Ferula assa-foetida* L.]: ... If malignant, evil-smelling ulcers are scarified and then the resin of asafoetida is put on them; it is beneficial). Hebr. *Nif'al* נִשְׂרַט is not attested for medieval medical literature. Zeraḥyah Ḥen translates Arab. شُرِطَ as נִשְׂרַט, just like Nathan, and Anonymous I renders the Arab. term as *Pu'al* שֹׂרַט.

שְׂרִיטָה · **scarification**: Arab. شرط · al-Rāzī, *K. fī al-Faṣd* · trans. Anonymous, *Ma'amar ba-Haqqazah* (Ms Parma, Biblioteca Palatina, Cod. Parm. 2283,4, fol. 96[b]): השער הארבעה עשר בתועלת כוסות המציצה עם שריטה ובלי שריטה (Ch. 14: On the usefulness of cupping with scarification and without scarification). Hebr. שְׂרִיטָה is not attested for medieval medical literature.

שָׂרַף • *Part.* **שׂוֹרֵף** • **הסם השורף** → **סַם**.

• **הרפואה השורפת** → **רְפוּאָה**.

• *Part. Pass.* **שָׂרוּף** · **calcined**: Arab. مكلّس (cf. WKAS 1:318f.) · Ibn Sīnā, *K. al-Qānūn* II · trans. Nathan ha-Me'ati, *Sefer ha-Qanun* (Ms Oxford, Bodleian Libraries, Can. Or. 88, fol. 89[a]): טלק ... השרוף ממנו יותר חזק ויותר רקיק ([Arab.] *ṭalq*: Talcum (mica): ... The calcined talcum is more potent and attenuant). Hebr. *Part. Pass.* שָׂרוּף does not feature in this sense in the current dictionaries. Zeraḥyah Ḥen translates Arab. مكلّس as נקי and Anonymous I has סיד.

שְׂרֵפָה • **שרפת המים החמים** · **scald**: Arab. حرق الماء الحار · Ibn Sīnā, *K. al-Qānūn* II · trans. Nathan ha-Me'ati, Sefer ha-Qanun (Ms Oxford, Bodleian Libraries, Can. Or. 88, fol. 108[r]: סוסן ... והפרדסי יותר משובח שבסמים לשרפת המים החמים (Lily (or iris) ...: The cultivated variety is most beneficial for scalds). Hebr. שרפת המים החמים is not attested in the current dictionaries. Zeraḥyah Ḥen translates Arab. حرق الماء الحار as כוית המים החמים and Anonymous I has שרפת המים החמים, just like Nathan.

שֹׁרֶשׁ • **שרש הרמון המדברי** · **root of the wild pomegranate tree**: Arab. عرق الرمان البري (cf. Ibn Sīnā, *Qānūn*, ed. Būlāq, I 364; MSh no. 219: أصل الرمان البري, now identified as: **root of glossostemon [*Glossostemon bruguieri* Desf.]**[401]) · i. Ibn Sīnā, *K. al-Qānūn*

401 Cf. Amin, Awad, Abd El Samad, and Iskander, 'Isolation of Estrone from Moghat Roots,' 295ff.

II · trans. Anonymous I, *Sefer ha-Qanun* (Ms Paris, BnF, héb. 1142, fol. 164[a]): מגאת מהות אמרו קצתם שהוא שרש[402] הרמון המדברי ואין זה מסכים למה שאמר שזרעו נאות לתאות המשגל ותניע אותה בחוזק ([Arab.] *mughāth*.[403] What is it? Some say that it is the root of the wild pomegranate tree; however, this does not fit what is said that its seed is good for (strengthens) sexual lust, and that it is a strong stimulant). Hebr. שרש הרמון המדברי is a non-attested calque from Arab. عرق الرمان البري. Nathan ha-Me'ati translates the Arab. term as גיד הרמון המדברי (see entry גִּיד) and Zeraḥyah Ḥen, mistakenly reading Arab. عرق as عَرَق, has זיעת הרמון המדברי.

· ii. *Shinnui ha-Shemot ha-Niqra'im Synonimi*, Mem 10 (Ms Florence, Biblioteca Medicea Laurenziana, Or. 17, fol. 82[b]): מגאת[404] הוא שורש רמון מדברי ([Arab.] *mughāth*;[405] i.e., root of the wild pomegranate tree).

• **מֻרְסָה → המורסות אשר בשורש האזנים.**

שָׁרְשִׁי · **original; real**: Arab. أصلي · Ibn Sīnā, *K. al-Qānūn* II · trans. Zeraḥyah Ḥen, *Sefer ha-Qanun* (Ms Oxford, Bodleian Libaries, Opp. Add. Fol. 12, fol. 247[b]): סַךְּ גַאלִיָה המהות הגאליה השרשיית היא הצינית הנעשית מן העפצים ובוסר הדקל על צד שנעשה האלרָאמִךְ ([Arab.] *sukk* [i.e., an astringent electuary containing musk (a.o.)];[406] [i.e., Arab.] *ghāliya* [i.e., a perfume composed of musk, ambergris, camphor, and ben oil, cf. SHS 1:413 (Pe 20)]. What is it? Real (original) *sukk* is the Chinese *sukk* that is made from gallnuts and unripe dates in the same manner as [Arab.] *al-rāmik*).[407] Hebr. שָׁרְשִׁי features in BM 7478 in the sense of 'radical,' in KT 4:162 as 'grundsätzlich, fundamental, hauptsächlich,' in HCD 83 as 'radical, basic, fundamental,' and in PESHAT as 'being the root of another number.'[408] Nathan ha-Me'ati translates Arab. أصلي as אמתי and Anonymous I has עקרי.

שִׁתּוּף · **sympathetic affection**: Arab. شركة (Gr. συνπάθεια; cf. UWS 2:368) · Ibn al-Jazzār, *Zād al-musāfir wa-qūt al-ḥāḍir* V.5 · trans. Moses ibn Tibbon, *Sefer Ṣedat ha-Derakhim*: ויתחייב ג"כ שיהיה השקוי מחולשת הכח המבשל כי הנה הפסד הדם אמנם יתילד מחולי הכח הזה כמו שבארנו. וכבר זכרנו בפתיחת המאמר הזה כי כאב הכבד לא ימלט מהיותו מתילד בכבד עצמו לבד או משתוף אבר אחר כמו האצטו' או הטחול או המעים או הכליות או הרחם או מה שדומה להם (Consequently, dropsy results from the weakness of the transforming faculty because the blood gets corrupted when it is weak, as I explained. I said in the beginning of the book that pain of the liver necessarily originates only from the liver itself or because it is sympathetically affected by another organ, such as the

402 שרש: Emend. ed. שרשי Ms שרשי הרמונים המדבריים Ms[1].
403 '*mughāth*': I.e., the root of glossostemon [*Glossostemon bruguieri* Desf.]; cf. MIG no. 546.
404 מגאת: Emend. ed. מאגת Ms.
405 See note 403.
406 Bos and Mensching, 'Arabic-Romance Medico-Botanical Glossaries,' 45.
407 For *rāmik*, an electuary prepared from gallnut and aromatic drugs, cf. IJZ 7:73f., n. 7.
408 https://peshat.org/display/peshat_lemmas_00075950 (accessed April 28, 2023).

stomach, spleen, intestines, kidneys, or the uterus or similar [organs]). Hebr. שִׁתּוּף is not attested for medieval medical literature. It features in the sense of a) 'commonality, something shared by two or more objects', b) 'common factor; factor that is common to two or more numbers', or c) 'homonymy, word used of two things that bear no relation to one another' in medieval philosophical literature; cf. PESHAT.[409] Do'eg ha-Edomi translates the Lat. parallel term *societas* as שְׁכוּנָה (see entry).

שֶׁתֶן • הזלת השתן → **הַזָּלָה.**

• הטפת השתן → **הַטָּפָה.**

• חולשת השתן → **חֻלְשָׁה.**

• הגיר השתן → **[נגר].**

• עורר השתן → **[עור].**

• עצירת השתן → **עֲצִירָה.**

• עוצר השתן → **עֹצֶר.**

• הרבה השתן → **[רבה].**

• שילוח השתן → **שִׁלּוּחַ.**

[שָׁתַף] • *Part. Puʿal* **מְשֻׁתָּף** · **mixed:** Arab. مخلوط · Ibn Sīnā, *K. al-Qānūn* II · trans. Anonymous II, *Sefer ha-Qanun* (Ms Parma, Biblioteca Palatina, Cod. Parm. 3045, fol. 30a): בישקו ... יצליח למורסות הנולדות מן הקור אחרי האוזן משותף עם זיעת[410] בטנים ושעוה ([Lat.] BYŠQW [i.e., Dat./Abl. from M. Lat. *viscum* or *viscus*]: Mistletoe (birdlime) [*Viscum album* L.]: ... Mixed with pine[411] resin and wax it is beneficial for cold swellings behind the ears). Hebr. *Part. Puʿal* מְשֻׁתָּף does not feature in this sense in the current dictionaries. Nathan ha-Me'ati, Zeraḥyah Ḥen, and Anonymous I translate Arab. مخلوط as מעורב.

---

409 https://peshat.org/display/peshat_lemmas_00011542 (accessed May 10, 2022).

410 זיעת בטנים: الراتينج a.

411 'pine resin': Trans. acc. to a.

ת

תַּאֲוָה • תאות אכילת החומר · **geophagy**: Arab. شهوة الطين · Ibn Sīnā, *K. al-Qānūn* II · trans. Nathan ha-Me'ati, *Sefer ha-Qanun* (Ms Oxford, Bodleian Libraries, Can. Or. 88, fol. 86[a]): חמאץ ... יועיל מן הירקון השחור מעורב עם יין וישקיט האצטו׳ ויסיר תאות אכילת החומר ([Arab.] *ḥummāḍ*: Sorrel [*Rumex acetosa* L.]: ... If taken with wine, it is useful for black jaundice; it relieves the stomach [of someone suffering from nausea]; it is effective against geophagy). In the sense of 'geophagy,' Hebr. תאות אכילת החומר is not attested in the current dictionaries. Zeraḥyah Ḥen translates Arab. شهوة الطين as תאות הטיט (see next entry).

• תאות הטיט · **geophagy**: Arab. شهوة الطين · Ibn Sīnā, *K. al-Qānūn* II · trans. Zeraḥyah Ḥen, *Sefer ha-Qanun* (Ms Oxford, Bodleian Libaries, Opp. Add. Fol. 12, fol. 213[b]): חֻמָּאץ׳ ... יועיל מן הירקון השחור עם היין וישכך הקרבונקלי ויאכל לתאות הטיט ([Arab.] *ḥummāḍ*: Sorrel [*Rumex acetosa* L.]: ... If taken with wine, it is useful for black jaundice; it gives relief from nausea; it should be ingested against geophagy). In the sense of 'geophagy,' Hebr. תאות הטיט is a non-attested calque from Arab. شهوة الطين. Nathan ha-Me'ati translates Arab. شهوة الطين as תאות אכילת החומר (see previous entry).

תֶּבֶן • תבן מגמלים · **camel grass (straw of Mecca)** [***Cymbopogon schoenanthus*** **(L.) Spreng.**]: Arab. إذخر (cf. MIG no. 181) · *Shinnui ha-Shemot ha-Niqra'im Synonimi*, Alef 7 (Ms Florence, Biblioteca Medicea Laurenziana, Or. 17, fol. 68[a]): אדכר[412] הוא סקוויננטי ונקרא תבן מגמלים ודומה לתבן שעורים ([Arab.] *idhkhir*, i.e., [Rom.] SQWYNNṬY [i.e., O. Ital. *squinante*], it is called [in Hebr.] *teven mi-gemallim* (lit. 'camel straw') and is similar to barley straw). Hebr. תבן מגמלים is a non-attested calque from Arab. إذخر.

תּוּגָה · **anxiety**: Arab. توحّش · Ibn Sīnā, *K. al-Qānūn* II · trans. Zeraḥyah Ḥen, *Sefer ha-Qanun* (Ms Oxford. Opp. Add. Fol. 12, fol. 230[b]):[413] לשון השור ... משמח מחזק הלב טוב לתוגה ולסינקופיץ ביין (Hebr.] *leshon ha-shor* [lit. 'ox tongue']: Borage [*Borago officinalis* L.]: ... [Taken] with wine, it gladdens and strengthens the heart [and] is good for anxiety and syncope). Hebr. תּוּגָה is not attested for medieval medical literature. In addition to תּוּגָה, Zeraḥyah translates Arab. توحّش as אֲנָחָה and מַחְשָׁבָה (see entries). Nathan ha-Me'ati and Anonymous I both render the Arab. term as הִשְׁתּוֹמְמוּת (cf. BCD 74 (NM 4:48) for an attestation from an anonymous trans. of Ibn Sīnā's *K. al-Adwiya al-qalbiyya* (i.e., *Sammim Libbiyim*)). For the term השתוממות השכל, which is also used by Nathan, see entry הִשְׁתּוֹמְמוּת.

תָּוֶךְ · **pulp**: Arab. جوف (cf. UW 600) · Ibn Sīnā, *K. al-Qānūn* II · trans. Nathan ha-Me'ati, *Sefer ha-Qanun* (Ms Oxford, Bodleian Libraries, Can. Or. 88, fols. 69[b]–70[a]): ... בטיך ינקה העור ויותר זרעו ותוכו כמו כן יועיל מהכתם הנקרא כלף ([Arab.] *biṭṭīkh*: Watermelon

---

412 אדכר: Emend. ed. אלדבר או אדבר Ms.

413 Zeraḥyah uses the same Hebr. term for Arab. توحّش on. fol. 235[b], entry מֹסְכּוּ 'MoSəKWu: Musk.'

[*Citrullus lanatus* (Thunb.) Matsum. & Nakai]: … It cleanses the skin, especially its seeds and pulp. It is also beneficial for freckles, called [in Arab.] *kalaf*). In the sense of 'pulp,' Hebr. תָּוֶךְ is a non-attested semantic borrowing from Arab. جوف. Zeraḥyah Ḥen translates the Arab. term as מה שבתוך.

תּוּת · **warty excrescence [esp. in the anal or genital regions]; genital wart**: Arab. توث (Gr. θύμος; cf. DDM 180; UW 301) · Ibn Sīnā, *K. al-Qānūn* II · trans. Zeraḥyah Ḥen, *Sefer ha-Qanun* (Ms Oxford. Opp. Add. Fol. 12, fol. 251[a]): סֶדֶאבְּ … עם הנתרון על הבהק הלבן ועל התלול והתות ויעביר ריח השומים והבצלים ויועיל מחולי השועל ([Arab.] *sadhāb*: Common rue [*Ruta graveolens* L.]: … It [is applied] with natron on the white variety of *bahaq*[414] (alphos), warts, and warty excrescences. It removes the unpleasant smell of garlic and onion and is useful for alopecia). In the sense of 'warty excrescence,' Hebr. תות is a non-attested calque from Arab. توث. Nathan ha-Me'ati renders Arab. توث as תותא and Anonymous I has *Plur.* תותים.

תַּחְבֹּשֶׁת • עשה תחבשת בחוטם → עָשָׂה.

תְּכוּנָה · **prescription**: Arab. صفة · al-Rāzī, *K. fī al-Faṣd* · trans. Anonymous, *Ma'amar ba-Haqqazah* (Ms Parma, Biblioteca Palatina, Cod. Parm. 2283,4, fol. 96[b]): השער הי"ג ברפו' השגגה הנופלת בהקזה: כאשר יקרה בהקזת הבסליק שיראה הדם אדום ויקפוץ וידלג אז ידע כי הוא מהשרין וצריך שיתרפא ברפו' גלי' אשר נאמ'[415] עליה שהיא טובה הרבה להפסיק הדם תכונתו (Ch. 13: On the remedy [to be applied] when a mistake occurs during bleeding: Whenever it happens, while bleeding the basilic vein, that you see blood bright and gushing, know that it is from an artery, and then it is necessary to use Galen's remedy of which it[416] is said that it is very good for stopping the blood. Its prescription …). Hebr. תְּכוּנָה is not attested in this sense in the current dictionaries. For its various meanings in (philosophical) lietrature, cf. PESHAT.[417]

תְּלָאָה • הוליד התלאה → [ילד].

תַּלְתַּלִּי · **curled**: Arab. جعد · Ibn Sīnā, *K. al-Qānūn* II · trans. Zeraḥyah Ḥen, *Sefer ha-Qanun* (Ms Oxford. Opp. Add. Fol. 12, fol. 230[a]): לוּף שַׁרְפֵּינְטַארַא … השרש מן התלתלי יטהר הכלף והבוהק והנמש … וכל שכן עם הדבש ([Arab.] *lūf*; [i.e., Rom.] ŠaRəPeYNəṬa'Ra': Arum [*Arum* sp., e.g., snakeshead [*Arum maculatum* L.]]: … The root of the curly variety clears freckles, *bahaq*[418] (alphos), and acne …, especially when applied with

---

414 '*bahaq* (alphos)': There are three varieties of the disease called *bahaq* acc. to Ibn al-Jazzār (cf. IJZ 7:108, n. 196): white, black, and dust-colored. The white variety is perhaps identical with *Vitiligo alba*, while the black variety is possibly a sort of melanoderma. Arab. *bahaq* stands for Gr. ἀλφός, cf. UW 97: 'weiße Hautflecken.' Durling, *Dictionary of Medical Terms*, 34, translates the Gr. term as: 'dull-white leprosy.' See entry בַּהַק: הבהק הלבן.

415 'נאמ': يقول a.

416 'It is said': 'he says' a.

417 https://peshat.org/display/peshat_lemmas_00004207 (accessed December 14, 2022).

418 '*bahaq* (alphos)': There are three varieties of the disease called *bahaq* acc. to Ibn al-Jazzār (cf. IJZ 7:108, n. 196): white, black, and dust-colored. The white variety is perhaps identical

honey). Hebr. תַּלְתַּלֵּי features in BM 7784 as part of the term כוכב התלתלי in the sense of 'comet' only. Nathan ha-Me'ati translates Arab. جعد as שאינו חלק and Anonymous I has *Part. Pass.* כָּווּץ (see entry כָּוַץ).

תְּנוּעָה • התנועה מאין חפץ · spasm; shivers; tetanus: Arab. كزاز (Gr. σπάσμα, τέτανος; cf. UW 626f., 671; WKAS 1:166: 'bad cold, shivers, ague;' DKT 503: 'tetanus') · Ibn Sīnā, *K. al-Qānūn* II · trans. Nathan ha-Me'ati, *Sefer ha-Qanun* (Ms Oxford, Bodleian Libraries, Can. Or. 88, fol. 112b): עקאר קרחא ... כלי הפרקים: כשמורחים בו ותבשילו ומשיחתו תועיל אל הרפיון הישן מהעצבים ומבטול הרגשתם וימנע תולדת התנועה מאין חפץ ובער׳ כזז ([Arab.] *ʿāqirqarḥā*: Pellitory [*Anacyclus pyrethrum* (L.) Lag.]: ... The joints: When it is rubbed [on the joints], likewise its decoction or oil, it is beneficial for chronic atony and loss of sensation in the nerves. It prevents tetanus, [called] in Arab. *kuzāz*). Hebr. התנועה מאין חפץ is a non-attested variant of the term התנועה אשר מבלי חפץ used by Nathan on fols. 73b–74a, entry גנדבא דסתר '[Arab.] *jandubīdastar*: Castoreum' (cf. NM 6:219f.). Zeraḥyah Ḥen transcribes Arab. كزاز as כזז (cf. ibid.) and Anonymous I renders the Arab. term as רפיון הנקרא כוזאז (cf. ibid. for רפיון).

• כבד התנועה → כָּבֵד.

תִּנְשֶׁמֶת · lizard (gecko): Arab. سامّ أبرص[419] · *Glossary* (Ms Moscow, Russian State Library, Guenzburg 573, fol. 156b): סאם אבראץ הוא תנשמת ([Arab.] *sāmm abraṣ*; i.e., [Hebr.] *tinshemet*). Hebr. תִּנְשֶׁמֶת is one of the unclean animals mentioned in Lev 11:30. Its identity is uncertain, it has been explained as 'chameleon' or a kind of 'lizard' (cf. KB 1765; BM 7826). The identification of תִּנְשֶׁמֶת as Arab. سامّ أبرص can be found in Sa'adya's trans. of Lev 11:30[420] and subsequently in Ibn Janāḥ's *K. al-Uṣūl*.[421]

תַּפּוּחַ • תפוח גן עדן · [lit. 'paradise apple']; banana: Arab. موز · Ibn Sīnā, *K. al-Qānūn* II · trans. Anonymous I, *Sefer ha-Qanun* (Ms Paris, BnF, héb. 1142, fol. 174b): מוז הנקרא תפוח גן עדן ([Arab.] *mawz*; called [in Hebr.] *tappuaḥ gan ʿeden* [lit. 'paradise apple']: Banana [*Musa paradisiaca* L.]). Hebr. תפוח גן עדן features in BM 7847, quoting LF 2:254, where it features as a trans. of Menahem de Lonsano's *pomo di paradiso*.

---

with *Vitiligo alba*, while the black variety is possibly a sort of melanoderma. Arab. *bahaq* stands for Gr. ἀλφός, cf. UW 97: 'weiße Hautflecken.' Durling, *Dictionary of Medical Terms*, 34, translates the Gr. term as: 'dull-white leprosy.' See entry בַּהַק: הבהק הלבן.

419 *sāmm abraṣ* (سامّ أبرص) 'lizard (gecko)': Cf. Aristotle, PA660b6–7: οἱ σαῦροι (cf. LSG 1586); idem, *K. al-Ḥayawān* (ed. Kruk, 55: السام أبرص); Lane 188, s.v. سامّ أبرص: 'the species of lizard described above, voce بُرْص: A species of the lizard called gecko, of a leprous hue;' FL 2:349: 'lacerta magnae species;' JAD 2:23: 'Lexicologists state that it is one of the large kinds of geckos;' ibid. n. 1: 'A species of gecko. In Egypt gen. Ptyodactylus;' D 1:680: 'salamandre.'

420 Cf. Derenbourg (ed.), *Targum Ḥamishah Ḥumshei Torah be-Lashon 'Aravit le-Rabbeinu Sa'adyah Ga'on ben Yoseph ha-Fayyumi*, 158.

421 Col. 464.

תָּפַר · **to suture**: Arab. خيّط · Ibn Sīnā, *K. al-Qānūn* II · trans. Nathan ha-Me'ati, *Sefer ha-Qanun* (Ms Oxford, Bodleian Libraries, Can. Or. 88, fol. 115^{a-b}): פרביון ... אמרו קצתם כי מי שנשכו דבר מן השרצים אם יבקעו עור ראשו ומה שכנגדו עד שתראה הגלגלת וממלאים מהשרף הזה שחוק ותופרים אותו לא יארע לו שום היזק ([Arab.] *furbiyūn* [from Gr. εὐφόρβιον]: Resin spurge [*Euphorbia resinifera* O. Berg.]: ... According to some people: If the skin of the head of a person, who is bitten by a snake or an insect, is given an incision until the cranium becomes visible and the pulverized gum [of resin spurge] is put therein and [the wound] is sutured, he will not suffer any harm). Hebr. תָּפַר does not feature in this sense in this sense in the current dictionaries. Anonymous I renders Arab. خيّط as תָּפַר, just like Nathan.

[תקן] • *Part. Pu'al* מְתֻקָּן · **perfumed**: Arab. مطيّب · Ibn Sīnā, *K. al-Qānūn* II · trans. Zeraḥyah Ḥen, *Sefer ha-Qanun* (Ms Oxford. Opp. Add. Fol. 12, fols. 248^{b}–249^{a}): סוּסַן גְ'לְיוּ ... ושמנו יותר מתיר ויתר מחליק בין שיהיה מתוקן או אינו מתוקן ([Arab.] *sawsan*; [i.e., Rom.] ǦiLYWu [i.e., Ital.-Rom. *giglio*]: Lily [*Lilium* L.] or iris [*Iris* L.]: ... Its oil is very dissolvent and laxative, whether it is perfumed or not perfumed). Hebr. *Part. Pu'al* מְתֻקָּן does not feature in this sense in the current dictionaries. Nathan ha-Me'ati translates Arab. مطيّب as מבושם and Anonymous I renders the Arab. term as מבושם בבשמים.

תְּרוּפָה • *Plur.* תרופות בועיות • תרופות · **medicines that raise blisters (vesicatories; vesicants)**: Lat. *vesicae* (cf. ND 1189) · Guy de Chauliac, *Inventarium sive Chirurgia Magna* (cf. CMM 1:419, ll. 18–19) · trans. Anonymous (Ms Paris, BnF, héb. 1189, fol. 229^{a}): אמנם התרופות המבקעות שאינן מחדשות קלפה רק הבועיות (Medicines that induce rupture but do not cause eschar are those that raise blisters). Hebr. תרופות בועיות is not attested in the current dictionaries.

תַּרְנְגוֹל • תרנגול עוור · **[lit. 'blind rooster']; caltrop (tribulus) [*Tribulus terrestris* L.]**: Arab. حسك; Pers. شكوهج (cf. MIG nos. 228, 343, 357) · *Shinnui ha-Shemot ha-Niqra'im Synonimi*, Ḥet 20 (Ms Florence, Biblioteca Medicea Laurenziana, Or. 17, fol. 78^{a}): חסך[422] היא אלשכוהגב והוא תרנגול עוור ונק' בערבי חמץ אלמירי ([Arab.] *ḥasak*; i.e., [Arab.-Pers.] *al-shakūhaj*, i.e., [Hebr.] *tarnegol 'iwwer*, called in Arab. *ḥimmiṣ al-amīr* [lit. 'chickpea of the prince,' cf. MIG no. 357]). Hebr. תרנגול עוור (lit. 'blind rooster') is a non-attested calque from Ibero-Rom. **ghālluh jāquh* or **ghālluh jīquh*, corresponding to Mod. Span. *gallo ciego*, cf. MIG nos. 229, 343, 941; MSh no. 151.

422 חסך: Emend. ed. חמסך Ms.

Bibliography

Adams, F. (trans.), *The Seven Books of Paulus Ægineta: Translated from the Greek with Commentary Embracing a Complete View of the Knowledge Possessed by the Greeks, Romans, and Arabians on all Subjects Connected with Medicine and Surgery*, 3 vols. (London 1844–1847).

Alcalay, R., *Millon Ivri-Angli Shalem: The Complete Hebrew-English Dictionary* (Ramat Gan 1972).

Amin, El S., O. Awad, M. Abd El Samad, and M.N. Iskander, 'Isolation of Estrone from Moghat Roots and from Pollen Grains of Egyptian Date Palm,' *Phytochemistry* 8 (1969): 295–297.

Argenter, J.A., and J. Ferrer, 'Jewish Texts in Old Catalan,' in: *Manual of Judaeo-Romance Linguistics and Philology*, ed. by G. Mensching and F. Savelsberg, 99–128 (Berlin 2023).

Aristotle → Kruk, R. (ed.)

Bachour, N., 'Healing with Mercury: The Uses of Mercury in Arabic Medical Literature,' *Asia* 69, no. 4 (2015): 831–866.

Bertoni, G., 'Denominazioni del *ramarro* (lacerta viridis) in Italia,' *Romania* 42, no. 166 (1913): 161–173.

Blau, J., *A Dictionary of Mediaeval Judaeo-Arabic Texts* (Jerusalem 2006).

Bos, G. (ed. and trans.), *Ibn al-Jazzār on Sexual Diseases and Their Treatment* (London 1997).

Bos, G. (ed. and trans.), *Ibn al-Jazzār on Fevers* (London 2000).

Bos, G., and R. Fontaine, 'Medico-Philosophical Controversies in Nathan b. Yo'el Falaquera's *Sefer Ṣori ha-Guf*,' *Jewish Quarterly Review* 90 (1999): 27–60.

Bos, G., F. Lauschus, and F. Savelsberg, 'Substitute Drugs in the Hebrew Tradition,' in: *From Formal Linguistic Theory to the Art of Historical Editions: The Multifaceted Dimensions of Romance Linguistics*, ed. by N. Pomino, E.M. Remberger, and J. Zwink, 303–316 (Göttingen 2023).

Bos, G., and G. Mensching, 'Arabic-Romance Medico-Botanical Glossaries in Hebrew Manuscripts from the Iberian Peninsula and Italy,' *Aleph* 15, no. 1 (2015): 9–61.

Derenbourg, J. (ed.), *Targum Ḥamishah Ḥumshei Torah be-Lashon 'Aravit le-Rabbeinu Sa'adyah Ga'on ben Yoseph ha-Fayyumi: Version arabe du Pentateuque de R. Saadia Ben Iosef al-Fayyoûmî* (Repr., Hildesheim 1979).

Durling, R., *Dictionary of Medical Terms in Galen* (Leiden 1993).

Freudenthal, G., M.R. McVaugh, and K. Mesler, 'Twelfth-Century Latin Medicine in Hebrew Garb: Doeg the Edomite as a Cultural Intermediary,' *Medieval Encounters* 26 (2020): 226–284.

Galen → Kühn, K.G. (ed.)

Gaster, M. (ed.), *Sefer Sod ha-Sodot*, in *Studies and Texts in Folklore, Magic, Mediaeval Romance, Hebrew Apocrypha, and Samaritan Archaeology*, 3 vols., (Repr., New York 1971).

Goshen-Gottstein, M., *Syntax and Vocabulary of Mediaeval Hebrew as Influenced by Arabic*, rev. by S. Assif and U. Melammed (Jerusalem 2006) [Hebr.].

Ibn al-Jazzār → Bos, G. (ed. and trans.)

Ibn Janāḥ, Abū l-Walīd Marwān, *K. al-Uṣūl: The Book of Hebrew Roots*, ed. by A. Neubauer (Oxford 1875).

Ibn Sahl, Sābūr, *Dispensatorium Parvum (Al-Aqrābādhīn al-saghīr)*, ed. by O. Kahl (Leiden 1994).

Kühn, K.G. (ed.), *Claudii Galeni Opera Omnia*, 20 vols. (Repr., Hildesheim 1964–1965).

Kruk, R. (ed.), *The Arabic Version of Aristotle's* Parts of Animals, *Books XI–XIV of the K. al-Ḥayawān: A Critical Edition* (Amsterdam 1978).

Leibowitz, J.O., and S. Marcus (eds.), *Sefer Hanisyonot: The Book of Medical Experiences Attributed to Abraham ibn Ezra* (Jerusalem 1984).

Lewysohn, L., *Zoologie des Talmuds* (Frankfurt am Main 1858).

Malouf, A., *Muʿjam al-Ḥayawān (An Arabic Zoological Dictionary)* (Cairo 1932).

Meyerhof, M., 'Der Bazar der Drogen und Wohlgerüche in Kairo,' *Archiv für Wirtschaftsforschung im Orient* 34 (1918): 180–218.

Neubauer, A., *Catalogue of the Hebrew Manuscripts in the Bodleian Libraries* (Repr., Oxford 1994); *Supplement of Addenda and Corrigenda*, comp. by M. Beit-Arié and ed. by R.A. May (Oxford 1994).

Paul of Aegina → Adams, F. (trans.)

Penzig, O., *Flora Popolare Italiana*, 2 vols. (Genoa 1924).

Rapoport, Y., and E. Savage-Smith (eds.), *An Eleventh-Century Egyptian Guide to the Universe*: The Book of Curiosities (Leiden 2014).

al-Rāzī, Abū Bakr Muḥammad ibn Zakariyyāʾ, *On Phlebotomy*, edition, translation, and commentary by J. Björn (PhD diss., *Studia Orientalia Lundensa*) (Lund 2023).

Richler, B., *Hebrew Manuscripts in the Biblioteca Palatina in Parma: Catalogue*, with palaeographical and codicological descriptions by M. Beit-Arié (Jerusalem 2001).

Richler, B., 'Manuscripts of Avicenna's *Kanon* in Hebrew Translation: A Revised and Up-to-Date List,' *Korot* 8, nos. 3–4 (1982): 145–168.

Richter, P., 'Über die spezielle Dermatologie des ʿAlī ibn al-ʿAbbās (Haly Abbas) aus dem 10. Jahrhundert unserer Zeitrechnung,' *Archiv für Dermatologie und Syphilis* 113, no. 1 (1912): 849–864; Repr. in *Beiträge zur Geschichte der arabisch-islamischen Medizin: Aufsätze*, vol. 3: *Aus den Jahren 1909–1913*, ed. by F. Sezgin, in collaboration with M. Amawi, D. Bischoff, and E. Neubauer, 465–480 (Frankfurt am Main 1987).

Saʿadyah Gaʾon → Derenbourg, J. (ed.)

Steinschneider, M., *Die hebräischen Übersetzungen des Mittelalters und die Juden als Dolmetscher* (Berlin 1893).

Steinschneider, M., 'Eine medicinische hebraeische Handschrift,' *Magazin für die Wissenschaft des Judentums* 12 (1885): 182–216.

Wallis, F., *Medieval Medicine: A Reader* (Toronto 2010).

Wujastik, D., 'Mercury Tonics in Sanskrit Literature,' in: *Soulless Matter, Seats of Energy: Metals, Gems and Minerals in South Asian Religions and Culture*, ed. by F.M. Ferrari and T. Dähnhardt, 94–115 (Sheffield and Bristol 2015).

Zonta, M., 'Zeraḥyah: Philosopher and Translator and His Role in 13th Century Rome' (paper read in Jerusalem, January 1, 2007).

Zotenberg, H., (ed.), *Catalogues des manuscrits hébreux et samaritains de la Bibliothèque Impériale* (Paris 1866).

Corrections to BCD and NM 1 and 6

BCD 56 (NM 1:20) דְּחִיקָה · bandage: **corr.**: tightness, tightening
BCD 100 (NM 1:93f.): חָלָל · חלל העורף · nape of the neck: **corr.** hollow of the neck.
BCD 204 (NM 4:147): עֹמֶק · העומק אשר בעליון אחורי הצואר · the nape of the neck: **corr.** the hollow of the neck.

NM 1:20: 'You already know about the way of bandaging in general; that is that the bandage should be tighter over the point of the fracture'; **corr.**: 'You already know about the way of bandaging in general; that is that it should be very tight over the point of the fracture'.
Ibid.: **delete**: 'Another term for 'bandage' employed by Hillel is קֶשֶׁר'.
NM 6:18: אָמָה: **corr.** אַמָּה.

Index of Greek Terms

ἀγηράτος → λίθος
ἀγκύλη 61, 164, 194
αἰγιλώπιον 121
ἄκορον 165
ἅλς → ἄνθος
ἀλφός 25, 33, 34, 64, 87, 97, 105, 107, 200, 234, 235
ἀμβλυωπία 82, 83, 96, 100, 112, 152
ἀνατρέπω: ἀνατρέπω τὸν στόμαχον 57, 60
ἄνθος: ἄνθος ἁλός 174, 192
ἄνθραξ 22
ἄση 57, 60
ἀσώδης 57, 60
ἄφθα, *Plur.* ἄφθαι 222

γαγγραινώδης 18, 19
γαλακτίτης 10

διάκλυσμα 195
διαφορητικός 171
διουρητικός 128, 197
δοθίην 115
δυσεντερία 225

εἰλεός 17, 77, 187
ἐνουρεω 51, 53, 224
ἐντεροκήλη 33, 61, 193
ἐκταράσσω: ἐκταράσσω τὴν κοιλίαν 129
ἐπαφαίρεσις 73
ἐπινυκτίς 37, 182
ἐπουλόω 73, 137
ἑρμοδάκτυλος 170
ἐσχάρα 190
εὐφόρβιον 236

ἡμικρανία 94

θαλάττιος λαγωός 22
θύμος 234

ἰάομαι 73, 137
ἵδρωα 221
ἴκτερος 113
ἴονθος 102
Ἰουδαϊκος λίθος 10, 71
ἰχθυοκόλλα 44

καρδάμωμον 172
καρδιωγμὸς 180
κοιλία → ἐκταράσσω
κολλάω 73, 137
κολοκυνθίς 30, 169, 201

λάγως → θαλάττιος
λέπρα 26, 105, 200
λήμη 86
λίθος: λίθος ἀγηράτος 9
λίθος: λίθος ὀφίτης 12
λίθος: λίθος σεληνίτης 10
Plur. λίθοι: λίθοι οἱ ἐν τοῖς σπόγγοις 9
λοιμός 85

μελίκρατον 114

ναυτία 57, 60

ὀβολός 19,
ὀμφάκιον/ὀμφάκινον 226
ὀφίτης → λίθος

παραλύομαι 204, 205
πίτυρον 136
πράσιον 22, 186
πυρία 49, 70
πῶρος 43

ῥῆγμα 32, 33, 57, 78, 83, 106, 135, 176, 177, 203, 216
ῥῆξις 83, 135

σεληνίτης → λίθος
σκαμμωνία 89
σκίγκος 107
σμῆξις 85, 121
σπάσμα 235
σπόγγος → λίθοι
στόμαχος → ἀνατρέπω
στραγγουρία 51, 53, 224
στρόφος 94
στῦψις 154
συνάγχη 80, 111
συνπάθεια 223, 231

τέτανος 235
τρόμος 204

ὑδροκήλη 23, 50, 113
ὑπερικόν 64, 117, 118, 158
ὑπώπιον 83, 95, 222
Plur. ὑπώπια 83, 95, 222

φλύκταινα 14, 26
φοῦ 35

χαμαίδρυς 121
χίμεθλον 33

Index of Arabic/Persian Terms

إبرية 136
إبط 28
أبولوسة: أبولوسات ← أنولوسة
أثر 119, 218
آثار 138, 218
إثمد 13
أدرة: أدرة الماء 23, 50, 113, 114
إذخر 233
أذن ← دود، دويّ، سيلان، شدخ، ورم، وسخ
أربية 196
أرميني ← حَجَر
أرنب بحري 22
اسفنج ← حَجَر
اسقنقور 106, 107
أصل ← ورم
أصلي 231
أقاقيا 159
إقليميا: إقليميا الذهب 191
إقليميا الفضّة 192
أكّال ← دواء
متأكّل 18, 19
أنف ← سعط، نتن
إنفاق ← زيت
أنولوسة: أنولوسات 19, 20
أهلي 38
آفة 75, 76, 109
إيلاوس 17, 18, 77, 187

بثر: بثور 128, 151
البثور اللينة 151
بحّة: بحّة الصوت 130
بحوحة 131
بحري ← أرنب
بري ← عرق
برد ← شق
أبرص ← سامّ
بصل: بصل الخنزير 31
بطن ← (حرك)
بِلّة 29
بلح 29, 30
بلادة: بلادة الذهن 215
بلادة فهم 216
ابن: ابن عرس 72
بنت: بنات الليل 37, 182
بهق: البهق الأبيض 25, 26
بورقية 27, 98
بول ← حبس، (درّ)، إدرار، عسر، تقطير
بياض 104
أبيض ← بهق

ترك 55
ترياق 183
تفاح ← ربّ
توث 234

تثاؤب 197, 198, 216
ثؤلول: ثآليل 171
تثقيل 54
تثنية 73

(جبر) تجبّر 43
جبسين 38, 82
جبل ← زبيب
جبلي ← صمغ
جبن ← ماء
جحوظ 29, 56
جرب: الجرب المتقرّح 40
جراد 21, 71
← رجل
جرى 198, 199
جَعِد 97, 234, 235
مجفف ← دواء
جلد ← رطوبة، (قشر)
جلاء 85, 121
جنب ← ذات، وجع
جنة ← عنب
جوزة 16
جوف 36, 175, 233, 234
أجوف 202

حبّ: حبّ الرأس 182
حبّ الزلم 173
حبّ القرع 41
حبّ الملوك 41
حبس: حبس البول 161, 162, 163, 164
حبس الدم 162
احتباس: احتباس الحيض 161
احتباس دم الطمث 161
حبش ← حَجَر
حَبْل: حبل الذراع 92
حَبَل ← عسر
(حجر) تحجّر 9
حَجْر 61, 164, 194
حجر المفاصل 61, 164, 194
حَجَر: حجر أرميني 9, 179
حجر الاسفنج 4, 9
حجر الحبش 11
حجر الحية 12
حجر الرحى 13
حجر الاساكفة 9
حجر يطفأ بالزيت 11
حجر العاج 13
حجر القمر 10, 11
حجر اللبن 4, 10
حجر المثانة 12, 13
حجر اليهود 4, 10, 71, 147, 148
حجارة 11, 12
حجارة المعدن 11, 12
حديد 34, 53
← خبث
حديث: حديث النفس 71
حدقة 18, 24, 25, 36, 37
حار ← حرق
حرباء 79
حرذون 98
حرافة 82
حرق: حرق الماء الحار 96, 230
حرقة 96
محرق ← دواء
(حرك) حرّك البطن 129
حزاز: حزاز الصخر 89, 135
حسك 236
حسو 81
حشرجة 39, 40, 157
حشا: أحشاء 47

حصاة ← (فتّ)
حاضر ← وقت
حفر 81, 82
حفظ 226
حقن 168
حقنة 168
محتقن ← رطوبة
محكك ← دواء
تحليل 61, 62
احتلام 49, 74, 75
حمّى: الحمّيات ذوات الأدوار 185
الحمّيات الدائرة 186
الحمّيات المفارقة 185, 186
الحمّيات المقلعة 186
حمودة 80
محمر ← دواء
حمول 55, 56, 137
احتناق: احتناق الرحم 81
حية ← حَجَر
حيض ← احتباس، نزف

خبث 174
خبث الحديد 174, 204
ختم 73, 137, 138
خاتم ← دواء
إختثار 145, 221
(خدر) تخدير 27
خَدَر 27, 95
مخدر← دواء
أخدع: أخدعان 179
خشكريشة 136, 190, 191
خشكريشات 136
مخشّن ← دواء
خطّ: خطوط 71
خفقان 180
خلط 65, 208, 211
مخلوط 232
اختلاف 75
اختلاف الدم 75
خمار 28, 137
خَمْل 12, 38, 215
خنزير ← بصل
خنفس 81
خانوق: خوانيق 80, 111, 112
مختنق ← رحم
اختيار 49
(خيط) خيّط 236
خيل ← ذنب

دبغ 154
(درّ) أدرّ البول 128, 155, 197
أدرّ الطمث 26, 155, 156
إدرار: إدرار البول 52, 155
دسومة 227
دشبد 43, 44
دقيق ← علم
دالية 76, 177
دوال 76, 177
دم ← حبس، احتباس، اختلاف، (سهل)، كهوبة، نفث
دمعة 46
(دمل) أدمل 73, 137, 153
اندمال 153
مدمل 138
دمّل 115
دماميل 115

إدمال 49, 73
مدمل ← دواء
دهنية 227
دود: الدود في الأذن 94
دور ← حمّى
دائر ← حمّى
دوسنطاريا 53, 225
دويّ: الدويّ في الأذن 94
دواء: الدواء الأكّال 139, 140, 205
الدواء المجفف 142, 143, 144, 210
الدواء المحرق 150, 214, 215
الدواء المحكك 141, 208
الدواء المحمر 138, 139, 205
الدواء الخاتم 142, 209
الدواء المخدر 140, 149, 205, 206
الدواء المخشّن 144, 145, 210
الدواء المدمل 140, 144, 145, 207, 208
الدواء المرخي 214
الدواء الرادع 129, 206, 207, 219
الدواء المزلق 143, 208, 209, 210
الدواء المسدّد 139, 145, 210
الدواء العاصر 146, 147, 214
الدواء المعفن 146, 211
الدواء المغري 142, 149
الدواء الغسّال 149, 213, 214
الدواء المغلظ 143, 145, 211
الدواء المفتّت 147, 148, 212
الدواء المفتّح 147, 148, 212
الدواء المفجّج 147, 211, 212
الدواء القابض 213
الدواء (ال)مقرح 144, 207
الدواء القاشر 148, 172, 190, 213
الدواء (ال)مقطّع 142, 208, 209
الدواء المقوي 141, 207
الدواء الكاسر الرياح 149, 150, 214
الدواء الكاوي 143, 209
الدواء الملطّف 206
الدواء الملين 208
الدواء المملس 141, 208
الدواء المنبت للحم 148, 212, 213
الدواء المنضج 140, 141, 206
الدواء المنفخ 144, 210
الدواء الهاضم 145, 146, 211
الدواء الموسّخ 142, 209
ديودار ← شير

ذراح: ذراريح 42, 183, 184
ذراع 19, 93
← حَبْل
ذقن 67
ذنب: ذنب الخيل 66
ذنب العين 66
ذهب ← إقليميا، لحام، لصاق
ذهن ← بلادة
ذو: ذوات الأدوار ← حمّى
مذيب 64, 65, 117, 118
ذات: ذات الجنب 76, 134, 163

رأس ← حبّ
ربّ 114, 115, 159, 196
ربّ التفاح 115
مربّى 38, 196, 218
مربّب 196
ربو 40, 163, 192, 194, 227, 228
رتيلاء 150, 151
رجل: رجل الغراب 197

أرجل الجراد 197
رحم ← احتناق، سيال، انضمام، نزف، انضمام
الرحم المختنق 199
رحى ← حجر
استرخاء 202
مرخي ← دواء
مسترخٍ 204, 205
رادع 129, 206, 207, 219
← دواء
رطوبة ← سيال
الرطوبات المحتقنة تحت الجلد 105, 200
رعشة 204
رعافي ← نزف
راعي ← مزمار
رفادة: رفائد 215
رمد 203
رماد 48
رمص 86, 87
رملي 72
← مكان
رمان ← عرق
رياح ← دواء، طرد، فشّ، مفشّش، كسر
ريحي 198, 201
ريق: على الريق 202

زئبق: زئبق مقتول 100, 101
زبيب: زبيب الجبل 182
زبد 74, 191
زجّاج ← ملح
زكام 52, 116
زلق 54, 119
مزلق ← دواء، شيء
زلم ← حبّ

مزمار: مزمار الراعي 66, 111
مزمن 22, 53, 91, 186, 187
زنبور 42, 124
زنابير 42, 184
زنجبيل: زنجبيل الكلب 67
زنخ 47, 91, 166, 185, 201
زهر(ة): زهر(ة) الملح 174, 192
زهرة النحاس 175
زائد ← شعر، لَحْم
زيت ← حَجَر
زيت الإنفاق 226

سحج 32, 45, 58, 105, 106, 189
سحج (الأمعاء) 128
مسدّد ← دواء
سذاب ← صمغ
سعط 70, 130, 167
سعط في الأنف 70, 130, 167, 168, 228
سُعِطَ 167, 168, 228
سعوط 53, 167, 168
سعفة 136
ساعي ← قرح، ورم
(سقط) أسقط 132
سقط 57
إسقاط 57
سقورديون 221
استسقاء: الاستسقاء اللحمي 76
سكب 188
اساكفة ← حَجَر
(سكن) سكّن 223, 224
تسكين 223
مسكن 117

سلّ 80, 111, 195
سمّ: سموم 150
سامّ: سامّ أبرص 193, 235
سمك ← غراء
مسمن 226
سمّان 224
سنّ ← قلع، وسخ
(سهل) أسهل 225
أسهل الدم 225, 226
استواء 59
سويق 189
سيلان: سيلان الأذن 49
سيال: سيالان الرحم 50, 51
سيالان رطوبات الرحم 50, 51

شأن: من شأنه أن 47, 85, 117
تشبّك 73, 220
مشتبك 220
شدخ: شدخ الأذن 106, 203, 216
شدخ العضل 106, 204
شرسام 121
شرسوف 126
(شرط) شُرِطَ 230
شَرْط 230
شريف ← عضو
شركة 223, 231
شرى 37, 182, 217, 218
شط: شطوط 229
شعبة 158
شعر 59, 60, 132, 228
← انتشار 59, 60, 132
شعر زائد 229
شعر العين 228, 229
الشعرى العبور 96, 97
← طلوع 97
شق: شقاق 32
شقاق البرد 33, 34
شقيقة 94
شقرة 179, 180
شكوهج (Pers.) 236
شهدي ← قرح، ورم
شهوة: شهوة الطين 233
مشه: مُشهٍّ للطعام 16
شوصة 77, 122
شوك: شوكة مصرية 188
شوكة يهودية 187, 188
شيء: الأشياء المزلقة 143, 208
شير: شير ديودار (Pers.) 74

صؤاب: صئبان 28
صبّاغ 179
صبّاغون 116, 167, 170, 179
← عرق، فوة، ملح
صخر ← حزاز
صدأ 190
تصديع 54
صدف 109
أصداف 82, 109
مصارع 14, 158
مصارعون 14, 158
مصعد 119, 157
صفيحة 217
صفرة 23
أصفر ← ماء
صمغ 38, 39, 67
صمغ السذاب الجبلي 39

مصنوع 168, 169, 179
صوت ← بحّة

ضربان 46
ضربان العين 46, 47, 69
اضطراب 182
ضرس 102
أضراس 102, 103
انضمام: انضمام فم الرحم 21
ضماد 70

مطبوخ 125
طبقة 111
طبقات 111
مطبق 43
طحلب 90
طرد: طرد الرياح 171, 224, 225
طرفة 87, 88
طعام ← مش
طاعون 44, 85, 124
طواعين 44, 85, 124
(طفأ) ← حَجَر
طمث ← احتباس، (درّ)
طلوع: طلوع الشعرى العبور 97
طلق 12
مطيّب 236
طين ← شهوة

ظلمة ← غشاوة
ظلمة (البصر) 82, 83, 112

مستعدّ 65
عدشية: عدشيات 155

(عدل) عدّل 92, 120, 221
معتدل 92
معدن ← حَجَر
عرس ← ابن
معرفة ← تقدمة
عرق: عرق الرمان البري 39, 230, 231
عروق الصباغين 167
عرطنيثا 169
عسر: عسر البول 79, 164
عسر الحبل 78, 162, 163
عسر النفس 160, 161, 163
عشا 152
عشاوة 79
عصب 69, 177, 178, 181
← التواء
عاصر ← دواء
عضل ← شدخ
عضو: عضو نفيس 15,16
أعضاء الشريفة 16
أعضاء الغذاء 14
الأعضاء النفيسة 15, 16
أعضاء النفض 14, 15
عطرية 35, 36
عطش 181
عفونة 160
معفن ← دواء
عقدة 165, 195
عقد 165, 195
تعقّد 61, 164, 194
انعقاد 61
عقل 160, 161
عاقل 162
اعتلف 29

علق 130

عليق: عليق الكلب 151

علك 44

علم: العلوم الدقيقة 74

(عمل) استعمل 152

عنب: عنب الجنة، الحية 158

عنكبوت ← نسج

عاج 13, 162, 227

← تحَجّر

عين ← ذنب، شعر، ضربان، كمودة، كهوبة، نتوء

غثيان 193

مغث 91, 193

غذاء ← عضو

غرب 121

غراب ← رجل

غرض 125

غراء: غراء السمك 44

تغرية 86, 183

مغرّ 42, 86, 142, 149, 183

مغري ← دواء

غسّال ← دواء

مغشوش 173

غشاوة 83, 100, 151, 152

تغضّن 67

مغلظ ← دواء

غمّ 112

تغيّر 160

(فتّ) فتّت 174, 175, 178

فتّت الحصاة 174

مفتّت ← دواء

مفتّح ← دواء

فتور 55, 176

فتق 33, 34, 61, 193

انفتال 177, 178

مفجّج ← دواء

فُرفُرِي 171

فارسي ← نار

استفراغ 85

مفارق ← حمّى

فسخ 32, 33, 57, 58, 78, 84, 135, 176, 177

فشّ 172

فشّش الرياح 220

مفشّش 171, 172

مفشّش للرياح 172

مفصل: مفاصل 61, 164, 175, 176, 194

← تحْجّر

فضّة ← إقليميا

فضل 25, 59

فضلي 110, 111, 154, 155

فم: فم الرحم ← انضمام

فهم ← بلادة

فواق 57, 61

فوة: فوة الصباغين 170

قابض 160, 213

← دواء

مقتول ← زئبق

تقدمة: تقدمة المعرفة 58

قُرَاد 99, 100, 176, 187

قرح: القروح الساعية 123

القروح الشهدية 127

مقرح ← دواء

متقرّح ← جرب

تقريح 59, 69, 70, 127

قرصعنة 187
قرع ← حبّ
مقرّنة 31, 54
قسط 53, 54
(قشر) تقشّر الجلد 189
قاشر ← دواء
تقشير 189
مقشّر 149, 172, 189, 190, 213
اقشعرار 150
قشعريرة 150
تقطير: تقطير البول 51, 52, 53, 224
قطران 156
مقطّع ← دواء
مقطوف 31
قلب: قلب المعدة 56, 60
تقلب: تقلب النفس 57, 60, 61
قلع: قلع الأسنان 165, 169
قلاع 182, 222
مقلع ← حمّى
قمر ← حَجَر
قمع 99, 128, 129, 165, 172, 173, 174, 180, 181, 187, 190
مقوي ← دواء
قيلة 23, 114

اكتحال 98, 99
كاذب 97, 98
(كرب) كرّب 89
تكرّب 89
(كرج) تكرّج 42, 43, 221
متكرّج 30
تكريج 159, 160
كزاز 235

كسر: كسر الرياح 171, 220
كاسر ← دواء
كعب 164
كعك 106
كلب ← زنجبيل، عليق
مكلّس 230
كلف 34, 102
كماد 49, 70, 71
كمودة: كمودة العين 83, 95, 222, 223
تكميد 201
كهوبة: كهوبة الدم تحت العين 53, 56, 99
كوارة 28
كوائر 28
مكان: الأماكن الرملية 72
كاوي ← دواء

لازورد 104
لبّ 36, 104, 175
لبن ← حَجَر
(لحم) ألحم 137, 138
لَحْم 36, 104, 148, 175, 212, 213
← دواء
لحم زائد 36
لحام: لحام الذهب 42, 69
لحمي ← استسقاء
لزوجة 51
لصاق: لصاق الذهب 41, 69
لصوق 43
لَطُوخ 52, 86, 107, 108, 124, 125, 200, 201
لُطُوخ 52, 86
ملطّف ← دواء
لم ← ما
لمع 35

- تلميع 35
  - تلميعات 35
- التواء: التواء العصب 177, 178, 181
- ليفي 30, 31
- ليل ← بنت
- (لين) ليّن 78, 202, 203
- لَيّن ← بثر
- مليّن ← دواء

- ما: ما لم 216
- مأق 45, 66, 110
  - مأقان 45, 66, 110
- مالقراطن 114
- تمتين 61
- مثانة ← حَجَر
- تمدّد 60, 126
- امتداد 60, 126
- مخاطية 131
- مرّي 110
- مسح 191
- مصري ← شوك
- معدة ← قلب
- معى ← سحج
- (مغص) أمغص 94, 165, 166
- مَغْص 94, 170
- مضمض 224
  - تمضمض 120, 195
- مضمضة 195, 200
- مقلة 37
- ملح ← زهر(ة)
  - ملح الزجّاجين 116
  - ملح الصبّاغين 116
- تمليح 115, 116
- مملس ← دواء
- ملك: ملوك ← حبّ
- موز 235
- ماء ← أدرة، حرق
  - ماء الجبن 114
  - ماء القراطن ← مالقراطن
  - الماء الأصفر 113
- ميبختج 158, 159
- ميويزج 181, 182

- منبت ← دواء
- نتوء: نتوء العين 90
- نتن 24
  - نتن الأنف 24, 153
- نحاس ← زهر(ة)
- نزف: نزف الحيض 50, 51
  - نزف الرحم 229, 230
  - النزف الرعافي 229
- (نزل) نزول 90
- ناسور 123
  - نواسير 123
- نسج: نسج العنكبوت 21, 22, 188
- نشارة 131
- انتشار 89, 90, 176
  - انتشار الشعر 59, 60, 132
- تنشيف 133
- انتصاب ← نفس
  - انتصاب النفس 58, 120, 134
- منضج ← دواء
- نفث: نفث دم 217
- نفخ 131, 132
- نفاخة: نفاخات 14
- منفخ ← دواء

نفس ← حديث، عسر، تقلب، انتصاب
نفس الانتصاب 76, 134, 163
نفيس ← عضو
نفض ← عضو
نافض 192, 201
(نفط) تنفّط 14, 26
نفطية 131
نفع 53, 181
نقرة 77, 132, 133
نقرس 115, 170
نقيع 125
نمش 34, 102
نمى 43
نوبة 58
نار: النار الفارسي 22

هتك 32, 58, 78, 83, 135, 176, 177
هاضم ← دواء
هامّة: هوامّ 65, 166
هوائية 17
هيضة 225

وجع: وجع الجنب 95
وجع الجنبين 95
توحّش 20, 60, 112, 233
ورل 20
ورم: الورم الساعي 123
الأورام الساعية 123
الأورام الشهدية 127
الأورام التي في أصل الأذن 123, 124
وسخ: أوساخ الأذن 64, 87, 107
أوساخ الأسنان 64, 87, 107
موسخ ← دواء
صفة 234
وعاء 77
أوعية 77
وقت: الوقت الحاضر 65
تهمة 112
وهن 32, 57, 78, 84, 135, 176, 177

ينبوت 63
يهود(ي) ← حَجَر، شوك

Index of Latin/Romance Terms

abstertivus → *medicina*
acacia 159
addo 70
agglutinatio 51
agnus castus 74, 172
ameos 57, 61, 93
amido(n)/amidó 75
amidum 75
anatra 38, 223
aniso 82
antras/anthrax 44, 85, 124
aqua: aqua ferrata 112
Armenus → *lapis*
asparagus, Plur. *asparagi/esparagi* 62
asperge/esparge/esperge 62
auxilium 156

borais 42, 69, 179
bursa: *bursa pastoris* → *capsella*

cancrosus 153
caperi/capperi 135
capsella: *capsella bursa pastoris* 99
caramida 174
carota, Plur. *carotae/carote* 162
cassia: cassia lignea 54
catapucia 94, 165
catarrosus 129
cauterium 96
cauterizacio 96
cavilla: *caville manuum* 92
  caville pedum 92
centaurea 85
cicatrix, Plur. *cicatrices* 218
ciner 48
clavilis 117
colica/colice 77, 101, 187
colloquintida 30, 169, 201
collum: *collum matricis* 180
colocyntis 30, 169, 201
concavitas 78
coniunctiva 70
consolido, Part. *consolidans*, Plur. *consolidantes* 43
constipatio 160, 161
contentus → *membrum*
continens → *membrum*
contineo 72
corrosivus 18, 19
cresteri/crestiri/cristeri/cristiri 168
crusta/cruste 136, 191
crustosus 191
cura 156
curatio 215
cyclamen 57

dieta 118
discurro 198
dissolvo: dissolvor 121

eruca/ruca 138
eruge 130
escar 190
espica 180
esquilla/squilla 31
estafizagra 114, 182
estorac 54
evaporo 17

ferratus → *aqua*
ferrugine 204
ferrugo 191, 204
ferrum → *scoria*
fissura, Plur. *fissurae/fissure*: *fissure labiorum* 138
flatus → *strictura*
flos: *flos eris* 175
fluxus: *fluxus sanguinis de naribus* 204
foeniculum: foeniculum romanum 82
forceps 118
furfures 136

galbano 155
galbanum 155
gallo ciego 236
gena: Plur. *genae* 217
giglio 96, 236
glutinativus 183
glutino, Part. *glutinans*, Plur. *glutinantes* 43
glutinosus 44
gummi 39

hemicrania 94
herba: herba serpentina 33, 97
homoplate 121

infeccio, Plur. *infecciones* 102
infectus 101
intentio 125
interior, Plur. *interiora* 47
inviscativus: inviscativa medicina 43
  inviscativa seu lenificativa medicina 141

labium → *fissura*
lacca 180
lacrimalis 46
lamina 217
lapis: lapis alagi 14
  lapis antimonii 13
  lapis Armenus 9, 104
  lapis qua extinguit in oleo 11
  lapis vesive 12, 13
laureola 136, 172, 189
lenificativus → *inviscativus*
lignàloe/lignaloe 25
lucertòn/lucertone/lucirtòn 20

manus → *cavilla*
marrubium 22, 186
matrix → *collum*
medicina → *inviscativus*
  medicina abstertiva 208
mellilota 127
membrum, Plur. *membra: membra contenta* 15
  membra continentia 15
  membra procidentia 15
mentha 110, 155
minaria 12
mira/mirra 113
mollicies 202
mortifico 55
mundificatio 85
muries 110
myrrha 113

naris → *fluxus*
nebulosus 166
nitrositas 35
nitrosus 35, 98

oleo → *lapis*

pallior 194
pannus, Plur. *panni* 25
pastenaga 55
pastor → *capsella*
pes → *cavilla*
plagella 101
plata 217
podagra 170
porrum, Plur. *porra* 171
procidens → *membrum*
pronosticon 58
punctura 170
purgatio 85
pustula, Plur. *pustulae* 26

rancid 185
repercussivum, Plur. *repercussiva* 218
rigor 192, 201
ruca → *eruca*
ruta 70, 132, 170

sanguis → *fluxus*
sapa 159
scoria: *scoria ferri* 191
serosus 228
serum 114
sincopis 180
sitis 181
societas 223, 232
sordidus 64
sorditia 14
squilla → *esquilla*
squinante 233
stincus 81, 107
strictura: *strictura in flatu* 192
suffumigo 188

tenta 177
  tentae 215
tuellum 154, 178

ulcerosus 127

vesica, Plur. *vesicae* 236
vesicans, Plur. *vesicancia* 30
viscum 232
viscus 232
vulneratus 127

www.ingramcontent.com/pod-product-compliance
Lightning Source LLC
LaVergne TN
LVHW010439051026
849527LV00002B/588